Intracytoplasmic Sperm Injection

Gianpiero D. Palermo • E. Scott Sills

Editors

Intracytoplasmic Sperm Injection

Indications, Techniques and Applications

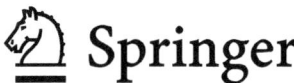 Springer

Editors
Gianpiero D. Palermo, MD, PhD
Center for Reproductive Medicine
Weill Cornell Medical College
New York, NY, USA

E. Scott Sills, MD, PhD
Center for Advanced Genetics
San Clemente, CA, USA

ISBN 978-3-319-70496-8   ISBN 978-3-319-70497-5   (eBook)
https://doi.org/10.1007/978-3-319-70497-5

Library of Congress Control Number: 2017961315

Printed on acid-free paper

This Springer imprint is published by Springer Nature
The registered company is Springer International Publishing AG
The registered company address is: Gewerbestrasse 11, 6330 Cham, Switzerland

Preface

This is a truly uncommon book. It is a comprehensive presentation of the male factor infertility experience, such as has never before been compiled in a single volume. Using intracytoplasmic sperm injection (ICSI) as the centerpoint for its varied content, the chapters which follow describe ICSI and its surrounding clinical landscape—from the background of pretreatment sociological features associated with male factor infertility to the molecular genetics of male gametogenesis. It is gratifying to see how these contributors have provided such an outstanding summary of their own expertise in an up-to-date and easy-to-access manner.

Since the initial success of in vitro fertilization in 1978, the field of assisted human reproduction has been transformed by an accelerating stream of discovery and technological progress. Such events have resulted in the expansion of ICSI indications, well beyond traditional severe male infertility. This relatively new clinical terrain periodically requires a new guide, and these chapters offer a fresh consolidation of current knowledge regarding all aspects of male infertility.

Indeed, here the reader will find descriptions of current practices, diagnostic and therapeutic, along with some newer and progressive ones including nuclear transplantation and genetic engineering. Developed for maximal accessibility by reproductive endocrinologists, embryologists, geneticists, research fellows, nurses, and sociologists, this book will also be useful to legislators and health policy leaders who consider wider regulatory implications of the assisted reproductive technologies.

We are grateful for the support of the publisher and look forward to the comments of readers, who we hope will find this new work beneficial.

New York, NY, USA   Gianpiero D. Palermo, MD, PhD
San Clemente, CA, USA   E. Scott Sills, MD, PhD

In Memoriam: Queenie V. Neri

Queenie V. Neri was a leading researcher in the field of male infertility and assisted fertilization for the past 18 years at the Ronald O. Perelman and Claudia Cohen Center for Reproductive Medicine, Weill Cornell Medicine, New York. In January 2015, Queenie was diagnosed with acute myeloid leukemia. After a brave battle for a year, she breathed her last on February 7, 2016, 9 days before her 42nd birthday. I take this opportunity to commemorate her life's achievements.

To her family, Queenie was a devoted daughter, aunt, sister, and friend who exuded joy, warmth, and kindness. She was no different in her professional life. Her diligence was inspiring, her curiosity was insatiable, her drive was enthusing, and her penchant for teaching was incredible. Queenie's technical prowess at performing gamete micromanipulation and extensive searches of testicular tissue for sperm were virtually unrivaled. Her comprehension of complex molecular genetics and stem cell biology consistently surpassed the knowledge of even the most established researchers. Queenie's work culminated in numerous scientific presentations at prestigious global meetings, several of which received awards from national organizations such as the American Society for Reproductive Medicine and the Society for Male Reproduction and Urology, as well as international organizations such as the European Society of Human Reproduction and Embryology. Queenie was courageous enough to present her prize paper work in October 2015 even in the middle of chemotherapy treatments.

Prior to her sudden demise, Queenie was actively engaged in her PhD work pertaining to therapeutic implications of spermatogonial stem cells. It is imperative to mention that Queenie had no formal training in the sciences prior to her work at Weill Cornell. In fact, her first responsibilities were as an editorial assistant. Her attempts at creating graphs or slides would invariably invoke scientific and mechanistic questions, and this zeal for learning reproductive biology transformed her into a nascent scientific investigator.

Those who knew Queenie would likely have their own interesting anecdote about her. However, there would be unanimous agreement that Queenie's charisma and exuberance was infectious. Even on the busiest of days, she mustered the energy to smile and laugh. No question was too hard; no task was too cumbersome; Queenie did it all with outmost vigor, grace, and of course a smile on her face. During my early days at Weill Cornell, I vividly remember dictating a minute-long, verbose scientific statement to Queenie. She typed intermittently but attentively. I looked at the screen of my laptop and found only a single sentence. I asked Queenie why the sentence was so short, to which she grinned and replied "I wrote down only the important parts." Her talent at distilling even the most complicated problems into the simplest parts was par excellence.

It pains me to write this eulogy for Queenie. Although her flourishing career was cut short abruptly, her work, essence, and spirit will never be forgotten. She will remain an inspiration to many, and her memory will be etched in our hearts. I'm certain that Queenie is smiling down from the heavens as we embark on this scientific endeavor.

New York, NY, USA   Gianpiero D. Palermo, MD, PhD

Contents

1   **Male-Factor Infertility: Factoring in the Male Experience**   1
Diederik F. Janssen

2   **Intracytoplasmic Sperm Injection: History, Indications,**
Technique, and Safety   9
Nigel Pereira and Gianpiero D. Palermo

3   **The Role of Reproductive Genetics in Modern Andrology**   23
Douglas T. Carrell, Timothy G. Jenkins, Benjamin R. Emery,
James M. Hotaling, and Kenneth I. Aston

4   **Effect of Paternal Age on Reproductive Outcomes:**
Data from Intracytoplasmic Sperm Injection
and Oocyte Donation   39
Lena Sagi-Dain and Martha Dirnfeld

5   **New Paradigms in De Novo Creation of Functional Human**
Spermatozoa: A Review of Biological Progress Towards
Clinical Application   49
Nina Neuhaus, Tim Pock, Stefan Schlatt, and Verena Nordhoff

6   **Assessment of Sperm DNA Integrity and Implications**
for the Outcome of ICSI Treatments   63
Preben Christensen and Anders Birck

7   **Sperm Evaluation Using the Comet Assay**   85
Océane Albert and Bernard Robaire

8   **Automated Morphology Detection from Human Sperm Images**   99
Seyed Abolghasem Mirroshandel and Fatemeh Ghasemian

9   **Clinical Approaches to Male Factor Infertility**   123
Omer A. Raheem and Tung-Chin Hsieh

**10 Intracytoplasmic Morphologically Selected
     Sperm Injection (IMSI): An Overview** 143
     Daniel Luna Origgi and Javier García-Ferreyra

**11 Implications of Sperm Source on ICSI Outcome:
     Assessment of TESE and Other Surgical Sperm
     Retrieval Methods** 157
     Nikita Abhyankar, Samuel Ohlander, and Martin Kathrins

**12 Intracytoplasmic Sperm Injection (ICSI):
     Applications and Insights** 169
     Toru Suzuki and Anthony C.F. Perry

**13 The Human Y-chromosome: Evolutionary Directions
     and Implications for the Future of "Maleness"** 183
     Darren K. Griffin and Peter J.I. Ellis

Index 193

Contributors

Nikita Abhyankar, MBChB, BMedSc Department of Urology, University of Illinois at Chicago, Chicago, IL, USA

Océane Albert, PhD Department of Pharmacology and Therapeutics and of Obstetrics and Gynecology, McGill University, Montreal, QC, Canada

Kenneth I. Aston, PhD Department of Surgery (Urology Division), University of Utah School of Medicine, Salt Lake City, UT, USA

Anders Birck, PhD SPZ Lab A/S, Copenhagen OE, Denmark

Douglas T. Carrell, PhD Andrology & IVF Laboratory Division, Department of Surgery (Urology) and Human Genetics, University of Utah School of Medicine, Salt Lake City, UT, USA

Department of Surgery (Urology Division), University of Utah School of Medicine, Salt Lake City, UT, USA

Preben Christensen, PhD SPZ Lab A/S, Copenhagen OE, Denmark

Martha Dirnfeld, MD Division of Fertility-In Vitro Fertilization, Department of Obstetrics and Gynecology, Carmel Medical Center, Faculty of Medicine, Technion University, Haifa, Israel

Peter J.I. Ellis, MA, PhD School of Biosciences, University of Kent, Canterbury, Kent, UK

Benjamin R. Emery, MPhil Department of Surgery (Urology Division), University of Utah School of Medicine, Salt Lake City, UT, USA

Javier García-Ferreyra, DSc FERTILAB Laboratory of Assisted Reproduction, Lima, Peru

Fatemeh Ghasemian, PhD Department of Biology, University of Guilan, Rasht, Guilan, Iran

Darren K. Griffin, BSc, PhD, DSc School of Biosciences, University of Kent, Canterbury, Kent, UK

James M. Hotaling, MD, MS Department of Surgery (Urology Division), University of Utah School of Medicine, Salt Lake City, UT, USA

Tung-Chin Hsieh, MD Department of Urology, University of California San Diego Health, San Diego, CA, USA

Diederik F. Janssen, MD, BA Independent Researcher, Nijmegen, The Netherlands

Timothy G. Jenkins, PhD Department of Surgery (Urology Division), University of Utah School of Medicine, Salt Lake City, UT, USA

Martin Kathrins, MD Harvard Medical School, Brigham and Women's Hospital, Boston, MA, USA

Seyed Abolghasem Mirroshandel, PhD Department of Computer Engineering, University of Guilan, Rasht, Guilan, Iran

Nina Neuhaus, PhD Centre of Reproductive Medicine and Andrology, University Hospital of Münster, Münster, Germany

Verena Nordhoff, PhD Centre of Reproductive Medicine and Andrology, University Hospital of Münster, Münster, Germany

Samuel Ohlander, MD Department of Urology, University of Illinois at Chicago, Chicago, IL, USA

Daniel Luna Origgi, BS FERTILAB Laboratory of Assisted Reproduction, Lima, Peru

Gianpiero D. Palermo, MD, PhD The Ronald O. Perelman and Claudia Cohen Center for Reproductive Medicine, Weill Cornell Medicine, New York, NY, USA

Nigel Pereira, MD The Ronald O. Perelman and Claudia Cohen Center for Reproductive Medicine, Weill Cornell Medicine, New York, NY, USA

Anthony C.F. Perry, PhD Laboratory of Mammalian Molecular Embryology, Department of Biology and Biochemistry, University of Bath, Bath, UK

Tim Pock, MSc Centre of Reproductive Medicine and Andrology, University Hospital of Münster, Münster, Germany

Omer A. Raheem, MD, MSc Department of Urology, University of Washington, Seattle, WA, USA

Bernard Robaire, PhD Department of Pharmacology and Therapeutics and of Obstetrics and Gynecology, McGill University, Montreal, QC, Canada

Lena Sagi-Dain, MD Division of Fertility-In Vitro Fertilization, Department of Obstetrics and Gynecology, Carmel Medical Center, Faculty of Medicine, Technion University, Haifa, Israel

Stefan Schlatt, PhD Centre of Reproductive Medicine and Andrology, University Hospital of Münster, Münster, Germany

E. Scott Sills, MD, PhD Reproductive Research Section, Center for Advanced Genetics, Carlsbad, CA, USA

Toru Suzuki, PhD Laboratory of Mammalian Molecular Embryology, Department of Biology and Biochemistry, University of Bath, Bath, UK

Chapter 1
Male-Factor Infertility: Factoring in the Male Experience

Diederik F. Janssen

1.1 Introduction

Male infertility is an often chronic reproductive health condition affecting millions of men worldwide [1]. Although figures are difficult to compare and definitions vary, one recent overview estimates the number of men affected by subfertility or infertility worldwide to be at least 30 million, with the highest rates reported in Africa and Eastern Europe [2]. Studies report infertility to be attributable to male factors in the wide range of 20–70% of reported cases, with the prevalence of men reported infertile varying from 2.5 to 12%. Internationally, 20–31% of fertility specialists identify the main cause of infertility as "male factor," and 17–29% as "both female and male factor" [3].

Many barriers in access to care for male-factor infertility are known to exist even where such care is available and affordable, which may lead to an underestimation of the problem [4]. Moreover, infertility research has long focused on women, leaving the male perspective under-examined in social scientific and social psychological research [5, 6]. The topic of male infertility thus has been underdeveloped in health psychology, medical sociology, medical anthropology, and clinical sexology [4, 7, 8]. Book-length studies published since the early 1990s do illustrate a growing interest in gendered dimensions of fertility and reproduction, especially as they inform men's experiences across culturally diverse settings [9–13]. This interest in positioning men in the global reproductive realm reflects a broader and international scholarly focus on men's reproductive and sexual health, masculinities, sexualities, and changing parenting roles since the early 1990s [14]. This has invited researchers to follow up on early research impressions such as the one documented in a 1988 article, that "men and women in American society interpret and react to infertility in radically different ways [such] that understanding the influence of gender on

D.F. Janssen (✉)
Independent Researcher, Nijmegen, The Netherlands
e-mail: diederikjanssen@gmail.com

© Springer International Publishing AG 2018   1
G.D. Palermo, E.S. Sills (eds.), *Intracytoplasmic Sperm Injection*,
https://doi.org/10.1007/978-3-319-70497-5_1

infertility is crucial to understanding how couples experience infertility" [15]. Men have since been shown to be a unique demographic in global infertility research, from knowledge and perceptions related to childlessness, infertility diagnoses, and assisted reproductive technologies (ARTs) to counselling and treatment experiences. This chapter provides a concise introduction to the literature on men's experiences of especially male-factor infertility, with an emphasis on recent contributions.

1.2   Male Fertility: Mapping Global Expectations and Knowledge Gaps

Appreciating today's experience of male infertility requires a culture-sensitive, historical and research-based interest in changeable and varying conceptions of men's reproductive health, among both men and women, and among both ART providers and ART beneficiaries. Historians have pointed out that male fertility research has only recently begun to take stock of the outcomes of decades of progressive efforts to "classify, standardize, and normalize" male bodies, their health, and especially their reproductive health, as the German and Taiwanese experiences illustrate [16, 17]. Medicalization of reproduction has had divergent outcomes for men. Qualitative researchers suggest that while in some contexts the medicalization of infertility incites stigma for men, in others men are found to be able to deploy medical parlance and routine as a technology to insulate and bolster, rather than necessarily diminish, their sense of masculinity in the otherwise feminized context of reproduction [18, 19]. A likely correlated factor is how men construe their own role across the various dimensions of fertility treatment trajectories and vis-à-vis the topic as such. In one study on Chilean men's assisted reproduction narratives, for instance, men portrayed themselves as secondary and nonactive characters, whereas in narratives about adoption, men centered themselves as co- or equal actors [20].

Men's infertility experiences equally require being located in rapidly changing transnational, transjurisdictional, and online contexts for the communication of both professional expertise and consumer knowledge. For instance, research suggests that gender is an important aspect of men's cross-border treatment experiences and that both traditional and emergent gender identities are expressed by treatment-seeking men [21]. Inhorn recently characterized ICSI a particularly compelling "masculine hope technology" for infertile Muslim male "reprotravelers" to Dubai, an emergent ICSI depot [22]. Such developments seem driven not least by men's expectations of treatment options. Studies on young men in Western countries commonly report a combination of high expectancy for having children in the future and considerable fertility-related knowledge gaps, including overestimations of success rates of ART [23]. Illustratively, recent research reports that almost all Australian male participants wanted to have at least two children but underestimated the impact of age on male and female fertility, overestimated the ability of assisted reproductive technology to overcome age-related fertility decline, and considered it acceptable for men to become fathers in their sixth decade of life [24]. Poorer understanding about fertility treatment outcomes and about the relationship between age and fertility appeared to be associated with socioeconomic disadvantage (no postsecondary education or health insurance) while greater acceptance of later-in-life fatherhood was related to circumstances including being older, childless, unpartnered, and higher educated.

1.3 Cultural Dimensions of Fertility, Masculinity, and Sexuality

Documenting the implications of gaps between expectations and knowledge, and mapping the factors that contribute to them, are essential in approaching male fertility across different ethnographic and social contexts. Understanding popular concepts of male (in)fertility is key to this analysis. British research on media representations of male infertility suggests that such representations may depend on a narrow range of stereotypically masculine reference points [25]. This is echoed by researchers warning for the dangers of practitioners stereotyping, and/or assuming homogeneity of, men irrespective of fertility status, as well as of professionals and researchers being unaware of their own culturally entrenched expectations and projections [26].

The experience of involuntary childlessness indeed importantly varies within and between research contexts. Fatherhood, especially first-time fatherhood, has been observed to have a complex, multistranded and ever-shifting relation to the sense of manhood [27–29]. Unsurprisingly, infertility often appears to be a thoroughly but complexly gendered experience. Even conceptualizations of sperm are known to be heavily imbued with gendered significations across a number of contexts [30–32]. Nevertheless, fertility and masculinity are variously intertwined concepts and the experience of male fertility and infertility varies across ethnographic and historical settings, in part depending on the availability of ART [10, 33]. Male infertility and the use of ICSI have understandably drawn the most extensive anthropological attention in pronatalist societies where male infertility is reported to impinge significantly on constructions of manhood and their symbolic purchase on national identity [13, 19, 22, 34–36].

1.4 Experiences of Infertility

Qualitative and quantitative research suggests that for many men, infertility is a predominantly negative experience, with men reporting feeling ignored, stigmatized and isolated, and a sense of loss of manhood [5, 37–39]. Few longitudinal studies examining quality of life in men with involuntary childlessness exist, however [40]. While women have generally been reported to experience more infertility stress than men, it has proven to be of overriding importance to explore qualitative differences in the ways that men and women are affected by and cope with infertility, all the more when observed across highly variable sociocultural settings [41]. Literature reviews report significant gender differences in coping with infertility at couple level, particularly in terms of coping styles [42, 43].

Regrettably, many studies do not examine the effect of infertility specifically of male factor etiology. Investigators who do compare groups of men and of couples classified on the basis of the cause of infertility commonly report no significant differences in men's coping [44]. Some early data suggested that US men's responses to infertility approximated those of women only when the infertility was attributable to a male factor [45]. More recent studies from Canada, the UK, Sweden, and Taiwan were more typical in reporting that men with a male-factor infertility diagnosis reacted in ways comparable to men in couples where the diagnosis was female, mixed, or of unexplained origin [46–49]. Within-gender differences may often exceed between-gender ones; some Western studies report substantial numbers of both men reporting perceived losses and men reporting perceived gains, in partner relationship quality and sexual satisfaction [50]. Causality remains a notable problem in male infertility research, however. The relationship between sexual dysfunction and male infertility may be bidirectional, for instance, and this may extend to psychological factors including self-reported stress [51–53]. Refinement of research designs at this point is invariably recommended.

1.5   Treatment Experiences

Systematic literature reviews focusing on men's psychological adaptation to infertility treatment and to negative treatment outcomes suggest that in many men, rates of clinically significant mental health problems are no higher than in the general population [44, 54]. One study involving men in couples about to begin their first IVF or ICSI treatment suggested that men are generally well-adjusted with regard to a first IVF/ICSI treatment cycle, independent of gender infertility diagnoses [46]. Research also suggests that men quite variably deal with fertility treatment in relation to role concepts, control beliefs, social support, and infertility cause [55]. Men often express a need for personal face-to-face meetings, dialogue, and opportunities to ask questions, in efforts to process information and exit the "maze" of technology they often find themselves in [44, 56]. Addressing this need may have nontrivial implications for treatment success. For instance, slow progressive sperm motility was negatively associated with anxiety in men proposed to a first, though not a multiple, ART experience [57].

1.6 Implications

While some authors report little evidence demonstrating the utility of social support for men adjusting to an infertility diagnosis [5], others have perhaps more aptly concluded that too little is yet known about men's counselling needs, which may be as specific as they may be varied, such that, when addressed adequately in an appropriate setting, high uptake rates may well be achieved [38, 58]. Underutilization of infertility counselling by men may variably be related to suboptimal levels of public awareness, lack of high-visibility individuals willing to discuss the problem, and men's general avoidance of mental health services [59].

Mapping such mediating factors both in diverse samples and on a per-case basis may be mandatory in tackling this now increasingly recognized problem. The finding of decreasing quality of life in men with the use of more invasive methods in treatment further indicates the need for more attention to psychosocial services in fertility clinics [60]. One study found that some two-thirds of Danish men undergoing fertility treatment reported a need for a deeper dialogue between nursing staff (rarely a counsellor) and the infertile man, the latter preferably to be viewed by health professionals as a stakeholder on equal terms with their female partner [61]. In addition, researchers cite online resources as providing helpful, often anonymous, platforms especially for men dealing with infertility issues [62–64]. Moreover, the arrival of ART services to hitherto ART-deprived settings can have a major, positive impact on gender relations, especially in infertile marriages, and is cited to lead to increased male adoption of ART, especially for male-factor infertility [1].

References

1. Inhorn MC, Patrizio P. Infertility around the globe: new thinking on gender, reproductive technologies and global movements in the 21st century. Hum Reprod Update. 2015;21(4):411–26.
2. Agarwal A, Mulgund A, Hamada A, Chyatte MR. A unique view on male infertility around the globe. Reprod Biol Endocrinol [Internet]. 2015 Dec [cited 2016 Nov 4];13(1). Available from: http://www.rbej.com/content/13/1/37
3. Audibert C, Glass D. A global perspective on assisted reproductive technology fertility treatment: an 8-country fertility specialist survey. Reprod Biol Endocrinol [Internet]. 2015 Dec [cited 2016 Nov 7];13(1). Available from: http://www.rbej.com/content/13/1/133
4. Mehta A, Nangia AK, Dupree JM, Smith JF. Limitations and barriers in access to care for male factor infertility. Fertil Steril. 2016;105(5):1128–37.
5. Arya ST, Dibb B. The experience of infertility treatment: the male perspective. Hum Fertil. 2016;26:1–7.
6. Culley L, Hudson N, Lohan M. Where are all the men? The marginalization of men in social scientific research on infertility. Reprod Biomed Online. 2013;27(3):225–35.
7. Bechoua S, Hamamah S, Scalici E. Male infertility: an obstacle to sexuality? Andrology. 2016;4(3):395–403.
8. Hanna E, Gough B. Experiencing male infertility. SAGE Open. 2015;5(4). https://doi.org/10.1177/2158244015610319.
9. Mason M-C. Male infertility—men talking. New York: Routledge; 1993.

10. Inhorn MC, Tjørnhøj-Thomsen T, Goldberg H, la Cour Mosegaard M, editors. Reconceiving the second sex: men, masculinity, and reproduction, Fertility, reproduction and sexuality, vol. vi. New York: Berghahn Books; 2009. p. 392.

11. Barnes LW. Conceiving masculinity: male infertility, medicine, and identity. Philadelphia: Temple University Press; 2014. 211 p

12. Daniels CR. Exposing men: the science and politics of male reproduction. Oxford. New York: Oxford University Press; 2006. 259 p

13. Inhorn MC. The new Arab man: emergent masculinities, technologies, and Islam in the Middle East. Princeton: Princeton University Press; 2012.

14. Marsiglio W, Lohan M, Culley L. Framing men's experience in the procreative realm. J Fam Issues. 2013;34:1011. https://doi.org/10.1177/0192513X13484260.

15. Greil AL, Leitko TA, Porter KL. Infertility: his and hers. Gend Soc. 1988;2(2):172–99.

16. Kampf A. Tales of healthy men: male reproductive bodies in biomedicine from "Lebensborn" to sperm banks. Health (N Y). 2013;17(1):20–36. https://doi.org/10.1177/1363459312447251.

17. Wu C-L. Managing multiple masculinities in donor insemination: doctors configuring infertile men and sperm donors in Taiwan: managing masculinities in donor insemination in Taiwan. Sociol Health Illn. 2011;33(1):96–113.

18. Bell AV. "I don''t consider a cup performance; I consider it a test': masculinity and the medicalisation of infertility. Sociol Health Illn. 2016;38(5):706–20.

19. Inhorn MC. Middle Eastern masculinities in the age of new reproductive technologies: male infertility and stigma in Egypt and Lebanon. Med Anthropol Q. 2004;18(2):162–82.

20. Herrera F. "Men Always Adopt" infertility and reproduction from a male perspective. J Fam Issues. 2013;34(8):1059–80.

21. Hudson N, Culley L. The bloke can be a bit hazy about what's going on': men and cross-border reproductive treatment. Reprod Biomed Online. 2013;27(3):253–60.

22. Inhorn MC. Medical cosmopolitanism in global Dubai: a twenty-first-century transnational intracytoplasmic sperm injection (ICSI) depot. Med Anthropol Q. 2016;31:5. https://doi.org/10.1111/maq.12275.

23. Ulla Christensen RS. Desire for parenthood, beliefs about masculinity, and fertility awareness among young Danish men. Reprod Syst Sex Disord [Internet]. 2013 [cited 2016 Nov 7];3(1). Available from: http://www.omicsonline.org/desire-for-parenthood-beliefs-about-masculinity-and-fertility-awareness-among-young-danish-men-2161–038X-3–127.php?aid=22328

24. Holton S, Hammarberg K, Rowe H, Kirkman M, Jordan L, Mcnamee K, Bayly C, Mcbain J, Sinnott V, Fisher J. Men's fertility-related knowledge and attitudes, and childbearing desires, expectations and outcomes: findings from the understanding fertility management in contemporary Australia survey. Int J Men's Health. 2016;15(3):215–28.

25. Gannon K, Glover L, Abel P. Masculinity, infertility, stigma and media reports. Soc Sci Med. 2004;59(6):1169–75.

26. Crawshaw M. Male coping with cancer-fertility issues: putting the "social" into biopsychosocial approaches. Reprod Biomed Online. 2013;27(3):261–70.

27. Pleck JH. Fatherhood and masculinity. In: The role of the father in child development, ed. ME Lamb. Hoboken, NJ: John Wiley, 2010. p. 27–57. http://psycnet.apa.org/record/2010-04805-002

28. Finn M, Henwood K. Exploring masculinities within men's identificatory imaginings of first-time fatherhood. Br J Soc Psychol. 2009;48(3):547–62.

29. Miller T. Falling back into gender? Men's narratives and practices around first-time fatherhood. Sociology. 2011;45:1094. https://doi.org/10.1177/0038038511419180.

30. Martin E. The egg and the sperm: how science has constructed a romance based on stereotypical male-female roles. Signs. 1991;16(3):485–501.

31. Moore LJ. Sperm counts: overcome by man's most precious fluid, Intersections: transdisciplinary perspectives on genders and sexualities. New York: New York University Press; 2007. 203 p.

32. Shand A. Semen anxiety: materiality, agency and the internet. Anthropol Med. 2007;14(3):241–50.

33. Bledsoe CH, Lerner S, Guyer JI. Fertility and the male life-cycle in the era of fertility decline, International studies in demography, vol. x. New York: Oxford University Press; 2000. p. 376.
34. Inhorn MC, Wentzell EA. Embodying emergent masculinities: men engaging with reproductive and sexual health technologies in the Middle East and Mexico. Am Ethnol. 2011;38(4):801–15.
35. Inhorn MC. "The Worms Are Weak": male infertility and patriarchal paradoxes in Egypt. Men Masculinities. 2003;5(3):236–56.
36. Inhorn MC, Birenbaum-Carmeli D. Assisted reproductive technologies and culture change. Annu Rev Anthropol. 2008;37(1):177–96.
37. Hinton L, Miller T. Mapping men's anticipations and experiences in the reproductive realm: (in)fertility journeys. Reprod Biomed Online. 2013;27(3):244–52.
38. Wischmann T, Thorn P. (Male) infertility: what does it mean to men? New evidence from quantitative and qualitative studies. Reprod Biomed Online. 2013;27(3):236–43.
39. Miall CE. Community constructs of involuntary childlessness: sympathy, stigma, and social support. Can Rev Sociol Can Sociol. 1994;31(4):392–421.
40. Schanz S, Häfner H-M, Ulmer A, Fierlbeck G. Quality of life in men with involuntary childlessness: long-term follow-up. Andrologia. 2014;46(7):731–7.
41. Greil AL, Slauson-Blevins K, McQuillan J. The experience of infertility: a review of recent literature. Sociol Health Illn. 2010;32(1):140–62.
42. Ying LY, LH W, Loke AY. Gender differences in experiences with and adjustments to infertility: a literature review. Int J Nurs Stud. 2015;52(10):1640–52.
43. Jordan C, Revenson TA. Gender differences in coping with infertility: a meta-analysis. J Behav Med. 1999;22(4):341–58.
44. Fisher JR, Hammarberg K. Psychological and social aspects of infertility in men: an overview of the evidence and implications for psychologically informed clinical care and future research. Asian J Androl. 2012;14(1):121–9.
45. Nachtigall RD, Becker G, Wozny M. The effects of gender-specific diagnosis on men's and women's response to infertility. Fertil Steril. 1992;57(1):113–21.
46. Holter H, Anderheim L, Bergh C, Moller A. The psychological influence of gender infertility diagnoses among men about to start IVF or ICSI treatment using their own sperm. Hum Reprod. 2007;22(9):2559–65.
47. Dhillon R, Cumming CE, Cumming DC. Psychological well-being and coping patterns in infertile men. Fertil Steril. 2000;74(4):702–6.
48. Peronace LA, Boivin J, Schmidt L. Patterns of suffering and social interactions in infertile men: 12 months after unsuccessful treatment. J Psychosom Obstet Gynecol. 2007;28(2):105–14.
49. Lee T-Y, Sun G-H, Chao S-C. The effect of an infertility diagnosis on the distress, marital and sexual satisfaction between husbands and wives in Taiwan. Hum Reprod. 2001;16(8):1762–7.
50. Hammarberg K, Baker HWG, Fisher JRW. Men's experiences of infertility and infertility treatment 5 years after diagnosis of male factor infertility: a retrospective cohort study. Hum Reprod. 2010;25(11):2815–20.
51. Beretta G. Sexual problems and infertility. In: Cavallini G, Beretta G, editors. Clinical management of male infertility [Internet]. Cham: Springer International Publishing; 2015 [cited 2016 Nov 4]. p. 179–83. Available from: http://link.springer.com/10.1007/978-3-319-08503-6_19
52. Nargund VH. Effects of psychological stress on male fertility. Nat Rev Urol. 2015;12(7):373–82.
53. Nordkap L, Jensen TK, Hansen ÅM, Lassen TH, Bang AK, Joensen UN, et al. Psychological stress and testicular function: a cross-sectional study of 1,215 Danish men. Fertil Steril. 2016;105(1):174–187.e2.
54. Martins MV, Basto-Pereira M, Pedro J, Peterson B, Almeida V, Schmidt L, et al. Male psychological adaptation to unsuccessful medically assisted reproduction treatments: a systematic review. Hum Reprod Update. 2016;22(4):466–78.
55. Schick M, Rösner S, Toth B, Strowitzki T, Wischmann T. Exploring involuntary childlessness in men—a qualitative study assessing quality of life, role aspects and control beliefs in men's perception of the fertility treatment process. Hum Fertil. 2016;19(1):32–42.

56. Sylvest R, Fürbringer JK, Schmidt L, Pinborg A. Infertile men's needs and assessment of fertility care. Ups J Med Sci. 2016:1–7.
57. Bártolo A, Reis S, Monteiro S, Leite R, Montenegro N. Psychological adjustment of infertile men undergoing fertility treatments: an association with sperm parameters. Arch Psychiatr Nurs. 2016;30(5):521–6.
58. Wischmann T. "Your count is zero"—counselling the infertile man. Hum Fertil. 2013;16(1):35–9.
59. Petok WD. Infertility counseling (or the lack thereof) of the forgotten male partner. Fertil Steril. 2015;104(2):260–6.
60. Schick M, Rösner S, Toth B, Strowitzki T, Jank A, Kentenich H, et al. Effects of medical causes, role concepts and treatment stages on quality of life in involuntary childless men. Andrologia. 2016;48(9):937–42.
61. Mikkelsen AT, Madsen SA, Humaidan P. Psychological aspects of male fertility treatment. J Adv Nurs. 2013;69(9):1977–86.
62. Malik SH, Coulson N. The male experience of infertility: a thematic analysis of an online infertility support group bulletin board. J Reprod Infant Psychol. 2008;26(1):18–30.
63. Hanna E, Gough B. Searching for help online: an analysis of peer-to-peer posts on a male-only infertility forum. J Health Psychol. 2016;1359105316644038. https://doi.org/10.1177/1359105316644038.
64. Richard J, Badillo-Amberg I, Zelkowitz P. "So Much of This Story Could Be Me" men's use of support in online infertility discussion boards. Am J Mens Health. 2016;11:663. https://doi.org/10.1177/1557988316671460.

Chapter 2
Intracytoplasmic Sperm Injection: History, Indications, Technique, and Safety

Nigel Pereira and Gianpiero D. Palermo

2.1   Introduction

The pioneering of intracytoplasmic sperm injection (ICSI) has been heralded as one of the major breakthroughs in the field of reproductive medicine. In the years since the first live births with ICSI were reported in 1992 [1], this technique has been deployed as a powerful tool to treat almost all forms of male infertility, and also to overcome fertilization failure [2]. ICSI, in conjunction with in vitro fertilization (IVF), has been integral in many millions of advanced reproductive treatments, resulting in the birth of over five million babies so far. In this chapter, we review the history of assisted reproductive technologies (ART) before the inception of ICSI, with special emphasis on the shortcomings of earlier techniques developed to treat male factor infertility. We highlight the advantages of ICSI and enumerate its various indications, including non-male factor infertility. Finally, we appraise the safety of ICSI by evaluating recent studies that have assessed the medical and reproductive health of children conceived using this technique.

2.2   History

2.2.1   ART Before ICSI

ART is a general term used to describe any reproductive technique or treatment which involves handling of oocytes and/or embryos [3]. Such technologies include gamete intrafallopian transfer (GIFT), zygote intrafallopian transfer (ZIFT), or IVF,

N. Pereira • G.D. Palermo (✉)
The Ronald O. Perelman and Claudia Cohen Center for Reproductive Medicine,
Weill Cornell Medicine, New York, NY, USA
e-mail: nip90760@med.cornell.edu; gdpalerm@med.cornell.edu

© Springer International Publishing AG 2018
G.D. Palermo, E.S. Sills (eds.), *Intracytoplasmic Sperm Injection*,
https://doi.org/10.1007/978-3-319-70497-5_2

which accounts for approximately 99% of all ART cycles [3]. It must be noted that treatments such as intrauterine insemination which only involve handling of sperm, or even female treatments such as ovarian stimulation or ovulation induction that do not involve handling of oocytes, are not included in the definition of ART [3].

The first live birth using ART, specifically IVF, was achieved in 1978 in a patient with tubal factor infertility [4]. It soon become evident that IVF could be used in patients with various types of infertility and that oocyte retrieval did not have to be limited to the natural (monofollicular) menstrual cycle as originally described. As early as 1984, several clinics reported the use of gonadotropins or antiestrogens to stimulate the growth of multiple follicles, from which multiple oocytes could be recovered [5, 6]. When fertilized, these oocytes could generate several good-quality embryos, which could be transferred in utero. Interestingly, it was noted that transferring two or more embryos could increase the efficacy of IVF [5, 7]. Using this protocol, the Bourn Hall clinic reported that their implantation rates increased from 16.5% to 30%, with over 118 live births occurring until 1984 [5]. Similarly, in Norfolk, 105 pregnancies were reported using a comparable protocol in 319 patients between 1981 and 1983 [8]. Also, during the same 3-year interval, the pregnancy rate was 19% and 25% per cycle and per transfer, respectively [8].

Despite early success in several clinics, IVF was inundated by poor fertilization or complete fertilization failure (CFF) even in the presence of an adequate number of oocytes. Several investigators had indicated that poor or absent fertilization occurred in up to 40% of IVF cycles and was especially common in couples where the male partner had suboptimal semen parameters [9, 10]. Thus, a substitute to conventional in vitro insemination was urgently needed which could fertilize oocytes irrespective of semen parameters.

2.2.2 Assisted Fertilization Techniques Before ICSI

Many embryologists sought to decrease the incidence of poor fertilization or CFF in IVF cycles by increasing in vitro sperm concentrations [11]. This was achieved most often by changing the volume of the inseminating medium so as to facilitate the co-mingling of gametes [11]. Others focused on enhancing the quality of sperm by using swim-up, sedimentation methods, or multilayer density gradients techniques aiming to increase the fraction of highly motile and morphologically normal spermatozoa available for in vitro insemination [9]. Methods such as using motility enhancers or removing the cumulus-corona cells were also attempted [12, 13]. While these methods were able to increase in vitro fertilization rates in men with mild-to-moderate oligozoospermia or asthenozoospermia, success remained very limited in men with complete teratozoospermia or severe oligo-asthenozoospermia. This was not surprising given that spermatozoa with diminished motility or poor morphology could not penetrate the thick glycoprotein coat of the oocyte, the zona pellucida (ZP), to achieve fertilization.

The focus then switched to assisted fertilization, i.e., assisting the spermatozoon to penetrate the ZP to achieve fertilization. Early investigations aimed at complete removal of the ZP to aid fertilization; however, such attempts resulted in polyspermy and abnormal embryo development. To overcome the shortcomings of complete zona removal, attempts were made to bypass the ZP by enzymatic "softening" with pronase or trypsin [14], or by very localized chemical treatment with acid Tyrode's solution before sperm exposure [15]. The latter technique, known as zona-drilling (ZD), involved exposure to a low pH solution, and increased the risk of chemical damage to the ooplasm in addition to the aforementioned risk of polyspermy [15]. ZD was therefore modified by creating a partial opening of the zona using mechanical force only; this technique was called partial zona drilling (PZD) [16]. Preliminary data showed that PZD achieved monospermic fertilization and that 10/16 (63%) of the PZD oocytes showed normal embryo cleavage [16]. Despite these encouraging results, investigators noted that spermatozoa still required assistance to interact with the cytoplasm of the oocyte when utilizing PZD [16, 17]. This necessity paved the way for another technique called sub-zonal insemination (SUZI) [18]. In this refined technique, up to three spermatozoa were brought with a pipette through the zona and deposited into the perivitelline space [18]. SUZI showed promising results; in one study of 43 couples with a history of CFF with IVF, SUZI achieved a fertilization rate of 30.9% (433 total oocytes) [19]. The cleavage rate of the fertilized oocytes was 80%, with 7 patients achieving pregnancy [19]. SUZI was also able to achieve fertilization in patients with more impaired semen parameters and control the incidence of polyspermy [11]. Yet, overall fertilization rates still remained low because the spermatozoa needed to undergo a complete acrosome reaction for fusion with the oolemma [19]. Given the shortcomings of complete zona removal, ZD, PZD, and SUZI, efforts continued to develop a microsurgical method to inject spermatozoa directly into the oocyte, without compromising the integrity of the ZP or the fertilization potential of the spermatozoon.

2.3 ICSI

2.3.1 Background and Development

It is thought that micromanipulation of gametes was attempted as early as the 1940s. However, in the 1960s, systematic studies in sea urchin [20, 21] and mouse [22] models showed that fertilization could be achieved with sperm microinjection. However, initial sperm microinjection strategies in human oocytes showed a high incidence of oocyte damage and poor embryo implantation [23], likely due to the impreciseness of the micromanipulator equipment. Evidence mounted that sperm microinjection in human oocytes would require intricate tools to pierce the ZP and oolemma, without damaging either. A considerable amount of time and effort was spent at the Free University of Brussels to convert crude micromanipulator equipment into smoother ones, including the tubing for the microinjector to deliver a constant pressure to a 5 μ diameter microneedle. Other changes included the use of appropriate dishes for micromanipulation, as well as newer holding and injecting pipettes [2].

It was while performing SUZI that a single spermatozoon inadvertently pierced the oolemma of an oocyte. Instead of being discarded, the oocyte was re-examined the following day, only to reveal two pronuclei, thus confirming fertilization [2]. This moment was perhaps the birth of ICSI. The technique not only bypassed the zona, but it also allowed for precise injection of a single spermatozoon within the ooplasm. The possibility emerged that ICSI might be capable of fertilizing nearly every mature oocyte injected, irrespective of spermatozoa characteristics [24–26]. As with SUZI and PZD, ICSI allowed documentation of pronuclear development, as well as the first embryonic cleavage without the visual obstruction of cumulus cells [27, 28]. Early studies using ICSI were also instrumental in revealing the genetics of abnormal human fertilization, specifically the pathogenesis of 1pn and 3pn embryos, leading to the evidence that the human sperm centrosome controls the first mitotic divisions after fertilization [29, 30].

2.3.2   Popularity of ICSI

Initial comparisons of ICSI with SUZI demonstrated fertilization rates of 44% and 18% with ICSI and SUZI, respectively [24]. However, further research showed that aggressive sperm immobilization by permanently crimping the sperm flagellum between the midpiece and the rest of the tail could increase fertilization rates [31]. In one study of 837 cycles, ICSI after aggressive sperm immobilization was associated with a higher fertilization and pregnancy rate of 82% and 82.4%, respectively, compared to a fertilization and pregnancy rate of 48.3% and 51.4%, respectively, with standard sperm immobilization and ICSI [31].

Following several refinements, ICSI has become a powerful tool to overcome suboptimal semen parameters and fertilization defects, thereby allowing infertile men to reproduce at rates that previously would have been deemed improbable [27]. In a recent retrospective, cross-sectional survey, the International Committee for Monitoring Assisted Reproductive Technologies (ICMART) reported data from >4,461,309 ART cycles initiated in 61 countries between 2008 and 2010 [32]. ICSI was utilized in 66% of all ART cycles during this period. Interestingly, the committee reported vast geographical variations in ICSI utilization. For example, ICSI utilization was 55% in Asia and 65% in Europe, but 100% in the Middle East [32]. In the USA, the use of ICSI has increased from 36.4% in 1996 to 76.2% in 2012 [33]. At our center, the utilization of ICSI has steadily increased from 32.2% in 1993 to 48.8% in 1995 to approximately 76.2% currently. During the past 23 years, we have performed a total of 39,918 ART cycles. The mean ages of female and male patients undergoing ICSI at our center is 37.3 ± 5 and 39.9 ± 8 years, respectively, while those undergoing IVF is 36.6 ± 4 and 39.5 ± 7 years, respectively. Between 1993 and 2016, 18,863 couples were treated with ICSI at our center. The total number of oocytes retrieved was 349,560 of which 279,361 (80%) were metaphase II oocytes available for ICSI. Of the oocytes injected, 206,110 developed two pronuclei, indicating a fertilization rate of 73.8%.

2.4   Indications

Conventional IVF was first utilized in patients with bilateral tubal occlusion or blockage that was not amenable to surgery. However, refinements in ovarian stimulation and embryology laboratory protocols coupled with the desire of infertile patients to achieve a pregnancy resulted in the utilization of IVF in patients with non-tubal infertility such as endometriosis, mild male-factor infertility, as well as unexplained infertility. Yet, several thousand patients with severe male-factor infertility could not be treated with IVF, and these patients would have to rely on donor sperm or adoption [11]. ICSI addressed these shortcomings of IVF and revolutionized the treatment of patients with severe male-factor infertility in whom the male partners were presumed to be the cause of repeated failed attempts at IVF or whose semen parameters were unacceptable for conventional IVF [11, 25]. ICSI has also become the mainstay of treating men with obstructive azoospermia (OA) [34, 35] or non-obstructive azoospermia (NOA) [36, 37] who require surgical retrieval of sperm. It has also been applied successfully in genetic conditions such as Klinefelter's syndrome [38], as well as other conditions such as anejaculation [39] and azoospermia due to chemotherapy [40].

ICSI has been used for several non-male factor indications. One such indication is the fertilization of poor-quality or dysmorphic oocytes, as determined by morphologic assessment [41]. Investigators have also proposed that ICSI should be used in poor responders to maximize fertilization rates in the oocytes available for injection [42]. ICSI may also be warranted for cryopreserved oocytes given that vitrification-thaw process can cause zona hardening [43]. Figure 2.1 summarizes various clinical indications of ICSI.

It must be noted that ICSI is being increasingly utilized by several clinics even in the presence of normal semen parameters [44]. For example, in the USA the application of ICSI for non-male factor infertility increased from 15.4% in 1996 to 66.9% in 2012 [33]. Interestingly, this increased utilization was not associated with any apparent benefit. Studies have also shown that ICSI for the sole indication of advanced maternal age or unexplained infertility provides no obvious therapeutic gain compared to conventional IVF [45, 46]. Currently, the American Society for Reproductive Medicine and the Society for Assisted Reproductive Technology confirm that there is insufficient evidence to support the routine use of ICSI in patients without male factor infertility [47]. Thus, it is important that the utilization of ICSI is personalized to the reproductive history of the couple undergoing ART.

While some of the clinical indications of ICSI have been debated, there are certain circumstances in which the use of ICSI should be strongly discouraged. ICSI

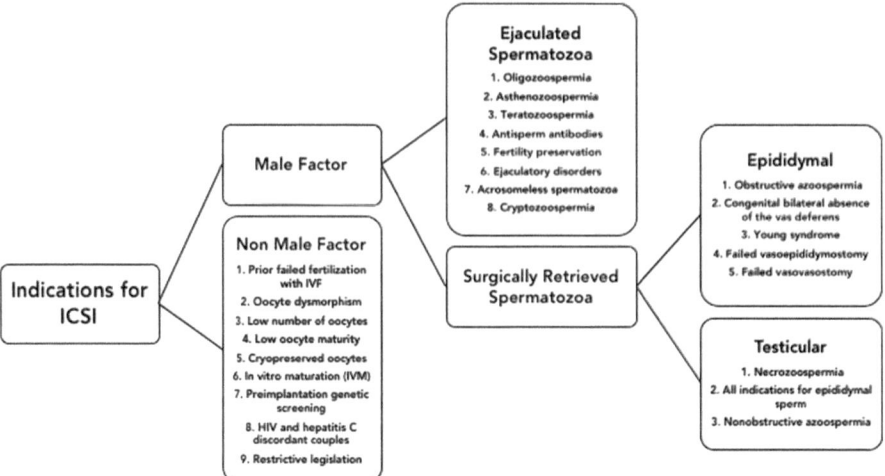

Fig. 2.1 Simplified flowchart depicting the male-factor and non-male factor indications for intra-cytoplasmic sperm injection (ICSI)

requires specialized technical skills and training [27] and has to be performed in a laminar flow hood setting, on a heated stage outside of the incubator in a highly regulated laboratory environment. More importantly, ICSI has to be performed expeditiously. Of note, early adopters of ICSI were able to improve pregnancy rates significantly by simply adhering to stringent laboratory conditions [27]. Thus, ICSI should not be performed when any of the aforementioned requirements cannot be met. ICSI should also not be used to reinseminate oocytes that do not fertilize following after conventional IVF, i.e., rescue ICSI [27]. Embryos generated from rescue ICSI have high rates of polyploidy [48] and often arrest at early developmental stages [49–51].

2.5   Technique

Details regarding oocyte collection and preparation of ejaculated and surgically retrieved sperm for ICSI have been described elsewhere [26, 31, 52]. However, details of the equipment and ICSI technique are given here.

2.5.1   Equipment

- A micromanipulation system (NAI-2P, Narishige International USA, Inc), which includes a hydraulic microinjector (IM-6), modified with a metal syringe, air-filled injector (IM-9C), and BDH oil—for loading the injector (BDH Laboratory Supplies; Dorset UK).

- An inverted microscope with polarized optics CFI S Plan Fluor (20× and 40× objectives) and CFI Apo (2×, 4×, and 10× objectives)
- A custom-designed horseshoe shaped heated stage (Easteach Laboratory; Maspeth New York, USA)
- Microtool requirements include injection pipettes (4–6 μm ID; 30° bend angle), injection pipettes (5–6 μm ID; 30° bend angle), and holding pipettes (120 μm OD; 30° bend angle).
- Oocyte transfer and denudation pipettes (hand-pulled, flame-polished Pasteur pipettes)
- ICSI dish (BD Falcon 351,006; Becton, Dickinson & Co., Franklin Lakes, New Jersey, USA)
- Stereomicroscope
- Repetitive pipette for dispending ICSI media
- Electronic repeating pipette for dispensing oil
- Pipetman P20 (F123600, Gilson, Inc.) for PVP and sperm loading

2.5.2 Tool Settings

The holding and injection pipettes are inserted into their respective micromanipulation tool holders that are mounted on an inverted microscope. The coarse motorized controllers are used to position the pipettes in the center of the microscopic field at 20×, after which the magnification is gradually increased by adjusting the hydraulic controllers. Under 400× magnification, correct pipette positioning is accomplished by using the hydraulic joysticks in such a way that both pipettes should be able to course through the entire optical field. The distal bent portions of both microtools should be kept slightly above parallel to prevent the elbows of the micromanipulation apparatus from touching the bottom of the dish and interfering with the control. These steps ensure prompt immobilization and visual control of the spermatozoon inside the injection pipette. Once the pipettes are properly aligned, they are raised using the coarse motorized controllers to allow placement of the ICSI dish on the microscope stage.

2.5.3 Preparation of the ICSI DISH

Nine drops containing 8 μl of injection medium are placed in a petri dish, with one in the center radially surrounded by the other eight. It is important that the drops are as close together as possible to allow full visualization within the 20 mm opening on the heated stage. The drops should then be gently overlaid with culture oil to prevent evaporation. Using a red non-embryo toxic wax pencil, the 12 o'clock position is marked, a circle drawn around the central drop, and the drops are sequentially numbered starting from the 12 o'clock position, moving counterclockwise. This allows easy navigation between droplets during ICSI. These dishes are stored at 37°C until use.

2.5.4 Loading of Gametes

Immediately before sperm injection, the central drop is removed and replaced with 1 μl of sperm suspension diluted in 4 μl of 7% PVP. Metaphase II oocytes devoid of cumulus cells are aspirated from the culture dish with a hand-pulled Pasteur pipette and a single oocyte is placed in each drop.

2.5.5 Sperm Immobilization

The spermatozoon is positioned at 90° with respect to the pipette tip, which is gently lowered to compress the principal piece of the tail by rolling the posterior flagellum over the bottom of the Petri dish. If initial attempts at immobilization are unsuccessful, the procedure is repeated until the tail is clearly kinked, looped, or convoluted. It is important to note that a misshapen tail may adhere to the dish or to the inner surface of the pipette. Following immobilization, the spermatozoon is aspirated tail first. The injection needle is lifted slightly via the two control knobs of the joystick to avoid damaging the needle spike. The microscope stage is then repositioned until the injection needle enters the oocyte drop. Of note, the difference in media consistency (PVP vs. culture medium) may allow the sperm to move distally into the pipette and become loose.

2.5.6 Sperm Injection

The magnification is briefly lowered to 200× to locate the oocyte within the drop. Once the oocyte is positioned centrally in the field, the magnification is returned to 400×. Next, the oocyte is held in place by suction through the holding pipette. Using both microtools, the oocyte is rotated slowly to locate the polar body and the area of cortical rarefaction (or polar granularity). The equatorial plane of the oocyte is located and the depth of the holding pipette is adjusted to have its internal opening in the same plane, which allows for greater support of the holding pipette in a position opposite to the injection site. In general, it is ideal to have the inferior pole of the oocyte touching the bottom of the dish, as it provides a more secure grip of the oocyte during injection. The injection pipette is then lowered and focused with the outer right border of the oolemma on the equatorial plane at 3 o'clock. The spermatozoon is positioned near the beveled opening of the injection pipette, which is brought to the zona. The pipette is pressed into the zona to penetrate it, followed by a gentle forward thrust to the inner surface of the oolemma at 9 o'clock. A break in the oolemma should occur at the approximate center of the oocyte. Such a break is denoted by a sudden quivering of the convexities of the oolemma (at the site of invagination) above and below the injection point, as well as by the proximal flow of ooplasmic organelles and the spermatozoon back into the pipette. The spermatozoon is then ejected with the ooplasmic component. To optimize interaction with the ooplasm, the spermatozoon should be ejected past the tip of the pipette to ensure a close intermingling with the ooplasmic lattices, which help maintain the spermatozoon in place while withdrawing the pipette. Additional ooplasm is aspirated back and forth with the injection pipette to induce oocyte activation. It is extremely important to avoid leaving behind residual medium with the spermatozoon as well as closing the breach of penetration. This is generally achieved by applying a mild suction while removing the pipette. Once the pipette is retracted from the oocyte, the injection point margins should maintain a funnel shape with the tip towards the center of the oocyte. If the border of the oolemma becomes everted, the cytoplasmic organelles can leak out and the oocyte may lyse. The average time required to perform ICSI per oocyte is approximately 30–40 s.

2.6 Safety

Studies regarding the safety of ICSI, as manifested in the perinatal outcomes and the medical and psychological health of the conceived children, have been ongoing since the early 1990s. Following the initial 3 years of ICSI application, investigators at the Free University of Brussels reported that the obstetric outcomes of the first 424 ICSI pregnancies were similar to the outcomes of the pregnancies conceived with IVF and other ART methods [53]. The same investigators then compared the outcomes of 904 consecutive ICSI pregnancies using ejaculated spermatozoa, epididymal spermatozoa, and testicular spermatozoa, and found no difference in the obstetric outcomes based on sperm source [54]. A follow-up study of pregnancies resulting from 987 ICSI cycles in New York showed no difference in the pregnancy outcomes of ICSI or IVF cycles [55]. No differences were also found in the frequency of miscarriages. Interestingly, the frequency of malformations in the ICSI group was lower than that observed in the IVF group [55]. When the medical and psychological health of 5-year-old ICSI children in Brussels, Gothenburg, and New York was investigated, it was found that ICSI did not adversely affect growth, psychological well-being, or cognitive development at age 5 [56, 57]. Another follow-up study demonstrated that ICSI offspring and their naturally conceived counterparts had similar motor skills and IQ at age 10 [58]. It is reassuring to note that a very recent study has confirmed that children born after ICSI or IVF had similar cognitive, motor, and language development as children born after natural (unassisted) conception [59].

The reproductive health of young adults conceived via ICSI has also been evaluated. In one study that compared 54 young men (18–22 years) conceived by ICSI due to male factor infertility to 57 naturally conceived peers, the authors found that the mean levels of follicle stimulating hormone, luteinizing hormone, testosterone, and inhibin B were comparable in both groups, even after controlling for age, body mass index, and season [60]. A follow-up study from the same center reported this group of 54 young men had lower median sperm concentration, total sperm count, and total motile sperm count than the naturally conceived peers [61]. However, the small sample size limited the generalization of these findings. The reproductive hormonal profiles of young ICSI-conceived women are currently awaited.

The aforementioned findings notwithstanding, the safety of ICSI has often come under scrutiny, and sometimes even criticism. This is predominantly due to the thought that ICSI involves arbitrary selection of sperm for injection, thereby bypassing physiologic in vivo sperm selection and fusion with the zona or oolemma [62, 63]. These concerns have been further perpetuated by studies claiming that ICSI increases the risk of imprinting disorders [64] or autism and mental retardation [65]. However, it is important to note that studies reporting concerns about the epigenetic and genetic implications of ICSI are often heterogeneous in methodology and are skewed by common confounders such as multiple gestations [66, 67]. Thus, single embryo transfer is essential in reducing the risk of adverse outcomes. It is also possible that infertility itself may be the larger issue that leads to adverse obstetric and health outcomes.

References

1. Palermo G, Joris H, Devroey P, Van Steirteghem AC. Pregnancies after intracytoplasmic injection of single spermatozoon into an oocyte. Lancet. 1992;340(8810):17–8.
2. Pereira N, Cozzubbo T, Cheung S, Palermo GD. Lessons learned in andrology: from intracytoplasmic sperm injection and beyond. Andrology. 2016;4(5):757–60.
3. https://www.cdc.gov/art/whatis.html. Accessed 9 Feb 2017.
4. Steptoe PC, Edwards RG. Birth after the reimplantation of a human embryo. Lancet. 1978;2(8085):366.
5. Edwards RG, Fishel SB, Cohen J, et al. Factors influencing the success of in vitro fertilization for alleviating human infertility. J In Vitro Fert Embryo Transf. 1984;1(1):3–23.
6. Jones GS, Garcia JE, Rosenwaks Z. The role of pituitary gonadotropins in follicular stimulation and oocyte maturation in the human. J Clin Endocrinol Metab. 1984;59(1):178–80.
7. Muasher SJ, Wilkes C, Garcia JE, Rosenwaks Z, Jones HW Jr. Benefits and risks of multiple transfer with in vitro fertilisation. Lancet. 1984;1(8376):570.
8. Jones HW Jr, Acosta AA, Andrews MC, et al. Three years of in vitro fertilization at Norfolk. Fertil Steril. 1984;42(6):826–34.
9. Cohen J, Edwards RG, Fehilly CB, et al. Treatment of male infertility by in vitro fertilization: factors affecting fertilization and pregnancy. Acta Eur Fertil. 1984;15(6):455–65.
10. Mahadevan MM, Trounson AO. The influence of seminal characteristics on the success rate of human in vitro fertilization. Fertil Steril. 1984;42(3):400–5.

11. Palermo GD, Kocent J, Monahan D, Neri QV, Rosenwaks Z. Treatment of male infertility. Methods Mol Biol. 2014;1154:385–405.
12. Yovich JM, Edirisinghe WR, Cummins JM, Yovich JL. Influence of pentoxifylline in severe male factor infertility. Fertil Steril. 1990;53(4):715–22.
13. Lavy G, Boyers SP, DeCherney AH. Hyaluronidase removal of the cumulus oophorus increases in vitro fertilization. J In Vitro Fert Embryo Transf. 1988;5(5):257–60.
14. Kiessling AA, Loutradis D, McShane PM, Jackson KV. Fertilization in trypsin-treated oocytes. Ann N Y Acad Sci. 1988;541:614–20.
15. Gordon JW, Talansky BE. Assisted fertilization by zona drilling: a mouse model for correction of oligospermia. J Exp Zool. 1986;239(3):347–54.
16. Cohen J, Malter H, Fehilly C, et al. Implantation of embryos after partial opening of oocyte zona pellucida to facilitate sperm penetration. Lancet. 1988;2(8603):162.
17. Malter HE, Cohen J. Partial zona dissection of the human oocyte: a nontraumatic method using micromanipulation to assist zona pellucida penetration. Fertil Steril. 1989;51(1):139–48.
18. Palermo G, Van Steirteghem A. Enhancement of acrosome reaction and subzonal insemination of a single spermatozoon in mouse eggs. Mol Reprod Dev. 1991;30(4):339–45.
19. Palermo G, Joris H, Devroey P, Van Steirteghem AC. Induction of acrosome reaction in human spermatozoa used for subzonal insemination. Hum Reprod. 1992;7(2):248–54.
20. Lin TP. Microinjection of mouse eggs. Science. 1966;151(3708):333–7.
21. Hiramoto Y. Microinjection of the live spermatozoa into sea urchin eggs. Exp Cell Res. 1962;27:416–26.
22. Hiramoto Y. An analysis of the mechanism of fertilation by means of enucleation of sea urchin eggs. Exp Cell Res. 1962;28:323–34.
23. Lanzendorf SE, Maloney MK, Veeck LL, Slusser J, Hodgen GD, Rosenwaks Z. A preclinical evaluation of pronuclear formation by microinjection of human spermatozoa into human oocytes. Fertil Steril. 1988;49(5):835–42.
24. Palermo G, Joris H, Derde MP, Camus M, Devroey P, Van Steirteghem A. Sperm characteristics and outcome of human assisted fertilization by subzonal insemination and intracytoplasmic sperm injection. Fertil Steril. 1993;59(4):826–35.
25. Palermo GD, Cohen J, Alikani M, Adler A, Rosenwaks Z. Intracytoplasmic sperm injection: a novel treatment for all forms of male factor infertility. Fertil Steril. 1995;63(6):1231–40.
26. Palermo GD, Neri QV, Schlegel PN, Rosenwaks Z. Intracytoplasmic sperm injection (ICSI) in extreme cases of male infertility. PLoS One. 2014;9(12):e113671.
27. Palermo GD, Neri QV, Rosenwaks Z. To ICSI or not to ICSI. Semin Reprod Med. 2015;33(2):92–102.
28. Palermo GD, Neri QV, Takeuchi T, Rosenwaks Z. ICSI: where we have been and where we are going. Semin Reprod Med. 2009;27(2):191–201.
29. Palermo G, Munné S, Cohen J. The human zygote inherits its mitotic potential from the male gamete. Hum Reprod. 1994;9(7):1220–5.
30. Palermo GD, Munné S, Colombero LT, Cohen J, Rosenwaks Z. Genetics of abnormal human fertilization. Hum Reprod. 1995;10(Suppl 1):120–7.
31. Palermo GD, Schlegel PN, Colombero LT, Zaninovic N, Moy F, Rosenwaks Z. Aggressive sperm immobilization prior to intracytoplasmic sperm injection with immature spermatozoa improves fertilization and pregnancy rates. Hum Reprod. 1996;11(5):1023–9.
32. Dyer S, Chambers GM, de Mouzon J, et al. International Committee for Monitoring Assisted Reproductive Technologies world report: Assisted Reproductive Technology 2008, 2009 and 2010. Hum Reprod. 2016;31(7):1588–609.
33. Boulet SL, Mehta A, Kissin DM, Warner L, Kawwass JF, Jamieson DJ. Trends in use of and reproductive outcomes associated with intracytoplasmic sperm injection. JAMA. 2015;313(3):255–63.
34. Schlegel PN, Palermo GD, Alikani M, et al. Micropuncture retrieval of epididymal sperm with in vitro fertilization: importance of in vitro micromanipulation techniques. Urology. 1995;46(2):238–41.

35. Schlegel PN, Cohen J, Goldstein M, et al. Cystic fibrosis gene mutations do not affect sperm function during in vitro fertilization with micromanipulation for men with bilateral congenital absence of vas deferens. Fertil Steril. 1995;64(2):421–6.
36. LM S, Palermo GD, Goldstein M, Veeck LL, Rosenwaks Z, Schlegel PN. Testicular sperm extraction with intracytoplasmic sperm injection for nonobstructive azoospermia: testicular histology can predict success of sperm retrieval. J Urol. 1999;161(1):112–6.
37. Palermo GD, Schlegel PN, Hariprashad JJ, et al. Fertilization and pregnancy outcome with intracytoplasmic sperm injection for azoospermic men. Hum Reprod. 1999;14(3):741–8.
38. Palermo GD, Schlegel PN, Sills ES, et al. Births after intracytoplasmic injection of sperm obtained by testicular extraction from men with nonmosaic Klinefelter's syndrome. N Engl J Med. 1998;338(9):588–90.
39. Chung PH, Palermo G, Schlegel PN, Veeck LL, Eid JF, Rosenwaks Z. The use of intracytoplasmic sperm injection with electroejaculates from anejaculatory men. Hum Reprod. 1998;13(7):1854–8.
40. Chan PT, Palermo GD, Veeck LL, Rosenwaks Z, Schlegel PN. Testicular sperm extraction combined with intracytoplasmic sperm injection in the treatment of men with persistent azoospermia postchemotherapy. Cancer. 2001;92(6):1632–7.
41. Alikani M, Palermo G, Adler A, Bertoli M, Blake M, Cohen J. Intracytoplasmic sperm injection in dysmorphic human oocytes. Zygote. 1995;3(4):283–8.
42. Moreno C, Ruiz A, Simón C, Pellicer A, Remohí J. Intracytoplasmic sperm injection as a routine indication in low responder patients. Hum Reprod. 1998;13(8):2126–9.
43. Practice Committees of American Society for Reproductive Medicine; Society for Assisted Reproductive Technology. Mature oocyte cryopreservation: a guideline. Fertil Steril. 2013;99(1):37–43.
44. Jain T, Gupta RS. Trends in the use of intracytoplasmic sperm injection in the United States. N Engl J Med. 2007;357(3):251–7.
45. Tannus S, Son WY, Gilman A, Younes G, Shavit T, Dahan MH. The role of intracytoplasmic sperm injection in non-male factor infertility in advanced maternal age. Hum Reprod. 2017;32(1):119–24.
46. Bhattacharya S, Hamilton MP, Shaaban M, et al. Conventional in-vitro fertilisation vs intracytoplasmic sperm injection for the treatment of non-male-factor infertility: a randomised controlled trial. Lancet. 2001;357(9274):2075–9.
47. Practice Committees of the American Society for Reproductive Medicine and Society for Assisted Reproductive Technology. Intracytoplasmic sperm injection (ICSI) for non-male factor infertility: a committee opinion. Fertil Steril. 2012;98(6):1395–9.
48. Tucker M, Elsner C, Kort H, Massey J, Mitchell-Leef D, Toledo A. Poor implantation of cryopreserved reinsemination-fertilized human embryos. Fertil Steril. 1991;56(6):1111–6.
49. Tsirigotis M, Nicholson N, Taranissi M, Bennett V, Pelekanos M, Craft I. Late intracytoplasmic sperm injection in unexpected failed fertilization in vitro: diagnostic or therapeutic? Fertil Steril. 1995;63(4):816–9.
50. Lundin K, Sjögren A, Hamberger L. Reinsemination of one-day-old oocytes by use of intracytoplasmic sperm injection. Fertil Steril. 1996;66(1):118–21.
51. Morton PC, Yoder CS, Tucker MJ, Wright G, Brockman WD, Kort HI. Reinsemination by intracytoplasmic sperm injection of 1-day-old oocytes after complete conventional fertilization failure. Fertil Steril. 1997;68(3):488–91.
52. Palermo GD, Neri QV, Monahan D, Takeuchi T, Schlegel PN, Rosenwaks Z. Intracytoplasmic sperm injection. In: Nagy ZP, Varghese A, Agarwal AC, editors. Practical manual of in vitro fertilization: advanced methods and novel devices. New York: Springer; 2012. p. 307–20.
53. Wisanto A, Magnus M, Bonduelle M, et al. Obstetric outcome of 424 pregnancies after intracytoplasmic sperm injection. Hum Reprod. 1995;10(10):2713–8.
54. Wisanto A, Bonduelle M, Camus M, et al. Obstetric outcome of 904 pregnancies after intracytoplasmic sperm injection. Hum Reprod. 1996;11(Suppl 4):121–9; discussion 130

55. Palermo GD, Colombero LT, Schattman GL, Davis OK, Rosenwaks Z. Evolution of pregnancies and initial follow-up of newborns delivered after intracytoplasmic sperm injection. JAMA. 1996;276(23):1893–7.
56. Ponjaert-Kristoffersen I, Tjus T, Nekkebroeck J, et al. Psychological follow-up study of 5-year-old ICSI children. Hum Reprod. 2004;19(12):2791–7.
57. Bonduelle M, Bergh C, Niklasson A, et al. Medical follow-up study of 5-year-old ICSI children. Reprod Biomed Online. 2004;9(1):91–101.
58. Leunens L, Celestin-Westreich S, Bonduelle M, Liebaers I, Ponjaert-Kristoffersen I. Follow-up of cognitive and motor development of 10-year-old singleton children born after ICSI compared with spontaneously conceived children. Hum Reprod. 2008;23(1):105–11.
59. Balayla J, Sheehy O, Fraser WD, et al. Neurodevelopmental outcomes after assisted reproductive technologies. Obstet Gynecol. 2017;129(2):265–72.
60. Belva F, Roelants M, De Schepper J, Van Steirteghem A, Tournaye H, Bonduelle M. Reproductive hormones of ICSI-conceived young adult men: the first results. Hum Reprod. 2017;32(2):439–46.
61. Belva F, Bonduelle M, Roelants M, et al. Semen quality of young adult ICSI offspring: the first results. Hum Reprod. 2016;31(12):2811–20.
62. Palermo GD, Neri QV, Takeuchi T, Squires J, Moy F, Rosenwaks Z. Genetic and epigenetic characteristics of ICSI children. Reprod Biomed Online. 2008;17(6):820–33.
63. Palermo GD, Neri QV, Rosenwaks Z. Safety of intracytoplasmic sperm injection. Methods Mol Biol. 2014;1154:549–62.
64. Lazaraviciute G, Kauser M, Bhattacharya S, Haggarty P, Bhattacharya S. A systematic review and meta-analysis of DNA methylation levels and imprinting disorders in children conceived by IVF/ICSI compared with children conceived spontaneously. Hum Reprod Update. 2014;20(6):840–52.
65. Sandin S, Nygren KG, Iliadou A, Hultman CM, Reichenberg A. Autism and mental retardation among offspring born after in vitro fertilization. JAMA. 2013;310(1):75–84.
66. Neri QV, Takeuchi T, Kang HJ, Lin K, Wang A, Palermo GD. Genetic assessment and development of children that result from assisted reproductive technology. Clin Obstet Gynecol. 2006;49(1):134–7.
67. Pereira N, Cozzubbo T, Cheung S, Rosenwaks Z, Palermo GD, Neri QV. Identifying maternal constraints on fetal growth and subsequent perinatal outcomes using a multiple embryo implantation model. PLoS One. 2016;11(11):e0166222.

Chapter 3
The Role of Reproductive Genetics in Modern Androlgy

Douglas T. Carrell, Timothy G. Jenkins, Benjamin R. Emery, James M. Hotaling, and Kenneth I. Aston

Abbreviations

CBAVD   Congenital bilateral absence of the vas deferens
CFTR   Cystic fibrosis transmembrane conductance regulator
CpGs   Cytosine-phosphate-guanine dinucleotides
MicroTESE Micro-surgical testicular sperm extraction
NSS   No sperm seen
YCMD   Y chromosome microdeletion

3.1 Introduction

Recent technological advances have accelerated our understanding of the genetic nature, causes, and therapies of disease. Genetic understanding of male infertility is ultimately based on improved and less expensive sequencing technologies, the development of novel analytical techniques, analytical advancements, and management of "big data" in the form of systems analyses, population databases, and

D.T. Carrell (✉)
Androlgy & IVF Laboratory Division, Department of Surgery (Urology) and Human Genetics, University of Utah School of Medicine, Salt Lake City, UT, USA

Department of Surgery (Urology Division), University of Utah School of Medicine, Salt Lake City, UT, USA
e-mail: douglas.carrell@hsc.utah.edu

T.G. Jenkins • B.R. Emery • J.M. Hotaling • K.I. Aston
Department of Surgery (Urology Division), University of Utah School of Medicine, Salt Lake City, UT, USA
e-mail: tim.jenkins@hsc.utah.du; bemery@hsc.utah.edu;
jim.hotaling@hsc.utah.edu; kiaston@utah.edu

© Springer International Publishing AG 2018
G.D. Palermo, E.S. Sills (eds.), *Intracytoplasmic Sperm Injection*,
https://doi.org/10.1007/978-3-319-70497-5_3

improved electronic healthcare records [1]. While the "genetics revolution" has now been heralded for decades, the emergence and progress of subcomponents of genetics, such as the fields listed above as well as other novel areas such as epigenetics, stem cell biology, and genome editing, have only relatively recently added to our knowledge of the genetic aspects of male infertility [2–4]. Therefore, in many respects the genetic revolution is still a young and accelerating phenomenon.

While the evaluation of the infertile male would ideally begin with an examination by a board certified male reproductive urologist/andrologist, the reality is that infertility care usually begins with the evaluation of the female by a reproductive endocrinologist, which often results in a nearly direct jump to therapy via in vitro fertilization (IVF), resulting in a potential loss of valuable genetic data to the patient and his family [5]. Intracytoplasmic sperm injection (ICSI) is revolutionary in its ability to treat many types of male infertility, but due to its success in leading to a pregnancy can contribute to the neglect of the proper care of underlying causes of infertility in the patient and in providing valuable information regarding the general health prospects of the patient and offspring due to associated genetic sequelae [6]. This is demonstrated by recent data that report that male infertility is also a marker of familial health with families of infertile men having a higher rate of pediatric cancer, testis cancer, and major congenital anomalies [7, 8].

It is estimated that approximately 30% of male infertility cases have known genetic causes, while approximately 40% remain idiopathic with presumed genetic etiologies. Therefore it is clear that care of the infertile male should currently involve a significant degree of genetic diagnostics and counseling which will continue to grow. While the promises of genetic medicine have not emerged as quickly as many may have assumed or wished, it is clear that the promises are beginning to be fulfilled and the pace of progress is increasing. The vision of obtaining genomic sequencing of patients with the practice of precision medicine is becoming closer [9]. However, it is important to consider that laboratory evaluations are presently available that can greatly aid in the care of the infertile male. Additionally, novel areas of genetic medicine, such as epigenetic evaluation of the patient's sperm, are advancing rapidly and currently of use in patient care. This chapter highlights current clinical guidelines regarding genetic issues in the care of infertile males, while also highlighting advancements towards personalized, genomic medical therapy.

3.2   Clinical Evaluation of the Infertile Male

The genetic evaluation of an infertile male begins with the clinical examination. Proper evaluation includes a detailed medical and reproductive history and physical exam by a reproductive urologist. The physical exam must document the presence or absence of the vas deferens, the quality of the epididymis, the longitudinal testis axis, any inguinal incisions, and evaluation of gynecomastia. Two semen analyses should be performed, and if No Sperm Seen (NSS) the pellet should be centrifuged and resuspended for further microscopic examination. A low volume acidic pH should prompt consideration of congenital absence of the vas deferens (CBAVD) and also prompt a post-ejaculatory urinalysis [10, 11]. Additionally, these men should have a bioavailable testosterone, FSH, LH, estradiol and, where indicated, prolactin and TSH [12–14].

It is also vital to inquire about environmental exposure such as wet heat, industrial solvents, pesticides, phthalates, and radiation both in early life and presently. All of these factors have been shown to have substantial and sustained impacts on spermatogenesis and, possibly, the sperm epigenetic profile [15]. Smoking, alcohol, and illicit drug use (anabolic steroids, cocaine, opioids, and marijuana) can also have an impact on male reproduction. Finally, obesity, an often-overlooked area in the male reproductive evaluation, has been shown to have a dose dependent impact on spermatogenesis, with obese men being significantly more likely to have poor quality sperm. Additionally, obesity modifies the sperm epigenome and has significant ramifications for future generations [16]. We have found that helping men understand that their lifestyle choices significantly impact the metabolic profile of their future progeny provides a powerful motivator for behavior change. Thus, we discuss this with all of our obese patients and encourage them to make the lifestyle changes necessary to improve their weight.

A karyotype and Y chromosome microdeletion (YCMD) is recommended by the American Urological Association and the European Academy of Andrology for all men with sperm concentration <5 M/ml and some international consortiums recommend genetic testing when the concentration is <10 M/ml [11, 17]. A standard G-band karyotype will usually identify Klinefelter's syndrome (47, XXY), a condition with a prevalence of 1:600 males and the most common cause of azoospermia detectable with basic genetic testing [18–20]. The gold standard for sperm retrieval in azoospermic men with Klinefelter's is microdissection testicular sperm extraction (microTESE). Typically, men with mosaic Klinefelter's syndrome are more likely than non-mosaic Klinefelter's to have sperm in the ejaculate and to have sperm identified at time of microTESE.

Although only a small number of men with Klinefelter's will have sperm in their ejaculate, it is imperative to obtain two semen analyses in all of these men to confirm azoospermia prior to performing a microTESE. Although controversial, many, including our group at University of Utah, are now advocating for microTESE just after puberty as some evidence indicates that spermatogenesis may be present initially in most adolescents with Klinefelter's [21–23]. A karyotype can also identify a number of translocations and deletions that can also negatively impact spermatogenesis. Fluorescent in situ hybridization (FISH) can be used to detect disomy or unbalanced chromosomal translocations in men with sperm aneuploidy or carriers of a known chromosomal translocation. These translocations in men with sperm aneuploidy can lead to a higher risk of non-euploid embryos and preimplantation genetic screening as well as genetic counseling is indicated [24]. Other karyo-typic abnormalities such as 47, XYY (present in 0.1% of male births) can also cause azoospermia/oligozoospermia [25].

Y chromosome microdeletion analysis is recommended for men with concentra-tions <5 M/ml or, for some international consortiums, <10 M/ml. AZFa, b, and c deletions can all cause azoospermia, with AZFa and AZFb generally being incompat-ible with spermatogenesis, although a recent report does indicate AZFb mutations may be associated with spermatogenesis in rare circumstances [26]. The presence of an AZFc microdeletion is clearly compatible with spermatogenesis and a micro-sur-gical testicular sperm extraction (microTESE) is indicated [14]. For azoospermic men with either absence of vas deferens on their exam or a low volume acidic ejacu-late without fructose and a post-ejaculatory urinalysis with NSS, cystic fibrosis trans-membrane conductance regulator (CFTR) genetic testing is indicated. CFTR mutations are the cause of cystic fibrosis, which has a prevalence of 1 in 1600 people of Northern European decent [27]. To have cystic fibrosis, men must have severe mutations in both copies of their CFTR genes. All men with cystic fibrosis have con-genital bilateral absence of the vas deferens (CBAVD). Further, 80% of the men with CBAVD have at least one CFTR mutation with a second less severe mutation pre-sumed to be present but not detected on initial screening. Men with CBAVD do not have the full manifestation of cystic fibrosis because they do not have the two severe mutations necessary to express the complete phenotype of the disease [28, 29].

At a minimum, a panel of common mutations and the 5 T allele should be tested. In men without vas deferens or where the wife is a known carrier, gene sequencing may be considered. If men present with only unilateral absence of the vas deferens, CFTR testing is indicated as well as a renal ultrasound as unilateral absence of the vas deferens is associated with unilateral renal embryogenesis [10]. If CFTR muta-tions are detected, these men should be counseled like any man with CFTR muta-tions. However, if renal agenesis is present, these men need to be counseled about the need to consider wearing flank protection during contact sports or limiting these injuries given that they only have one functional kidney. Perhaps the most important aspect of counseling for any man testing positive for a CFTR mutation is to have his wife evaluated for CFTR mutations as well.

A proper evaluation of the infertile male is vital to optimizing IVF/ICSI out-comes. As described below, anomalies in the fidelity, ploidy, and chemical modifi-cations to sperm DNA have direct influence in limiting embryogenesis potential in couples undergoing IVF. Further, as genetic and epigenetic testing allows identifica-tion of ever greater numbers of causative mutations of spermatogenic dysfunction, the reproductive urologist may be able to sub-phenotype men into categories of male infertility that have significant consequences for male fertility potential as well as individual and familial somatic health.

3.3 Laboratory Evaluation of Sperm

3.3.1 Sperm Aneuploidy

In many cases of male infertility, defects in stem cell progression, meiosis, or spermatogenesis affect resulting sperm DNA [30]. It has long been established that sperm aneuploidy, a numerical alteration in the number of chromosomes, is increased in many men with infertility or subfertility [31]. From early studies using sperm karyotyping [32], to the now common (but underutilized) interphase fluorescent in situ hybridization (FISH) technique [33], it has been established that there are populations of infertile men with an increased risk of transmitting sperm aneuploidies to the embryo [34, 35] (Fig. 3.1). The subtypes of infertile men with an increased risk of sperm aneuploidies that have been best characterized are men with balanced and unbalanced translocations, Klinefelter's syndrome, severe oligo-, astheno- and teratozoospermia, severely abnormal sperm morphology abnormalities (macrocephalic sperm, globozoospermia, or increased multi-flagellar sperm), non-obstructive azoospermia, and advanced paternal age. It should also be noted that men with oligoasthenoteratozoospermia (OAT) are at a higher relative risk than in isolated oligo, asthenozoospermia or teratozoospermia [36]. This is particularly relevant given that these populations are those most benefited by the use of ICSI for treatment of male-factor infertility.

The origin of these sperm-borne aneuploidies most commonly arises from non-disjunction events during meiosis [37], but may also occur as a result of structural abnormalities and/or an abnormal somatic karyotype [38]. Aneuploidies may also be increased due to the inter-chromosomal effect (ICE) of other structural anomalies,

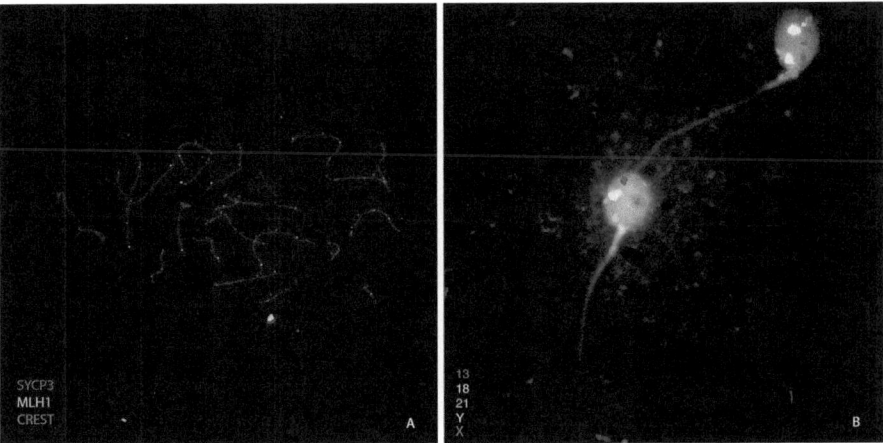

Fig. 3.1 Meiotic recombination and the formation of sperm aneuploidies. This figure demonstrates meiotic recombination foci (panel **a**) of pachytene stage spermatocytes. Aberrant synapsing of the chromatids can result to non-segregation errors, resulting in sperm aneuploidies visualized using FISH (panel **b**)

particularly translocations [39]. The diagnosis of these abnormalities using sperm FISH has revealed that the prevalence of aneuploidies does not match the theoretical risk [40]. Therefore, the use of sperm FISH in diagnosis and determining a care plan for couples considering ART is warranted for the pathologies described above.

Routine sperm FISH has evolved to routinely offer a panel of five chromosomes for testing (X, Y, 13, 18, 21). The methodology for this has been previously described [33]. Briefly, ejaculated or testicular sperm are concentrated onto a glass slide using centrifugation. The sperm are then slightly decondensed using either a heat or chemical treatment of dithiothreitol (DTT). Commercial probes are available for five-probe simultaneous hybridization, but more commonly used are those for hybridization of X, Y, and 18 and 13, 21 separately. The sperm nuclei (2–5000 nuclei per chromosome) are then evaluated in a highly labor-intensive manner to obtain a rate of aneuploidy for the sample provided. Automated platforms for evaluation of sperm aneuploidies are evolving and show promise in reducing the amount of time, and therefore cost, of sperm aneuploidy screening [34]. While there is currently not a best practice guideline or World Health Organization normal value set, it has been suggested that a total aneuploidy rate greater than 3%, in the five chromosome assay discussed herein, is of clinical significance and should be considered when ART is recommended [34, 40].

3.4 Sperm DNA Damage

Sperm DNA fragmentation is thought to arise from several factors, including abnormal histone to protamine exchange [41], abnormal protamine content and ratio [42], and oxidative stress in the seminal plasma [43, 44]. The assessment of sperm DNA damage has now been studied in many subfertile and infertile groups and there are several thorough reviews on the topic [30]. They show varying levels of support for the use of sperm DNA damage assays as a viable tool for prediction of ART success. There is currently support that there is a defined effect of sperm DNA damage on ART outcome and these assays should be incorporated into infertility diagnosis and treatment [45], while some reports are less favorable [46, 47]. A recent meta-analysis [45] does report a significant association between the two parameters, again supporting a role for sperm DNA damage screening. It remains to be seen if the use of ICSI helps in the selection of sperm for fertilization with a lower level of sperm DNA damage and therefore increased prognosis for a live birth.

3.5 Screening for Mutations, SNPS and CNVS

As previously discussed, routine genetic screening for men with obstructive azoospermia includes CFTR mutation screening, and screening for severe spermatogenesis impairment (NOA and severe oligozoospermia) includes AZF deletion screening and karyotype analysis. Unfortunately, while AZF deletions and karyotype abnormalities are responsible for a significant proportion of NOA and severe oligozoospermia, more than half of the cases that are screened are negative for known genetic anomalies. Likewise, an underlying cause for other forms of male infertility often cannot be identified.

The high proportion of idiopathic infertility cases significantly limits a clinician's ability to appropriately counsel patients in terms of treatment prognosis or to develop personalized treatment strategies. Additionally, without the identification of a definitive cause for the infertility, it cannot be determined whether resultant offspring will be subfertile or infertile or afflicted with other conditions related to the paternal infertility.

Significant efforts have been made to bridge this knowledge gap over the past few decades with modest success. Early efforts involved candidate gene sequencing studies in which sequencing of a single gene is performed in a group of patients and a group of controls in an effort to identify mutations or polymorphisms that occur at a higher frequency in patients compared with controls. This strategy has been employed in numerous independent studies. Generally, little concordance has been found between studies; however, association for a few SNPs has been replicated across multiple studies. These include SNPs in MTHFR, FSHB, and GSTM1 [48–50]. While the association is clear in these few cases, the very small effect size of these SNPs on male fertility render these polymorphisms not clinically actionable, so routine screening is not performed. Causal mutations have been identified in genes including KAL1, FGFR1, PROK2, and PROKR2 in about a third of Kallmann's syndrome patients [51]. This syndrome is associated with hypogonadotropic hypogonadism and NOA; however, the condition is exceedingly rare, and NOA patients are not routinely screened for these mutations.

As genomic technologies have advanced, so have genetic studies of male infertility (Fig. 3.2). Genome-wide analysis using genomic microarrays allowed the evaluation of thousands to a few million SNPs across thousands of genes, giving rise to the genome-wide association study. Microarrays also enabled the detection of genomic duplications and deletions (CNVs), opening the door to the identification of rare, larger and potentially more impactful genomic variants in addition to the relatively common SNPs included on arrays. These studies have been performed in numerous diseases including male infertility, with modest success [52–71]. Most importantly, microarray-based studies offered a first indication of the genomic architecture of male infertility on a genome-wide scale. From the handful of such studies, it is apparent that common polymorphisms contribute minimally to male infertility. Several GWAS that evaluated CNVs in addition to SNP associations identified an apparent increased genomic instability in infertile men [62, 64, 67]. In addition, several rare CNVs that are probably responsible for NOA have been reported. These include DMRT1 [67] and TEX11 [72]. Following the initial report of DMRT1 deletions in NOA men, subsequent studies reported increased mutation frequency of the gene in NOA men [73, 74]. A TEX11 deletion was initially detected in two NOA patients by array comparative genomic hybridization testing, and subsequent mutation screening by Sanger sequencing identified five additional NOA men with TEX11 mutations [72]. A subsequent study likewise identified apparent causal mutations in TEX11 in NOA men [75].

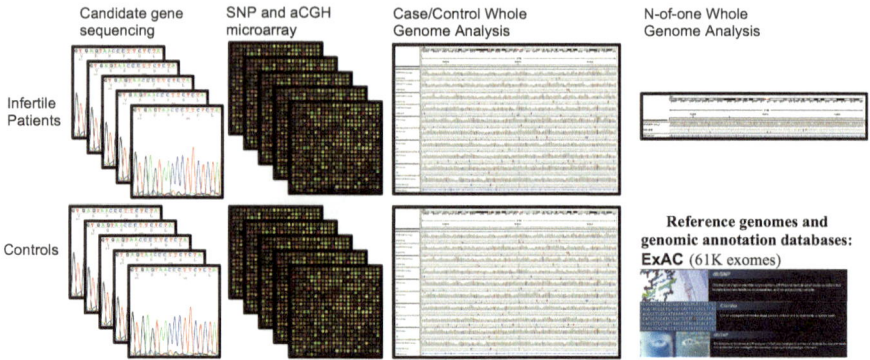

Fig. 3.2 The evolution of tools to characterize the genetics of male infertility. Early attempts to identify genetic lesions associated with infertility employed Sanger sequencing of candidate genes in populations of infertile men and fertile controls. Initial whole genome approaches utilized SNP or CGH arrays to identify genomic variants (SNPs and/or CNVs) across the genome in a case/control context. As next generation sequencing technologies matured, whole genome and whole exome sequencing in groups of cases and controls was performed. Cumulatively, data gathered using these approaches indicated that n-of-one analyses, wherein the genomic sequence of a single patient is compared against hundreds or thousands of reference sequences couples with comprehensive annotation data, are necessary to efficiently identify genomic variants contributing to male infertility. These analytical tools are currently being developed and refined

From the early GWAS it became increasingly apparent that assays capable of identifying rare or private mutations on a genome-wide scale would be necessary to identify novel causal mutations in infertile men. Rapidly declining DNA sequencing costs have enabled the application of whole exome and whole genome sequencing approaches to male infertility. Early successes in identifying causal mutations, particularly in consanguineous families with multiple infertile men, have demonstrated the potential for such approaches to uncover important genetic variants in male infertility. Examples include the identification of ZMYND10 mutations in men with primary ciliary dyskinesia [76], a homozygous mutation in INHBB in a man who was found to display uniparental disomy for chromosome 2 [67], and a TEX15 mutation in NOA men from a consanguineous family [77].

A primary challenge in whole exome and whole genome studies is data analysis and interpretation. Accumulating data suggest that the majority of undiscovered genomic variants that cause male infertility will be extremely rare or private variants, so classical case-control experimental design will be inadequate for the identification of male infertility variants. Current efforts are targeted at developing tools to identify important variants in the context of a single patient genome compared with a large number of fertile control genomes, coined "*n* of 1" analysis [78].

A recent whole genome sequencing study found that the human genome contains an average of more than 8500 novel genetic variants [79]. The reliable identification, functional annotation, and statistical prioritization of those variants from a single patient becomes a monumental task and requires the development of bespoke analytical tools specific to infertility. Progress is being made, but continued work, large consortium-based studies and concerted efforts for functional validation of novel findings are necessary before we can expect personalized genomic analysis to be routinely applied in the setting of reproductive medicine.

3.6 The Emerging Field of Sperm Epigenetics

While gene mutations, structural and numerical alterations of chromosomes, and damage to sperm DNA via strand breaks have long been known as causes of male infertility, the establishment of epigenetic anomalies as a cause of male infertility is relatively recent. The epigenome has progressively become a popular subject of research in many tissues throughout the body and the germ line is no exception. This is largely due to the recent evidence, which suggests that the sperm epigenome plays an important role in normal sperm development, mature sperm function, embryogenesis, and even potentially in offspring health [80–83]. Many key epigenetic regulators exist in sperm including DNA methylation at cytosine-phosphate-guanine dinucleotides (CpGs), nuclear proteins (including canonical and testes specific variants of histone proteins) and associated posttranslational modifications, as well as various forms of RNA (microRNA, piRNA, lncRNA, etc.). Each of these various facets of the germ line epigenome is important to the regular activity of sperm and is thus of interest in the andrology lab for both a basic understanding of cell biology and to identify potential areas where these important marks may be informative in the diagnosis and/or treatment of male infertility. A great deal of recent effort has been exerted toward this specific goal [80, 84–86].

3.6.1 DNA Methylation

A key epigenetic regulator in sperm is DNA methylation (Fig. 3.3). In many somatic cell types, this important epigenetic mark can be used to distinguish between different cell types and even between various abnormalities from a distinct tissue (cancer and other pathologies) [87]. Similarly, sperm DNA methylation signatures are markedly altered in samples with abnormal semen characteristics. Specifically, a recent study showed striking alterations between semen samples with "normal" sperm characteristics and those with various infertility phenotypes including low viability, low motility, and low count [83]. These regional methylation alterations tended to occur more frequently at sites important in meiosis and germ cell development pathways, suggesting that upstream misregulation exists in sperm development and that epigenetic signatures both reflect and help to drive these changes [83]. In addition, the sperm epigenome appears to be required for normal fertilization and embryogenesis. From evidence (both direct and indirect) it appears that altered sperm DNA methylation can affect a couple's capacity to become pregnant [84]. It is logical then to assume that these same marks may be informative in predicting the capacity of a sperm population from an ejaculate to generate viable embryos capable of generating healthy offspring through natural conception or in vitro

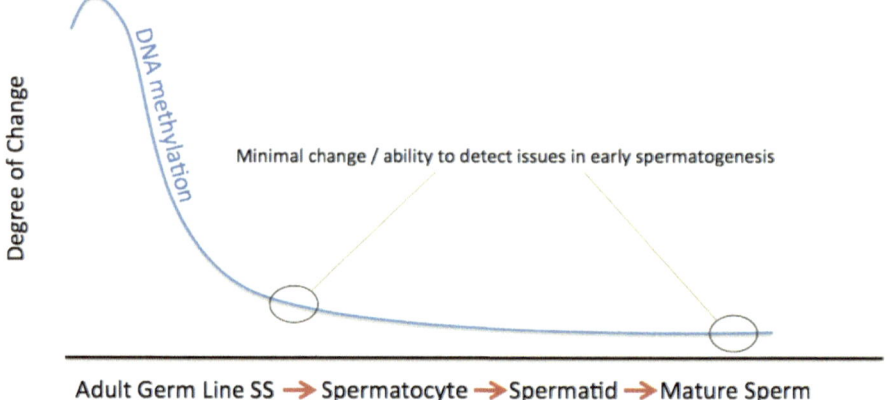

Fig. 3.3 Theoretical depiction of the degree of significant modifications that occur to the sperm methylome throughout stages of spermatogenesis. Because the methylome remains extremely stable from the adult germ line stem cell to the mature sperm in mammals, assessment of sperm DNA methylation provides a unique window into potential alterations that occurred in early spermatogenesis

fertilization. As evidence of this concept, recent work from our lab has shown that DNA methylation signatures are distinct enough to enable significant predictive power when determining the likelihood that a given sperm DNA methylation signature is taken from an IVF patient or a fertile donor [80]. Further, in the same study it was shown that sperm DNA methylation signatures might even be capable of predicting the quality of embryos should the couple in question pursue IVF, and a clinical assay has been introduced [80].

These emerging findings provide a great deal of promise to the potential of epigenetic diagnostic tests that can be developed and/or refined in the very near future. This potential is incredibly important to understand in the context of the current state of the art diagnostic techniques in the andrology lab that are notoriously limited in capacity to ascertain a man's reproductive potential [88]. Only some of the typically used semen analysis results suggest any associations with fecundity, and more often these results are insufficient and highly variable [89], thus making predictions in regard to fertility as well as making clinical decisions beyond general recommendations is very difficult with the currently used approaches. Taken together, it is important to note the potential of utilizing epigenetic data in a typical patient workup.

3.6.2   RNA Assessment

With the advent of new tools in next generation sequencing and beyond, many intriguing discoveries have taken place regarding the role of sperm RNAs in normal sperm function and even in embryogenesis [85, 86]. Because of the low amount of total RNA which can be found in the quiescent sperm cell analyses can be difficult, but intriguing (and still controversial) data suggest that specific RNAs in sperm are important in embryogenesis [90, 91]. An additional study has recently shown that there are multiple RNA "elements" in the sperm that are required to facilitate successful IVF outcomes [86] again suggesting that there sperm RNAs are important in the process of embryogenesis. Similar to some studies assessing DNA methylation signatures, this study in particular has the potential to affect diagnostics in the fertility clinic. In brief, the study demonstrated that the absence of even a single member of the 648 RNA "elements" identified decreased the likelihood of success with multiple forms of infertility treatment and in particular with IVF. There are limitations with the use of RNA as a diagnostic tool in sperm specifically and any contamination from somatic cells can be quite detrimental to the process as the sperm contains far less RNA than that of a somatic cell. Thus, any contamination (even in low amounts) can result in dramatically altered results. Despite this potential downside (which all epigenetic assessments in sperm share to varying degrees), the potential utility is clear and may help to drive novel diagnostic testing in the andrology lab that may have real implications in the future of reproductive healthcare.

3.6.3   Nuclear Protein Evaluation

Multiple forms of nuclear proteins exist in the mature sperm. Multiple histone variants exist and many of these can also possess posttranslational modifications to tails, which are considered to be epigenetic modifications, based on the classic definition. Some of these modifications (including H3K4 methylation and H3K27 methylation) have been shown in previous studies to be enriched at developmental promoters suggesting an important role in embryonic development [92]. In fact, some studies suggest that depletion of these marks at developmental promoters in sperm is found in some men with infertility [93]. When considering a more loose definition of epigenetics, and specifically taking into consideration the unique nature of the sperm, many categorize the location of histone proteins (both in consideration of and irrespective of posttranslational modifications) as a key regulator in the mature sperm and as a driver of important events in the early embryo [92, 94]. This is largely due to the unique nature of the histone to protamine transition, in which the vast majority of histone proteins are removed and replaced by protamine proteins to form a more tightly compact nucleus during spermiogenesis [94]. This important event in sperm development leaves only a small portion of genome histone bound and it is believed that this replacement is programmatic in nature thus facilitating a looser chromatin structure at areas important in embryonic development where the histones are retained. It is important for andrologists to consider this pattern and, in fact, this measure of chromatin compaction is something that has been assessed in fertility labs for many years with multiple approaches. Most of these approaches are not specific in nature and only assess general levels of histone retention in the mature sperm but these methods (such as analine blue staining) have been used to discover differences in chromatin defects in infertile populations [95].

Because the epigenome, in many ways, defines the differences between cell types and between various forms (healthy vs. abnormal) of individual tissues, it provides an excellent opportunity in diagnostics. While in most cases, the underlying etiology of an abnormality in sperm is multifactorial and is unlikely to be driven by epigenetics alone, the resultant alterations are often detectable in the epigenome as these are the key regulators for cell function that are often perturbed. Thus, assessing the sperm epigenome is a logical step in the pursuit of better options for diagnosing male fertility, and this effort already appears to be fruitful.

3.7 Summary

This chapter has described current guidelines regarding genetic analysis of the infertile male, as well as including emerging information on gene polymorphisms, copy number variations, and epigenetic variants that will be key in diagnosing male infertility. It is increasingly clear that most causes of male infertility are due to rare variants, solely or in combinations, that will be identified in a genetic screen that will be helpful in the broad healthcare of the patient. While it is likely that specific, targeted screens may be relevant in some cases, such as targeted epigenetic screens, the advancement of reproductive care will not be isolated to the field, rather it will likely be dependent on the introduction of personalized medicine paradigms in healthcare. In the meantime, and likely also after the advent of the changes described above, prudent use of available genetic assays should be implemented in an effort to provide accurate information on the success of potential therapies, the relevance of the patient's infertility to his health status, and to potentially provide information relevant to the health of the offspring.

References

1. Carrell DT, Aston KI, Oliva R, Emery BR, De Jonge CJ. The "omics" of human male infertility: integrating big data in a systems biology approach. Cell Tissue Res. 2016;363(1):295–312.
2. Hamazaki T, El Rouby N, Fredette NC, Santostefano KE, Terada N. Concise review: induced pluripotent stem cell research in the era of precision medicine. Stem Cells. 2017;35(3):545–50.
3. Jenkins TG, Aston KI, James ER, Carrell DT. Sperm epigenetics in the study of male fertility, offspring health, and potential clinical applications. Syst Biol Reprod Med. 2017;63(2):69–76.
4. Chira S, Gulei D, Hajitou A, Zimta AA, Cordelier P, Berindan-Neagoe I. CRISPR/Cas9: transcending the reality of genome editing. Mol Ther Nucleic Acids. 2017;7:211–22.
5. Mehta A, Nangia AK, Dupree JM, Smith JF. Limitations and barriers in access to care for male factor infertility. Fertil Steril. 2016;105(5):1128–37.
6. Glazer CH, Bonde JP, Eisenberg ML, Giwercman A, Haervig KK, Rimborg S, et al. Male infertility and risk of nonmalignant chronic diseases: a systematic review of the epidemiological evidence. Semin Reprod Med. 2017;35(3):282–90.
7. Hanson HA, Anderson RE, Aston KI, Carrell DT, Smith KR, Hotaling JM. Subfertility increases risk of testicular cancer: evidence from population-based semen samples. Fertil Steril. 2016;105(2):322–8 e1.

8. Anderson RE, Hanson HA, Patel DP, Johnstone E, Aston KI, Carrell DT, et al. Cancer risk in first- and second-degree relatives of men with poor semen quality. Fertil Steril. 2016;106(3):731–8.
9. Rehm HL. Evolving health care through personal genomics. Nat Rev Genet. 2017;18(4):259–67.
10. National Guideline C. The evaluation of the azoospermic male: AUA best practice statement.
11. National Guideline C. The optimal evaluation of the infertile male: AUA best practice statement.
12. Hotaling J, Carrell DT. Clinical genetic testing for male factor infertility: current applications and future directions. Andrology. 2014;2(3):339–50.
13. Hotaling JM, Patel Z. Male endocrine dysfunction. Urol Clin North Am. 2014;41(1):39–53.
14. Hotaling JM. Genetics of male infertility. Urol Clin North Am. 2014;41(1):1–17.
15. Bonde JP, Flachs EM, Rimborg S, Glazer CH, Giwercman A, Ramlau-Hansen CH, et al. The epidemiologic evidence linking prenatal and postnatal exposure to endocrine disrupting chemicals with male reproductive disorders: a systematic review and meta-analysis. Hum Reprod Update. 2016;23(1):104–25.
16. Craig JR, Jenkins TG, Carrell DT, Hotaling JM. Obesity, male infertility, and the sperm epigenome. Fertil Steril. 2017;107(4):848–59.
17. Foresta C, Ferlin A, Gianaroli L, Dallapiccola B. Guidelines for the appropriate use of genetic tests in infertile couples. Eur J Hum Genet. 2002;10(5):303–12.
18. Groth KA, Skakkebaek A, Host C, Gravholt CH, review BAC. Klinefelter syndrome—a clinical update. J Clin Endocrinol Metab. 2013;98(1):20–30.
19. Bojesen A, Gravholt CH. Klinefelter syndrome in clinical practice. Nat Clin Pract Urol. 2007;4(4):192–204.
20. Bojesen A, Juul S, Gravholt CH. Prenatal and postnatal prevalence of Klinefelter syndrome: a national registry study. J Clin Endocrinol Metab. 2003;88(2):622–6.
21. Aksglaede L, Wikstrom AM, Rajpert-De Meyts E, Dunkel L, Skakkebaek NE, Juul A. Natural history of seminiferous tubule degeneration in Klinefelter syndrome. Hum Reprod Update. 2006;12(1):39–48.
22. Plotton I, Giscard d'Estaing S, Cuzin B, Brosse A, Benchaib M, Lornage J, et al. Preliminary results of a prospective study of testicular sperm extraction in young versus adult patients with nonmosaic 47,XXY Klinefelter syndrome. J Clin Endocrinol Metab. 2015;100(3):961–7.
23. Paduch DA, Fine RG, Bolyakov A, Kiper J. New concepts in Klinefelter syndrome. Curr Opin Urol. 2008;18(6):621–7.
24. Kohn TP, Kohn JR, Darilek S, Ramasamy R, Lipshultz L. Genetic counseling for men with recurrent pregnancy loss or recurrent implantation failure due to abnormal sperm chromosomal aneuploidy. J Assist Reprod Genet. 2016;33(5):571–6.
25. Borjian Boroujeni P, Sabbaghian M, Vosough Dizaji A, Zarei Moradi S, Almadani N, Mohammadpour Lashkari F, et al. Clinical aspects of infertile 47,XYY patients: a retrospective study. Hum Fertil (Camb). 2017:1–6.
26. Stouffs K, Vloeberghs V, Gheldof A, Tournaye H, Seneca S. Are AZFb deletions always incompatible with sperm production? Andrology. 2017;5(4):691–4.
27. Liou TG, Rubenstein RC. Carrier screening, incidence of cystic fibrosis, and difficult decisions. JAMA. 2009;302(23):2595–6.
28. Southern KW. Cystic fibrosis and formes frustes of CFTR-related disease. Respiration. 2007;74(3):241–51.
29. Grzegorczyk V, Rives N, Sibert L, Dominique S, Mace B. Management of male infertility due to congenital bilateral absence of vas deferens should not ignore the diagnosis of cystic fibrosis. Andrologia. 2012;44(5):358–62.
30. Bach PV, Schlegel PN. Sperm DNA damage and its role in IVF and ICSI. Basic Clin Androl. 2016;26:15.
31. Harton GL, Tempest HG. Chromosomal disorders and male infertility. Asian J Androl. 2012;14(1):32–9.
32. Rudak E, Jacobs PA, Yanagimachi R. Direct analysis of the chromosome constitution of human spermatozoa. Nature. 1978;274(5674):911–3.

33. Emery BR. Sperm aneuploidy testing using fluorescence in situ hybridization. Methods Mol Biol. 2013;927:167–73.
34. Carrell DT. The clinical implementation of sperm chromosome aneuploidy testing: pitfalls and promises. J Androl. 2008;29(2):124–33.
35. Hwang K, Weedin JW, Lamb DJ. The use of fluorescent in situ hybridization in male infertility. Ther Adv Urol. 2010;2(4):157–69.
36. Gianaroli L, Magli MC, Cavallini G, Crippa A, Nadalini M, Bernardini L, et al. Frequency of aneuploidy in sperm from patients with extremely severe male factor infertility. Hum Reprod. 2005;20(8):2140–52.
37. Hassold TJ. Nondisjunction in the human male. Curr Top Dev Biol. 1998;37:383–406.
38. Shi Q, Martin RH. Aneuploidy in human spermatozoa: FISH analysis in men with constitutional chromosomal abnormalities, and in infertile men. Reproduction. 2001;121(5):655–66.
39. Anton E, Vidal F, Blanco J. Interchromosomal effect analyses by sperm FISH: incidence and distribution among reorganization carriers. Syst Biol Reprod Med. 2011;57(6):268–78.
40. Tempest HG. Meiotic recombination errors, the origin of sperm aneuploidy and clinical recommendations. Syst Biol Reprod Med. 2011;57(1–2):93–101.
41. Zhang X, San Gabriel M, Zini A. Sperm nuclear histone to protamine ratio in fertile and infertile men: evidence of heterogeneous subpopulations of spermatozoa in the ejaculate. J Androl. 2006;27(3):414–20.
42. Aoki VW, Emery BR, Liu L, Carrell DT. Protamine levels vary between individual sperm cells of infertile human males and correlate with viability and DNA integrity. J Androl. 2006;27(6):890–8.
43. Zini A, Garrels K, Phang D. Antioxidant activity in the semen of fertile and infertile men. Urology. 2000;55(6):922–6.
44. Koca Y, Ozdal OL, Celik M, Unal S, Balaban N. Antioxidant activity of seminal plasma in fertile and infertile men. Arch Androl. 2003;49(5):355–9.
45. Simon L, Zini A, Dyachenko A, Ciampi A, Carrell DT. A systematic review and meta-analysis to determine the effect of sperm DNA damage on in vitro fertilization and intracytoplasmic sperm injection outcome. Asian J Androl. 2017;19(1):80–90.
46. Collins JA, Barnhart KT, Schlegel PN. Do sperm DNA integrity tests predict pregnancy with in vitro fertilization? Fertil Steril. 2008;89(4):823–31.
47. Zini A, Sigman M. Are tests of sperm DNA damage clinically useful? Pros and cons. J Androl. 2009;30(3):219–29.
48. Tuttelmann F, Laan M, Grigorova M, Punab M, Sober S, Gromoll J. Combined effects of the variants FSHB -211G>T and FSHR 2039A>G on male reproductive parameters. J Clin Endocrinol Metab. 2012;97(10):3639–47.
49. Wei B, Xu Z, Ruan J, Zhu M, Jin K, Zhou D, et al. MTHFR 677C>T and 1298A>C polymorphisms and male infertility risk: a meta-analysis. Mol Biol Rep. 2012;39(2):1997–2002.
50. Song X, Zhao Y, Cai Q, Zhang Y, Niu Y. Association of the Glutathione S-transferases M1 and T1 polymorphism with male infertility: a meta-analysis. J Assist Reprod Genet. 2013;30(1):131–41.
51. Dode C, Hardelin JP. Clinical genetics of Kallmann syndrome. Ann Endocrinol (Paris). 2010;71(3):149–57.
52. Hu Z, Xia Y, Guo X, Dai J, Li H, Hu H, et al. A genome-wide association study in Chinese men identifies three risk loci for non-obstructive azoospermia. Nat Genet. 2012;44(2):183–6.
53. Zhao H, Xu J, Zhang H, Sun J, Sun Y, Wang Z, et al. A genome-wide association study reveals that variants within the HLA region are associated with risk for nonobstructive azoospermia. Am J Hum Genet. 2012;90(5):900–6.
54. Aston KI, Carrell DT. Genome-wide study of single-nucleotide polymorphisms associated with azoospermia and severe oligozoospermia. J Androl. 2009;30(6):711–25.
55. Aston KI, Conrad DF. A review of genome-wide approaches to study the genetic basis for spermatogenic defects. Methods Mol Biol. 2013;927:397–410.
56. Dalgaard MD, Weinhold N, Edsgard D, Silver JD, Pers TH, Nielsen JE, et al. A genome-wide association study of men with symptoms of testicular dysgenesis syndrome and its network biology interpretation. J Med Genet. 2012;49(1):58–65.

57. Qin Y, Ji J, Du G, Wu W, Dai J, Hu Z, et al. Comprehensive pathway-based analysis identifies associations of BCL2, GNAO1 and CHD2 with non-obstructive azoospermia risk. Hum Reprod. 2014;29(4):860–6.
58. Lu C, Xu M, Wang R, Qin Y, Ren J, Wu W, et al. A genome-wide association study of mitochondrial DNA in Chinese men identifies two risk single nucleotide substitutions for idiopathic oligoasthenospermia. Mitochondrion. 2015;24:87–92.
59. Hu Z, Li Z, Yu J, Tong C, Lin Y, Guo X, et al. Association analysis identifies new risk loci for non-obstructive azoospermia in Chinese men. Nat Commun. 2014;5:3857.
60. Yu J, Wu H, Wen Y, Liu Y, Zhou T, Ni B, et al. Identification of seven genes essential for male fertility through a genome-wide association study of non-obstructive azoospermia and RNA interference-mediated large-scale functional screening in drosophila. Hum Mol Genet. 2015;24(5):1493–503.
61. Ni B, Lin Y, Sun L, Zhu M, Li Z, Wang H, et al. Low-frequency germline variants across 6p22.2–6p21.33 are associated with non-obstructive azoospermia in Han Chinese men. Hum Mol Genet. 2015;24(19):5628–36.
62. Tuttelmann F, Simoni M, Kliesch S, Ledig S, Dworniczak B, Wieacker P, et al. Copy number variants in patients with severe oligozoospermia and sertoli-cell-only syndrome. PLoS One. 2011;6(4):e19426.
63. Song SH, Shim SH, Bang JK, Park JE, Sung SR, Cha DH. Genome-wide screening of severe male factor infertile patients using BAC-array comparative genomic hybridization (CGH). Gene. 2012;506(1):248–52.
64. Krausz C, Giachini C, Lo Giacco D, Daguin F, Chianese C, Ars E, et al. High resolution X chromosome-specific array-CGH detects new CNVs in infertile males. PLoS One. 2012;7(10):e44887.
65. Stouffs K, Vandermaelen D, Massart A, Menten B, Vergult S, Tournaye H, et al. Array comparative genomic hybridization in male infertility. Hum Reprod. 2012;27(3):921–9.
66. Eggers S, DeBoer KD, van den Bergen J, Gordon L, White SJ, Jamsai D, et al. Copy number variation associated with meiotic arrest in idiopathic male infertility. Fertil Steril. 2015;103(1):214–9.
67. Lopes AM, Aston KI, Thompson E, Carvalho F, Goncalves J, Huang N, et al. Human spermatogenic failure purges deleterious mutation load from the autosomes and both sex chromosomes, including the gene DMRT1. PLoS Genet. 2013;9(3):e1003349.
68. Jorgez CJ, Wilken N, Addai JB, Newberg J, Vangapandu HV, Pastuszak AW, et al. Genomic and genetic variation in E2F transcription factor-1 in men with nonobstructive azoospermia. Fertil Steril. 2015;103(1):44–52 e1.
69. Fruhmesser A, Vogt PH, Zimmer J, Witsch-Baumgartner M, Fauth C, Zschocke J, et al. Single nucleotide polymorphism array analysis in men with idiopathic azoospermia or oligoasthenozoospermia syndrome. Fertil Steril. 2013;100(1):81–7.
70. Halder A, Kumar P, Jain M, Iyer VK. Copy number variations in testicular maturation arrest. Andrology. 2017;5(3):460–72.
71. Dong Y, Pan Y, Wang R, Zhang Z, Xi Q, Liu RZ. Copy number variations in spermatogenic failure patients with chromosomal abnormalities and unexplained azoospermia. Genet Mol Res. 2015;14(4):16041–9.
72. Yatsenko AN, Georgiadis AP, Ropke A, Berman AJ, Jaffe T, Olszewska M, et al. X-linked TEX11 mutations, meiotic arrest, and azoospermia in infertile men. N Engl J Med. 2015;372(22):2097–107.
73. Lima AC, Carvalho F, Goncalves J, Fernandes S, Marques PI, Sousa M, et al. Rare double sex and mab-3-related transcription factor 1 regulatory variants in severe spermatogenic failure. Andrology. 2015;3(5):825–33.
74. Tewes AC, Ledig S, Tuttelmann F, Kliesch S, Wieacker P. DMRT1 mutations are rarely associated with male infertility. Fertil Steril. 2014;102(3):816–20. e3
75. Yang F, Silber S, Leu NA, Oates RD, Marszalek JD, Skaletsky H, et al. TEX11 is mutated in infertile men with azoospermia and regulates genome-wide recombination rates in mouse. EMBO Mol Med. 2015;7(9):1198–210.

76. Zariwala MA, Gee HY, Kurkowiak M, Al-Mutairi DA, Leigh MW, Hurd TW, et al. ZMYND10 is mutated in primary ciliary dyskinesia and interacts with LRRC6. Am J Hum Genet. 2013;93(2):336–45.
77. Okutman O, Muller J, Baert Y, Serdarogullari M, Gultomruk M, Piton A, et al. Exome sequencing reveals a nonsense mutation in TEX15 causing spermatogenic failure in a Turkish family. Hum Mol Genet. 2015;24(19):5581–8.
78. Wilfert AB, Chao KR, Kaushal M, Jain S, Zollner S, Adams DR, et al. Genome-wide significance testing of variation from single case exomes. Nat Genet. 2016;48(12):1455–61.
79. Telenti A, Pierce LC, Biggs WH, di Iulio J, Wong EH, Fabani MM, et al. Deep sequencing of 10,000 human genomes. Proc Natl Acad Sci U S A. 2016;113(42):11901–6.
80. Aston KI, Uren PJ, Jenkins TG, Horsager A, Cairns BR, Smith AD, et al. Aberrant sperm DNA methylation predicts male fertility status and embryo quality. Fertil Steril. 2015;104(6):1388–97 e1–5.
81. Hammoud SS, Low DH, Yi C, Carrell DT, Guccione E, Cairns BR. Chromatin and transcription transitions of mammalian adult germline stem cells and spermatogenesis. Cell Stem Cell. 2014;15(2):239–53.
82. Jenkins TG, Aston KI, Cairns BR, Carrell DT. Paternal aging and associated intraindividual alterations of global sperm 5-methylcytosine and 5-hydroxymethylcytosine levels. Fertil Steril. 2013;100(4):945–51.
83. Jenkins TG, Aston KI, Hotaling JM, Shamsi MB, Simon L, Carrell DT. Teratozoospermia and asthenozoospermia are associated with specific epigenetic signatures. Andrology. 2016;4(5):843–9.
84. Jenkins TG, Aston KI, Meyer TD, Hotaling JM, Shamsi MB, Johnstone EB, et al. Decreased fecundity and sperm DNA methylation patterns. Fertil Steril. 2016;105(1):51–7 e1–51–7 e3.
85. Jodar M, Selvaraju S, Sendler E, Diamond MP, Krawetz SA, Reproductive Medicine N. The presence, role and clinical use of spermatozoal RNAs. Hum Reprod Update. 2013;19(6):604–24.
86. Jodar M, Sendler E, Moskovtsev SI, Librach CL, Goodrich R, Swanson S, et al. Absence of sperm RNA elements correlates with idiopathic male infertility. Sci Transl Med. 2015;7(295):295re6.
87. Portela A, Esteller M. Epigenetic modifications and human disease. Nat Biotechnol. 2010;28(10):1057–68.
88. WHO. Laboratory Manual for the Examination an Processing of Human Semen Annali dell'Istituto superiore di sanita. 2010;5th ed(1).
89. Poland ML, Moghissi KS, Giblin PT, Ager JW, Olson JM. Variation of semen measures within normal men. Fertil Steril. 1985;44(3):396–400.
90. Yuan S, Tang C, Zhang Y, Wu J, Bao J, Zheng H, et al. mir-34b/c and mir-449a/b/c are required for spermatogenesis, but not for the first cleavage division in mice. Biol Open. 2015;4(2):212–23.
91. Liu WM, Pang RT, Chiu PC, Wong BP, Lao K, Lee KF, et al. Sperm-borne microRNA-34c is required for the first cleavage division in mouse. Proc Natl Acad Sci U S A. 2012;109(2):490–4.
92. Hammoud SS, Nix DA, Zhang H, Purwar J, Carrell DT, Cairns BR. Distinctive chromatin in human sperm packages genes for embryo development. Nature. 2009;460(7254):473–8.
93. Hammoud SS, Nix DA, Hammoud AO, Gibson M, Cairns BR, Carrell DT. Genome-wide analysis identifies changes in histone retention and epigenetic modifications at developmental and imprinted gene loci in the sperm of infertile men. Hum Reprod. 2011;26(9):2558–69.
94. Balhorn R. The protamine family of sperm nuclear proteins. Genome Biol. 2007;8(9):227.
95. Auger J, Mesbah M, Huber C, Dadoune JP. Aniline blue staining as a marker of sperm chromatin defects associated with different semen characteristics discriminates between proven fertile and suspected infertile men. Int J Androl. 1990;13(6):452–62.

Chapter 4
Effect of Paternal Age on Reproductive Outcomes: Data from Intracytoplasmic Sperm Injection and Oocyte Donation

Lena Sagi-Dain and Martha Dirnfeld

In recent decades, a prominent tendency for delayed childbearing has been noted [1]. This trend can be accounted for by several factors including gradually increased lifespan, more widespread contraceptive use, and changing female opportunities in society [2]. Yet advanced parental age does have its drawbacks, as it could unintentionally increase the risk of various adverse reproductive and postnatal outcomes. Numerous studies have explored the association between advanced maternal age and fertility. The decline in pregnancy rates begins at about 35 years for the female, sharply decreasing after 39 years [3, 4]. Adverse effects of maternal ageing add on throughout the pregnancy, expressed as higher risks for spontaneous abortions, congenital anomalies, intrauterine fetal demise, and various perinatal complications [5]. This negative influence is also reflected in assisted reproductive technology (ART) by decreased amount of recovered oocytes, lower fertilization rate, reduced embryo implantation efficiency, and decreased rates of pregnancy and live birth [6–8]. Two main processes accounting for this adverse effect on fertility include age-related decrease in the amount of available follicles and the parallel increase in the proportion of aneuploid oocytes [9].

Several theories have been suggested to account for the increased risk for chromosomal aberrations, including age-related degradation of meiotic spindle proteins taking part in chromosomal segregation (possibly related to accumulating environmental damage, e.g., free radicals), less effective functioning of intrinsic checkpoints monitoring the assembly of the mitotic spindle, and decrease in chiasmata, leading to less efficient stabilization of the homologues during chromosomal recombination [10, 11].

Similarly to maternal ageing, in the last decades a significant increase in births to fathers over age 35 has also been noted [12]. However, as opposed to advanced

L. Sagi-Dain (✉) • M. Dirnfeld
Division of Fertility-In Vitro Fertilization, Department of Obstetrics and Gynecology, Carmel Medical Center, Faculty of Medicine, Technion University, Haifa, Israel
e-mail: lenada@clalit.org.il; dirnfeld_martha@clalit.org.il

© Springer International Publishing AG 2018
G.D. Palermo, E.S. Sills (eds.), *Intracytoplasmic Sperm Injection*,
https://doi.org/10.1007/978-3-319-70497-5_4

maternal age influence, the relationship between male ageing and ART outcomes has received far less attention. The probable reason for this could be a seemingly milder effect of advanced paternal age on fertility, as conceptions have been reported even among males aged 70–80 years. The results of the few papers examining the effects of paternal age on reproductive outcomes are controversial. Several analyses have demonstrated an adverse effect of male ageing on fertility. For example, Klonoff-Cohen et al. conducted a prospective analysis of 221 in-vitro fertilization (IVF) and gamete intrafallopian transfer (GIFT) cycles [13]. The investigators reported increased odds of 11% for not achieving a pregnancy with each additional year of paternal age, with 12% odds of not having a successful live birth. de La Rochebrochard et al. retrospectively examined IVF cycles in 1938 fathers and noted increased rates of conception failure in males over 40 years [14]. In addition, male ageing has been associated with increased rates of spontaneous miscarriage [15]. However, other studies have not found any significant correlations between adverse ART outcomes and male ageing [16, 17]. In an attempt to summarize the literature on the subject, in 2010 we published a review that included ten published works [18]. Due to significant clinical and methodological diversity of the included studies, a meta-analysis could not be performed. We could not identify any meaningful association between advanced paternal age and various fertility measures, including fertilization, implantation, pregnancy, miscarriage, or live birth rates. The only two parameters in which some significance was noted with rising paternal age were decreased sperm volume and blastocyst formation [18].

Nevertheless, making conclusions based on studies examining patients undergoing autologous IVF cycles is quite problematic due to numerous biases. For example, ovarian hyperstimulation syndrome in some cycles can adversely affect endometrial receptivity and fetal development [19]. Moreover, one of the most important confounders deeply affecting IVF outcomes is maternal age, as older males tend to have older female partners. Several studies have tried to overcome this confounder by adjusting the examination for maternal age. However, a much more bias free analysis can be performed with studies using oocyte donation model, as oocyte donors are usually women under 35 years of age, minimizing the bias of advanced maternal age. Also, as ovum recipients typically undergo hormonal endometrial preparation, ovarian hyperstimulation is not expected to occur in these women.

Following these considerations, in 2015 we performed a systematic review of studies examining the effect of paternal age on the results of oocyte donation cycles [20]. Twelve articles were included in the analysis, encompassing a total of 12,538 oocyte donation cases [15, 17, 21–30]. No statistically significant correlation was shown by most studies between advanced paternal age and sperm characteristics such as concentration and morphology, except for decreased volume and possibly motility. In addition, no meaningful effect was noted in ART outcomes, including fertilization rates, embryo cleavage/development, implantation, pregnancy, spontaneous miscarriage, or live birth (see Table 4.1). Of note, overall quality of the evidence was rated as very low according to Grading of Recommendations Assessment, Development, and Evaluation criteria.

Table 4.1 Effects of paternal age on oocyte donation outcomes

First author (year)	Fertilization	Cleavage embryos	Blastocysts	Embryo quality	Implantation	Biochemical pregnancy	Clinical pregnancy	Miscarriage	Live birth rates
Medium quality studies									
Gallardo (1996)	NS	NS	–	NS	NS	–	NS	NS	–
Paulson RJ (2001)	NS	–	–	–	–	–	NS	–	NS
Frattarelli JL (2007)	NS	NS	Decrease	NS	NS	NS	–	Increase	Decrease
Girsh E (2008)	NS	–	–	–[a]	–	Decrease[a]	–	–	–
Luna M (2009)	Decrease[b]	–	Decrease	Decrease[c]	NS[d]	–	NS[e]	NS[e]	–
Gu L (2012)	NS	–	–	–	–	–	NS	NS	NS
Robertshaw I (2014)	–	–	–	–	–	–	–	–[f]	Decrease
High quality studies									
Bellver J (2008)	NS	NS	–	NS[g]	NS	NS[h]	–	NS	–
Campos I (2008)	NS	–	–	NS	NS[j]	–	NS[i]	NS	–
Duran EH (2010)	Decrease[k]	–	NS[l]	NS	NS	–	NS	NS	NS
Whitcomb BW (2011)	NS	NS[m]	–	–	–	–	NS	NS	NS
Begueria (2014)	NS	–	–	NS	–	NS	NS	NS	NS

NS no-significant

[a] Percentage of good quality day 3 embryos was lower in the nonpregnant group (26%) compared to the pregnant group (34%; $p = 0.01$). Also, paternal age was higher in the nonpregnant group (46.8 ± 7.8 years) vs. pregnant group (43.2 ± 8.1 years, $p = 0.003$)

(continued)

Table 4.1 (continued)

[b]Overall, fertilization rates significantly decreased with advancing age; however, when categorized by type of insemination (intra-cytoplasmic sperm injection vs. conventional), these rates were not different for age groups <40 years and 40–49 years, but were noted to be significantly lower for those cases that had undergone conventional insemination in group >50 years

[c]Decreased number of embryos with ≥7 cells on day 3

[d]Implantation rates were maintained in the three age groups (<40, 40–49, and >50 years). However, when men ≥50 years subdivided by age (50–59 years and >60 years), a significant decline in implantation rates ($p = 0.022$) was noted in the latter

[e]A trend toward a lower clinical pregnancy rates (72% vs. 50%, p = 0.14) and a higher loss rate (13% vs. 38%, $p = 0.17$) was noted for men >60 years

[f]Mean paternal age was significantly different among the 3 pregnancy outcome groups after controlling for donor age: nonpregnant (42.5 ± 1.1 years), spontaneous abortion (41.6 ± 1.1 years), and live birth (39.4 ± 0.5 years), $p = 0.02$

[g]Positive correlation was observed between embryo fragmentation 48 and 72 h after fertilization and paternal age, although r values were not clinically relevant. The correlations were below 0.3, being $r = 0.028$ and $r = 0.027$, respectively

[h]By logistic regression analysis, the variations in pregnancy rates for oocyte donation cycles induced by male age were significant ($P = 0.048$); nevertheless, the 95% confidence interval of the odds ratio included 1.0 and R2 value was very low (0.04), and therefore the model presented is not clinically relevant

[i]When corrected for recipients' age—"Only when both members were 'old,' we observed that age negatively affected pregnancy and implantation rates"

[k]In intra-cytoplasmic sperm injection group only

[l]Limited number of blastocyst transfers was examined ($n = 25$)

[m]No change in number of embryos frozen

Seven of 12 studies included both intra-cytoplasmic sperm injection (ICSI) and conventional IVF procedures; however, only one of these papers performed a separate analysis of ICSI cycles [26]. Only two investigations specifically focused only on ICSI cycles [24, 29].

The first manuscript to describe the effects of paternal age in ICSI cycles with donated oocytes was published by Girsh et al. in 2008 [24]. The investigators performed a retrospective analysis of 484 ICSI cycles, comparing male age and sperm parameters among 110 cycles resulting in a pregnancy to the 374 remaining cycles. The investigators found that men in the pregnancy group were significantly younger than in the nonpregnant group (43.2 ± 8.1 vs. 46.8 ± 7.8 years; $p = 0.003$). Of note, the percentage of day 3 "good" embryos, defined as six to eight blastomeres containing less than 10% fragmentation, was significantly higher in the pregnant group (34%) compared to the nonpregnant group (26%; $p = 0.01$). In addition, average male age was 43.2 ± 7.8 years in pregnancies progressing over 12 weeks, compared to pregnancies ending in spontaneous miscarriage (46.4 ± 2.1 years; p not published). Interestingly, a significant prevalence of teratozoospermia was noted in males of the nonpregnant group (29% vs. 11%, respectively). A significant correlation was found between worsening sperm morphology and male ageing: mean paternal age in normozoospermic patients was 44.8 years, compared to 47.9 years in mild teratozoospermia ($p = 0.02$), 48.4 years in moderate teratozoospermia ($p = 0.04$), and 51.9 years in severe teratozoospermia ($p = 0.001$). Quality of this study was defined as "medium" according to Newcastle-Ottawa Quality Assessment Scale, due to inadequate description of the derivation of the cohort (not mentioning whether all cases of oocyte donation during certain time period were selected) and inadequate adjustment for important confounders (such as recipients' age or any sperm parameters).

Another retrospective analysis of 519 ART cycles using donor oocytes was published by Duran et al. [26]. The analysis included 168 (32.4%) ICSI cycles. Males were arbitrarily categorized into three age groups: 25–38 years, 39–49 years, 50 years or older. Parameters included in the analysis for pregnancy prediction were recipient's age, male age, donor age, peak donor estradiol concentration, sperm concentration, motility, number of metaphase II oocytes, fertilization rate, embryo transfer day, total number of embryos transferred, embryo score for transferred embryos (ESTE), and mean ESTE. Thus, this study was rated as "high quality." A significant decline in fertilization rates was noted with advancing paternal age: 0.86 ± 0.15 vs. 0.82 ± 0.18 vs. 0.79 ± 0.23, respectively ($p = 0.04$). This correlation was also noted when performing a separate analysis for ICSI cycles, i.e., fertilization rates were higher in 25–38-years-old fathers, compared with those aged 50 years or more ($p = 0.008$ by one-way ANOVA with Bonferroni correction). However, pregnancy and live birth rates were not associated with male ageing and were only predicted by ESTE by binary logistic regression analysis. Clinical pregnancy rates in ICSI cycles were also predicted by recipient's age ($p = 0.005$). Of note, in this study deterioration in semen volume and sperm motility was noted with advancing paternal age.

The largest of 12 studies included in our systematic review was published in 2015 by Begueria et al. [29]. This retrospective cohort study included 4887 oocyte donation cycles, all fertilized by ICSI. In this study, a significant correlation was demonstrated between male age and all sperm parameters analyzed, including sperm volume, concentration, and motility. However, after adjustment for various confounders including donor and recipient age, fresh vs. frozen sperm, and number of transferred embryos (3 and 2 versus 1), no significant differences were found between different male age groups in any of the reproductive outcomes (biochemical pregnancies, miscarriage rates, clinical pregnancies, ongoing pregnancies, and live birth rates).

Thus, only three studies were found in the literature examining the effects of paternal age on fertility outcomes in oocyte donation cycles incorporating ICSI. While one medium quality study has demonstrated a significantly younger paternal age in cycles leading to clinical pregnancies, two high quality confounder-adjusted analyses did not show any meaningful correlation between male ageing and reproductive outcomes. Therefore, the available evidence in oocyte donation model implies that advanced paternal age does not adversely affect ART outcomes. However, by no means it can be concluded that older fathers undergoing ART require no specific age-adjusted counseling.

One crucial limitation that has to be noticed in all the abovementioned studies is lack of referral to additional crucial variables besides typical ART outcomes. For example, none of the papers has examined the influence of paternal ageing on the presence of congenital anomalies or delayed psychomotor development. One other factor not yet analyzed by any of the investigators is the incidence of specific autosomal dominant disorders known to be associated with advanced paternal age, including achondroplasia, neurofibromatosis type 1, craniosynostosis syndromes such as Crouzon syndrome, Noonan syndrome, and hereditary cancer predisposition syndromes such as retinoblastoma and multiple endocrine neoplasia types 2A and 2B [31–36]. These diseases are mostly caused by specific point mutations, and the involved fathers are frequently unaffected, leading to a thought that the mutations occur in the paternal germ cells during spermatogenesis.

Several hypotheses have been suggested to explain this increased rates of "paternal age effect" conditions. First, compared to ovarian germ cells, the male germ line has a higher predisposition to random mutational events. In particular, spontaneous point mutations and small deletions have been demonstrated two- to sevenfold more frequently in the male germ cells [37]. These types of mutations are generally created by two main mechanisms: intrinsic DNA replication errors, or mutations caused by external damage. Both types of mutational mechanisms are expected to occur at higher frequency among older fathers. As mitotic divisions of spermatogonial stem cells continue throughout many decades at an assumed rate of about 23 divisions per year [38], this process could explain the increased tendency for male DNA mutations, as opposed to the limited prenatal oocyte mitotic divisions. Similarly, lifetime accumulation of oxidative stress (such as free radical damage) and of exogenous mutagens, e.g., radiation exposure, could constitute an additional mutation source. In addition, advanced paternal age seems to be related to less effective DNA damage repair mechanisms and less efficient protection against oxidative stress, such as decreased activity of antioxidant enzymes in seminal plasma [39].

All these theories, while accounting for the general tendency for sperm DNA damage with advancing male age, do not explain the preponderance of specific mutations at defined DNA loci, causing the abovementioned genetic disorders related to male ageing. Classical hypothesis involved genomic DNA hotspots, causing hypermutability at particular loci. However, a recent theory has brought up the issue of a "selfish selection" mechanism, that is, an advantageous clonal expansion of mutated spermatogonia [40]. This process is similar in many aspects to malignancy inception, in which random genetic and epigenetic alterations derange DNA repair machinery, causing a continuing buildup of further genetic aberrations. Eventually, some of these mutations accidentally occur in genes responsible for cell survival and proliferation, leading to selective proliferation of these abnormal cells. In accordance with this theory, many of the genes responsible for paternal age related autosomal dominant diseases are either tumor suppressors or proto-oncogenes, functioning mainly through tyrosine kinase receptor/RAS signaling pathway. Thus, random mutations in these genes can be expected to lead to selective proliferation of abnormal cells, including paternal germ cells.

Additional disorders known to be associated with advancing paternal age are several neuropsychiatric and neurodevelopmental disorders including schizophrenia, epilepsy, autism, obsessive compulsive disorder, and Alzheimer disease [41–44]. In addition, higher risk for malignancy has been reported in the progeny of older fathers, such as breast cancer, brain tumors, prostate cancer, and hematologic malignancies [45–48]. However, none of the studies examining the implications of paternal age in ART cycles has referred to these longer-term disorders.

In summary, although the available evidence suggests that male ageing does not inflict any adverse effects on reproductive outcomes in an oocyte donation model using ICSI, this conclusion is based on conflicting results and limited sampling. Moreover, these studies have not examined the correlation between paternal age and various postnatal disorders known to be associated with male ageing, including autosomal dominant genetic diseases, neurodevelopmental disorders, and increased cancer risk. These issues should be discussed during pretreatment counseling of older couples, as well as of younger fathers considering postponing childbearing.

References

1. Hamilton BE, et al. Annual summary of vital statistics: 2010–2011. Pediatrics. 2013;131(3):548–58.
2. Mills M, et al. Why do people postpone parenthood? Reasons and social policy incentives. Hum Reprod Update. 2011;17(6):848–60.
3. Menken J, Trussell J, Larsen U. Age and infertility. Science. 1986;233(4771):1389–94.
4. Maheshwari A, Hamilton M, Bhattacharya S. Effect of female age on the diagnostic categories of infertility. Hum Reprod. 2008;23(3):538–42.

5. Heffner LJ. Advanced maternal age—how old is too old? N Engl J Med. 2004;351(19):1927–9.
6. Ziebe S, et al. Embryo quality and developmental potential is compromised by age. Acta Obstet Gynecol Scand. 2001;80(2):169–74.
7. Pantos K, et al. Influence of advanced age on the blastocyst development rate and pregnancy rate in assisted reproductive technology. Fertil Steril. 1999;71(6):1144–6.
8. Szamatowicz M, Grochowski D. Fertility and infertility in aging women. Gynecol Endocrinol. 1998;12(6):407–13.
9. Pellestor F, et al. Maternal aging and chromosomal abnormalities: new data drawn from in vitro unfertilized human oocytes. Hum Genet. 2003;112(2):195–203.
10. Mahmood R, et al. Mechanisms of maternal aneuploidy: FISH analysis of oocytes and polar bodies in patients undergoing assisted conception. Hum Genet. 2000;106(6):620–6.
11. Battaglia DE, et al. Influence of maternal age on meiotic spindle assembly in oocytes from naturally cycling women. Hum Reprod. 1996;11(10):2217–22.
12. Martin JA, et al. Births: final data for 2008. Natl Vital Stat Rep. 2010;59(1):1. 3–71
13. Klonoff-Cohen HS, Natarajan L. The effect of advancing paternal age on pregnancy and live birth rates in couples undergoing in vitro fertilization or gamete intrafallopian transfer. Am J Obstet Gynecol. 2004;191(2):507–14.
14. de La Rochebrochard E, et al. Fathers over 40 and increased failure to conceive: the lessons of in vitro fertilization in France. Fertil Steril. 2006;85(5):1420–4.
15. Frattarelli JL, et al. Male age negatively impacts embryo development and reproductive outcome in donor oocyte assisted reproductive technology cycles. Fertil Steril. 2008;90(1):97–103.
16. Spandorfer SD, et al. Effect of parental age on fertilization and pregnancy characteristics in couples treated by intracytoplasmic sperm injection. Hum Reprod. 1998;13(2):334–8.
17. Bellver J, et al. Influence of paternal age on assisted reproduction outcome. Reprod Biomed Online. 2008;17(5):595–604.
18. Dain L, Auslander R, Dirnfeld M. The effect of paternal age on assisted reproduction outcome. Fertil Steril. 2011;95(1):1–8.
19. Garcia-Velasco JA, et al. Factors that determine discordant outcome from shared oocytes. Fertil Steril. 2003;80(1):54–60.
20. Sagi-Dain L, Sagi S, Dirnfeld M. Effect of paternal age on reproductive outcomes in oocyte donation model: a systematic review. Fertil Steril. 2015;104(4):857–865 e1.
21. Gallardo E, et al. Effect of age on sperm fertility potential: oocyte donation as a model. Fertil Steril. 1996;66(2):260–4.
22. Paulson RJ, Milligan RC, Sokol RZ. The lack of influence of age on male fertility. Am J Obstet Gynecol. 2001;184(5):818–22. discussion 822–4
23. Campos I, et al. Effects of men and recipients' age on the reproductive outcome of an oocyte donation program. J Assist Reprod Genet. 2008;25(9–10):445–52.
24. Girsh E, et al. Male age influences oocyte-donor program results. J Assist Reprod Genet. 2008;25(4):137–43.
25. Luna M, et al. Paternal age and assisted reproductive technology outcome in ovum recipients. Fertil Steril. 2009;92(5):1772–5.
26. Duran EH, et al. Impact of male age on the outcome of assisted reproductive technology cycles using donor oocytes. Reprod Biomed Online. 2010;20(6):848–56.
27. Whitcomb BW, et al. Contribution of male age to outcomes in assisted reproductive technologies. Fertil Steril. 2011;95(1):147–51.
28. Gu L, et al. Effect of male age on the outcome of in vitro fertilization: oocyte donation as a model. J Assist Reprod Genet. 2012;29(4):331–4.
29. Begueria R, et al. Paternal age and assisted reproductive outcomes in ICSI donor oocytes: is there an effect of older fathers? Hum Reprod. 2014;29(10):2114–22.
30. Robertshaw I, et al. The effect of paternal age on outcome in assisted reproductive technology using the ovum donation model. Reprod Sci. 2014;21(5):590–3.
31. Shotelersuk V, et al. FGFR2 mutations among Thai children with Crouzon and Apert syndromes. J Craniofac Surg. 2003;14(1):101–4. discussion 105–7

32. Rannan-Eliya SV, et al. Paternal origin of FGFR3 mutations in Muenke-type craniosynostosis. Hum Genet. 2004;115(3):200–7.
33. Seemanova E, Zenker M. Mutagenic effect of advanced paternal age in neurocardiofaciocutaneous syndrome. Cas Lek Cesk. 2014;153(5):242–5.
34. Orioli IM, et al. Effect of paternal age in achondroplasia, thanatophoric dysplasia, and osteogenesis imperfecta. Am J Med Genet. 1995;59(2):209–17.
35. Liu Q, et al. Parental age and Neurofibromatosis type 1: a report from the NF1 patient registry initiative. Familial Cancer. 2014;
36. Choi SK, et al. Positive selection for new disease mutations in the human germline: evidence from the heritable cancer syndrome multiple endocrine neoplasia type 2B. PLoS Genet. 2012;8(2):e1002420.
37. Li WH, Yi S, Makova K. Male-driven evolution. Curr Opin Genet Dev. 2002;12(6):650–6.
38. Vogel F, Rathenberg R. Spontaneous mutation in man. Adv Hum Genet. 1975;5:223–318.
39. Kelso KA, et al. Lipid and antioxidant changes in spermatozoa and seminal plasma throughout the reproductive period of bulls. J Reprod Fertil. 1997;109(1):1–6.
40. Goriely A, Wilkie AO. Paternal age effect mutations and selfish spermatogonial selection: causes and consequences for human disease. Am J Hum Genet. 2012;90(2):175–200.
41. D'Onofrio BM, et al. Paternal age at childbearing and offspring psychiatric and academic morbidity. JAMA Psychiat. 2014;71(4):432–8.
42. Wu Y, et al. Advanced paternal age increases the risk of schizophrenia and obsessive-compulsive disorder in a Chinese Han population. Psychiatry Res. 2012;198(3):353–9.
43. Vestergaard M, et al. Paternal age and epilepsy in the offspring. Eur J Epidemiol. 2005;20(12):1003–5.
44. Bertram L, et al. Paternal age is a risk factor for Alzheimer disease in the absence of a major gene. Neurogenetics. 1998;1(4):277–80.
45. Choi JY, et al. Association of paternal age at birth and the risk of breast cancer in offspring: a case control study. BMC Cancer. 2005;5:143.
46. Urhoj SK, et al. Advanced paternal age and mortality of offspring under 5 years of age: a register-based cohort study. Hum Reprod. 2014;29(2):343–50.
47. Larfors G, Hallbook H, Simonsson B. Parental age, family size, and offspring's risk of childhood and adult acute leukemia. Cancer Epidemiol Biomark Prev. 2012;21(7):1185–90.
48. Zhang Y, et al. Parental age at child's birth and son's risk of prostate cancer. The Framingham Study. Am J Epidemiol. 1999;150(11):1208–12.

Chapter 5
New Paradigms in De Novo Creation of Functional Human Spermatozoa: A Review of Biological Progress Towards Clinical Application

Nina Neuhaus, Tim Pock, Stefan Schlatt, and Verena Nordhoff

5.1 De Novo Creation of Spermatozoa: A Distant Vision or a Near Reality?

The aim of scientists to create de novo specialized cells of the human body, especially gametes, is as old as research itself. However, it is only recently that we have learned that our cells, whether somatic or germ line, contain more than just the genomic blueprint. Recent studies have shown that genomic integrity and epigenetic regulations play an important role [1]. Epigenetic features of germ cells are especially important. Therefore, the goal is not merely the in vitro production of a cell that looks and functions like a spermatozoon, but a cell that has the same genomic integrity and epigenetic marks that would be produced in vivo.

Which types of patients would benefit from de novo creation of spermatozoa? Patients facing depletion or loss of germ cells due to chemotherapy or radiotherapy treatment for cancer represent an obvious group. Within this cohort, prepubertal patients would particularly benefit, as they do not have the option to cryopreserve spermatozoa as a fertility reserve prior to treatment. In addition, patients with germ cell arrest secondary to genetic defects including 47, XXY patients would benefit. Lastly, individuals whose testes are devoid of germ cells would also benefit, although experimental approaches using autologous germ line stem cells would not be possible for such patients. This chapter focuses on those experimental strategies employing germ line stem cells (spermatogonial stem cells) for the de novo generation of spermatozoa.

N. Neuhaus • T. Pock • S. Schlatt • V. Nordhoff (✉)
Centre of Reproductive Medicine and Andrology, University Hospital of Münster,
Münster, Germany
e-mail: nina.neuhaus@ukmuenster.de; tim.pock@ukmuenster.de;
stefan.schlatt@ukmuenster.de; verena.nordhoff@ukmuenster.de

© Springer International Publishing AG 2018   49
G.D. Palermo, E.S. Sills (eds.), *Intracytoplasmic Sperm Injection*,
https://doi.org/10.1007/978-3-319-70497-5_5

5.2   Introduction: Spermatogenesis and Spermiogenesis

In the immature testes, germ line stem cells (spermatogonia) are the most advanced germ cell type and are located at the basement membrane of the *tubuli seminiferi*. At puberty, spermatogenesis begins, resulting in the formation of haploid spermatozoa. The spermatogonial stem cells must fulfill the following tasks: (1) initiation and maintenance of sperm production, (2) creation of a reserve pool of stem cells, and (3) maintenance of DNA integrity as the genetic material is transferred to the next generation.

Human spermatogonia are divided into three types based on morphological and functional properties: A_{dark}, A_{pale}, and B spermatogonia. A_{dark} spermatogonia are the regenerative reserve of the testis. A_{pale} spermatogonia show a comparably high mitotic activity and make up the functional reserve. B spermatogonia mark the entry of differentiation and meiosis [2]. During puberty, A_{dark} spermatogonia are mitotically active and occupy the stem cell niches within the seminiferous tubules of the testis. In contrast, this stem cell population shows low mitotic activity in the adult testis and serves as the stem cell reserve, which is only activated upon damage of the germ cell epithelium. Meiosis starts with the differentiation of B spermatogonia into preleptotene primary spermatocytes. Following meiosis, spermiogenesis begins. This process involves morphological transformations including the formation of an acrosome and a flagellum. The formation of a typical sperm head requires condensation of chromatin, elongation of the nucleus, and the removal of cytoplasm.

Over the last few decades, two main strategies have been pursued for de novo production of spermatozoa. Many studies have attempted to reproduce this extremely complex process in vitro and to achieve spermatozoa from spermatogonia. Other studies have rather aimed to establish re-fertilization approaches based on spermatogonial stem cells seeking to achieve the in vivo maturation of immature germ cells [3, 4]; such spermatozoa could then be used in the frame of assisted reproductive treatments. Importantly, prior to that, functional properties including the genetic and epigenetic integrity of generated germ cells have to be ensured. Other studies have focused on protocols for the isolation and propagation of spermatogonial stem cells. These cells could be transplanted back into the donor's testis following successful cancer treatment. Employing this approach, even the re-fertilization of patients could be achieved as the spermatogonial stem cells have the capacity to migrate back into their niches within the testis and to reinitiate spermatogenesis. For approaches seeking to retransfer of either spermatogonial stem cells or entire testicular tissues to patients, the possibility of inadvertently transferring residual cancer cells in recovered cancer patients constitutes an additional concern. Therefore, this chapter outlines the hitherto experimental approaches for the de novo generation of spermatozoa as well as the functional tests that are available to assess integrity of in vitro generated germ cells (see Fig. 5.1).

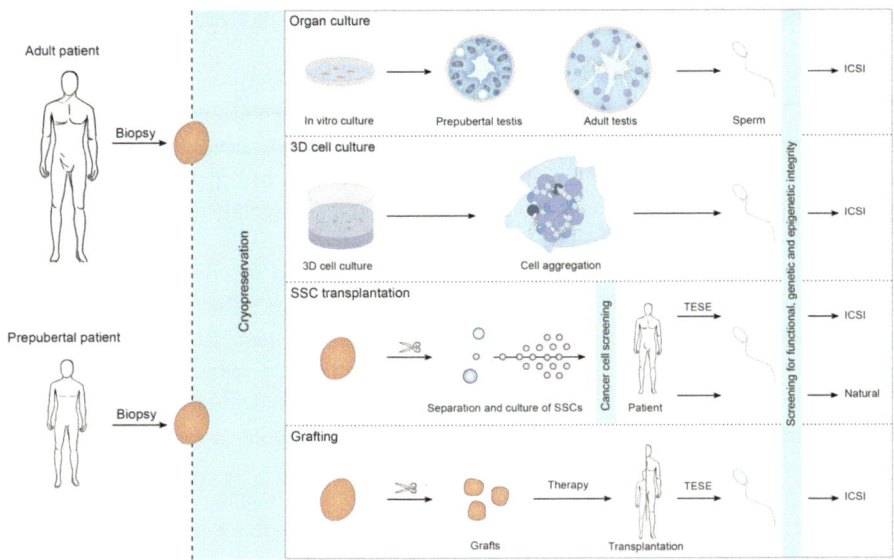

Fig. 5.1 Different approaches of de novo creation of spermatozoa from either adult or prepubertal patients: organ culture, 3D culture, spermatogonial stem cell (SSC) culture, and transplantation or grafting. *Note: TESE* testicular sperm extraction; *ICSI* intracytoplasmic sperm injection

5.2.1   In Vitro Spermatogenesis

5.2.1.1   In Vitro Spermatogenesis Using an Organ Culture Approach

While experiments to achieve in vitro spermatogenesis were performed more than a century ago [5], true scientific breakthroughs have only been achieved in recent years. Spermatogenesis is a complex process that is tightly regulated by the structure and soluble factors provided by a specialized compartmentalized microenvironment. Keeping the complex structural and functional properties of the testicular tissues intact is an advantage of the organ culture approach compared to in vitro cell culture systems (see Fig. 5.1). As a circulatory system to supply tissue with oxygen and nutrients cannot be maintained in vitro, mechanical dissociation of the starting material into small tissues fragments (1–3 mm in diameter) is crucial. Apart from that, culture at the interphase between culture medium and gas layer has long been considered the gold standard [6]. In 2011, Sato et al. showed for the first time that in vitro spermatogenesis could be achieved using immature neonatal mouse testes. Successful differentiation was observed specifically in those cultures that were supplemented with KnockOut Serum Replacement (KSR) instead of fetal calf serum (FCS), leading the authors to speculate that the latter may contain substances that inhibit spermatogenesis; KSR was thus used for subsequent experiments. Round spermatids were obtained from 3.5d post partum (dpp) old testes following 23 days of culture; sperm was isolated from 2.5dpp old tissues after 42 days, respectively.

To assess function, round spermatids and sperm were isolated and injected into oocytes using round spermatid injection (ROSI) and intracytoplasmic sperm injection (ICSI), respectively. Importantly, the resulting offspring were healthy and fertile [7]. As testicular tissues from pediatric cancer patients are cryopreserved for long-term storage, Sato et al. also applied this protocol to cryopreserved neonatal mouse tissue. Haploid cells were isolated after 43 days of organ culture and both round spermatids and spermatozoa were detected; offspring derived from these germ cells were healthy and fertile [8].

As epimutations are a concern for gametes produced in vitro, Yokonishi et al. investigated the differential methylation profile of 11 germ line regions including, *H19*, *Lit1*, *Meg1*, *Snrpn*. No differences were found among ROSI-derived, ICSI-derived, and control animals. This finding is an important validation for transferring this approach into a clinical setting; however, additional challenges need to be addressed, namely the difference in kinetics between mouse and human spermatogenesis. In mice, spermatogenesis requires only 35 days vs. 76 days in humans. Thus, longer term cultures will be necessary for human tissue. To establish conditions for long-term tissue culture, Komeya et al. [9] tested a microfluidic device wherein testicular tissue from neonatal mice was separated from flowing media by a porous membrane. Using this modified organ culture approach, Komeya et al. not only improved the efficiency of induction of spermatogenesis in vitro, but also extended the culture duration to 6 months. Importantly, the original organ culture approach reported in 2011 by Sato et al. has now been successfully used by a different research group to induce in vitro spermatogenesis in newborn (5dpp) Sprague-Dawley rats. Specifically, following 52 days of culture up to 0.8 ± 1.3% of seminiferous tubules contained acrosin-positive differentiated germ cells [10].

Based on these breakthroughs with mouse tissue, it is feasible that in vitro spermatogenesis using immature human testicular tissues as starting material may also be successful in the future. One advantage of in vitro generated spermatozoa is that these could be analyzed for epigenetic as well as genetic integrity and only single sperm cells would be needed for ICSI treatments. Consequently, the risk of reintroduction of residual cancer cells in oncological patients could essentially be eliminated.

5.2.1.2   Three-Dimensional Culture of Single Cells

To achieve in vitro differentiation of spermatogonia, three-dimensional soft agar or methylcellulose culture systems have also been investigated (see Fig. 5.1). This approach is based on two assumptions: (1) Spermatogonia require a three-dimensional structure for expansion and differentiation and (2) in vitro differentiation may be inhibited in intact testicular tissue structures. Therefore, testicular tissue is digested enzymatically to obtain a single cell suspension. Cell fractions enriched in spermatogonia and testicular somatic cells are then placed into different phases of the soft agar culture system, thereby facilitating the exchange of hormones and growth factors across different cell fractions. Using testicular tissue from immature mice, it was initially revealed that SSCs differentiated up to the level of postmeiotic germ cells in this soft agar culture system [11]. In a subsequent study, the same group revealed that even complete maturation into morphologically normal spermatozoa can be achieved. While in vitro maturation was not influenced by the type of matrix (e.g., soft agar vs. methylcellulose), complete maturation did depend on the presence of somatic cells and gonadotropin hormones [12, 13]. Unfortunately, the functionality of these in vitro generated spermatozoa remains unknown, due to the technical challenge of recovering spermatozoa from the matrices. This three-dimensional culture approach has meanwhile been applied to assess the in vitro differentiation of spermatogonia from immature rat testes. However, under the culture conditions tested, maturation has been achieved only up to the stage of pachytene spermatocytes [14]. More recently, this three-dimensional culture system was applied to a nonhuman primate species, *Macaca mulatta* [15]. Comparable to previous studies, soft agar and methylcellulose were used to generate 3D matrices. Testicular tissues from juvenile animals (13–33 months of age; $n = 6$) were used as the starting material. Following 30 days of culture, postmeiotic cells were observed whether or not hormones (FSH and testosterone) were present. It remains to be assessed which additional stimuli are required to achieve the final stages of germ cell differentiation in this primate model. Such studies would be especially relevant towards achieving in vitro spermatogenesis in humans.

5.2.2 In Vivo Maturation of Germ Cells

5.2.2.1 Propagation of Spermatogonial Stem Cells In Vitro for Autologous Germ Cell Transplantation and In Vivo Spermatogenesis

The germ cell transplantation assay was first introduced in 1994. For this approach, spermatogonial stem cells were isolated from donor mice and injected into the seminiferous tubules of sterile recipient testes. Following injection, donor cells migrated towards the basement membrane, repopulated the seminiferous tubules, and underwent spermatogenesis [16]. The functionality of these donor-derived sperm was proven. Of note, the recipient mice had a reduced natural fertility resulting in smaller litter sizes. Even after artificial insemination in a dish (in vitro fertilization, IVF), lower fertilization and formation of blastocysts were observed. A likely explanation for these findings is the reduced colonization of recipient testis, as only 50% of seminiferous tubules showed normal spermatogenesis [17]. In addition, the percentage of motile spermatozoa from recipient animals was lower and sperm cells showed quickly decreasing motility in culture. These limitations, however, can be overcome with ICSI treatment since neither cell number nor sperm motility has a direct effect on ICSI outcome. Accordingly, ICSI results in recipient and control animals were comparable [18].

To translate this germ cell transplantation approach to a clinical setting, additional requirements have to be fulfilled (see Fig. 5.1). Specifically, the number of SSCs in testicular tissue overall is limited, and in testicular biopsies especially so.

Therefore, protocols for the isolation and propagation of SSCs have to be established. Interestingly, mouse SSCs were shown to maintain a normal karyotype, an androgenetic imprinting pattern, as well as the ability to re-establish spermatogenesis following germ cell transplantation even after a 2-year culture period [19].

Protocols to enrich and culture spermatogonial stem cells from primates have also been developed in recent years. This is of fundamental importance because rodents and humans have different spermatogonial stem cell systems [2]. In contrast, the nonhuman primate model of the marmoset monkey shares many key characteristics with humans regarding testicular development and, notably, the spermatogonial stem cell system [20–24]. The nonhuman primate model provides easily accessible normal adult testicular tissue that can be used to establish culture conditions for spermatogonial stem cells. To date, short-term culturing of these cells has been successful; SSCs maintained their potential to home into their stem cell niches following germ cell transplantation [25]. Moreover, cells in culture maintained a stable androgenetic methylation profile throughout the culture period (Langenstroth Röwer et al., *in press*). In humans, a number of groups have reported the successful isolation and short-term culturing of adult [26–28] as well as prepubertal SSCs [29]. Developing culture protocols that also support the propagation and long-term culturing of human SSCs is currently the major focus in this research area.

5.2.2.2 Autologous Transplantation of Testicular Tissues

To achieve in vivo differentiation of immature testicular tissues, different transplantation approaches have been investigated: (1) autologous, (2) heterologous, and (3) xenotransplantation. In 2002, it was revealed that transplantation of neonatal mouse testicular tissues under the back skin of recipient mice resulted in differentiation of germ line stem cells into spermatozoa [30, 31]. Importantly, a subsequent study showed that these spermatozoa produced healthy and fertile offspring via ICSI [31].

Remarkably, transplantation of human fetal testicular tissue under the skin of mice (xenotransplantation) led to the differentiation of germ line stem cells into sperm. However, xenotransplantation using testicular tissue from 3-month-old boys resulted in differentiation only up to the stage of pachytene spermatocytes [32]. Comparable experiments with adult human tissues were even less successful, as most yielded only degenerated tissue with few remaining germ cells which could be retrieved [33]. In addition, the potential transfer of a murine virus constitutes an additional risk for the patient that has to be eliminated. Thus, homologous transplantation of testicular tissues presents the best option. For this approach, the patient's own tissue is cryopreserved for autotransplantation following gonadotoxic treatment (see Fig. 5.1). While several centers worldwide offer cryopreservation of prepubertal testicular tissue, thus far no successful autotransplantations have been performed. However, promising results have been reported using testicular tissues from a nonhuman primate model (*Macaca mulatta*). Juvenile testicular tissue was collected prior to irradiation and castration and cryopreserved.

Subsequently, thawed cryopreserved tissue was autologously grafted. To assess the impact of the graft environment, grafts were placed under the skin of the shoulder, the arm, or into the scrotum. Importantly, full germ cell maturation until the stage of spermatozoa was only observed in those grafts that had been placed into the scrotum, demonstrating the importance of the implantation site. Nevertheless, full germ cell differentiation was very low: only 3–7% of scrotal grafts showed full spermatogenesis 5 months after implantation [34]. In order to transfer this approach to the clinic, it needs to be determined how much immature tissue needs to be auto-grafted to ensure a high probability of spermatozoa retrieval. Also, as intact testicular tissues are employed for this approach, it cannot be excluded that malignant cells may exist in these tissues. Previous studies in rats have shown that as few as 20 leukemic cells were sufficient to cause a cancer relapse [35]. Thus, such an approach can only be considered for patients for whom the transfer of residual tumor cells can be ruled out.

5.3   Proof of Functionality

5.3.1   Tests for the Functional Properties of De Novo Generated Spermatozoa

5.3.1.1   ICSI

As spermatozoa carry the paternal genetic information forward to the next generation, screening for functionality and genetic integrity is an imperative. For morphological integrity, staining methods recommended by WHO [36] can be easily applied. However, even morphologically abnormal sperm can fertilize and result in healthy offspring regardless of which reproductive technique is used [37–40]. Round spermatids can also result in healthy babies, but at a lower frequency [41]. Apart from morphology, a spermatozoon should be screened for vitality. Vitality is a prerequisite for successful ICSI, as injection of a dead or disintegrated sperm will result in fertilization failure.

Considering all in vitro production studies, it becomes evident that the amount of de novo created spermatozoa will be very low, enough only for ICSI treatment. The most obvious sign of vitality is motility. However, in cases of de novo generated spermatozoa it is quite likely that sperm will be immotile. Vitality can also be evaluated by eosin staining—vital and non-vital spermatozoa can be easily differentiated as only living cells exclude the dye [36]. However, clinical use of spermatozoa for ICSI after this diagnostic analysis should be avoided. If spermatozoa are intended for clinical use with ICSI, either the hypo-osmotic swelling test (HOS test) or laser-assisted immotile sperm selection (LAISS) should be performed. During the HOS test, spermatozoa are (partially) transferred to a hypo-osmotic medium and tail swelling is observed only in living spermatozoa [42, 43]. During LAISS, targeted laser energy induces curling of the flagellum tip of viable sperm only [44–46]. More problematic is the inability of the spermatozoon to activate the oocyte after injection. Suboptimal sperm may fail to induce naturally occurring calcium oscillations within the oocyte, e.g., due to sperm-related deficiencies in the phospholipase C-zeta cascade [47, 48]. Methods can be used to induce oocyte calcium oscillations including mechanical stimulation, electrical activation, and the use of chemicals [49–55].

5.3.1.2 IUI or IVF

For conventional fertilization of oocytes by intrauterine insemination (IUI) or IVF, the normality of the acrosome reaction has to be tested. The acrosome reaction takes place after sperm bind to the *zona pellucida*. To penetrate the zona and fuse with the oocyte's plasma membrane, the acrosome reaction is an absolute prerequisite. To evaluate the binding function of spermatozoa to *zona pellucida*, the hemizona assay can be used [56]. Alternatively, disaggregated human *zona pellucida* proteins can be used to check for normal acrosome function [57, 58]. Zona-intact oocytes from other mammals cannot be used for this test as binding is hampered by species differences [59–61]. To assess if de novo generated spermatozoa can fuse with an oocyte, the hamster oocyte penetration (HOP) test can be performed. Properly acrosome-reacted human spermatozoa will fuse at their equatorial region with the hamster oocyte plasma membrane. However, one has to keep in mind the possibility of false negatives, i.e., spermatozoa unable to fuse with the hamster oocyte but able to fuse with a human oocyte [62].

5.3.2 Tests for Epigenetic Integrity of De Novo Generated Spermatozoa

Chromosomal integrity has been evaluated in two generations of mice following germ cell transplantation, finding no chromosomal anomalies [63]. In addition, litter development was normal with regard to animal size and weight [64]. More challenging than establishing ploidy status is proving epigenetic stability. Histone modification, noncoding RNAs and DNA methylation changes are covalent alterations that do not change the base sequence itself [1]. Nevertheless, epigenetic properties are essential for activating and inhibiting gene expression. Epigenetic marks are set early during development and are passed on to the next generations. During early testis development, DNA methylation marks are erased and re-established [65]. After spermatozoon-oocyte fusion and the onset of cellular division, the developing embryo undergoes a wave of genome-wide demethylation, with one exception: imprinted genes. Imprinted genes are methylated biallelic genes expressed in a monoallelic maternal or paternal manner [66]. The maintenance of imprinting is important as changes can lead to disorders [67]. After implantation into the uterus, a second wave of demethylation takes place, but this time only in primordial germ cells. Any epigenetic marks not demethylated in the first wave now undergo demethylation during this second wave, thus establishing a sex-specific DNA methylation pattern [65, 68, 69]. Changes or disturbances in the male gamete specific epigenetic pattern due to the artificial de novo creation of spermatozoa may influence not only spermatogenesis, but the offspring as a whole. It is important to note that factors disturbing epigenetic mechanisms in sperm may affect reproductive outcomes directly [70].

In a previous study, three genes were assessed in the two generations following germ cell transplantation. Reassuringly, these epigenetic marks showed no differences compared to control animals [64]. In a clinical setting, however, global screening of epigenetic integrity in human spermatogonia before germ cell transplantation is prudent, as epigenetic changes in spermatozoa appear to play a role in male infertility [65, 71–80]. This is further supported by a meta-analysis of aberrant methylation in two imprinted genes in the spermatozoa of infertile men [81]. Spermatozoa in the semen of oligoasthenozoospermic men present epigenetic mosaicism, likely arising from errors during imprint erasure [70, 82].

5.4 Conclusion

Considerable progress has been made in the de novo generation of spermatozoa in recent years. Based on these new findings, it appears more probable than ever that the de novo generation of human spermatozoa from immature germ cells will be possible in the future. This would especially benefit patients with germ cell arrest or prepubertal patients facing germ cell loss due to gonadotoxic treatment. If successful, de novo generation of spermatozoa would enable such patients to father their own children in the future. As de novo generated spermatozoa transfer genetic material to the next generation, screening of in vitro generated cells for functionality as well as genetic and epigenetic integrity is an imperative.

References

1. Berger SL, Kouzarides T, Shiekhattar R, Shilatifard A. An operational definition of epigenetics. Genes Dev. 2009;23(7):781–3.
2. Ehmcke J, Wistuba J, Schlatt S. Spermatogonial stem cells: questions, models and perspectives. Hum Reprod Update. 2006;12(3):275–82.
3. Staub C. A century of research on mammalian male germ cell meiotic differentiation in vitro. J Androl. 2001;22(6):911–26.
4. Georgiou I, Pardalidis N, Giannakis D, Saito M, Watanabe T, Tsounapi P, et al. In vitro spermatogenesis as a method to bypass pre-meiotic or post-meiotic barriers blocking the spermatogenetic process: genetic and epigenetic implications in assisted reproductive technology. Andrologia. 2007;39(5):159–76.

5. Goldschmidt R. Some experiments on spermatogenesis in vitro. Proc Natl Acad Sci U S A. 1915;1(4):220–2.
6. Trowell OA. The culture of mature organs in a synthetic medium. Exp Cell Res. 1959;16(1):118–47.
7. Sato T, Katagiri K, Gohbara A, Inoue K, Ogonuki N, Ogura A, et al. In vitro production of functional sperm in cultured neonatal mouse testes. Nature. 2011;471(7339):504–7.
8. Yokonishi T, Sato T, Komeya M, Katagiri K, Kubota Y, Nakabayashi K, et al. Offspring production with sperm grown in vitro from cryopreserved testis tissues. Nat Commun. 2014;5:4320.
9. Komeya M, Kimura H, Nakamura H, Yokonishi T, Sato T, Kojima K, et al. Long-term ex vivo maintenance of testis tissues producing fertile sperm in a microfluidic device. Sci Rep. 2016;6:21472.
10. Reda A, Hou M, Winton TR, Chapin RE, Söder O, Stukenborg JB. In vitro differentiation of rat spermatogonia into round spermatids in tissue culture. Mol Hum Reprod. 2016;22(9):601–12.
11. Stukenborg J-B, Wistuba J, Luetjens CM, Elhija MA, Huleihel M, Lunenfeld E, et al. Coculture of spermatogonia with somatic cells in a novel three-dimensional soft-agar-culture-system. J Androl. 2008;29(3):312–29.
12. Stukenborg JB, Schlatt S, Simoni M, Yeung CH, Elhija MA, Luetjens CM, et al. New horizons for in vitro spermatogenesis? An update on novel three-dimensional culture systems as tools for meiotic and post-meiotic differentiation of testicular germ cells. Mol Hum Reprod. 2009;15(9):521–9.
13. Abu Elhija M, Lunenfeld E, Schlatt S, Huleihel M. Differentiation of murine male germ cells to spermatozoa in a soft agar culture system. Asian J Androl. 2012;14(2):285–93.
14. Reda A, Hou M, Landreh L, Kjartansdóttir KR, Svechnikov K, Söder O, et al. In vitro spermatogenesis - optimal culture conditions for testicular cell survival, germ cell differentiation, and steroidogenesis in rats. Front Endocrinol (Lausanne). 2014;5:1–11.
15. Huleihel M, Nourashrafeddin S, Plant TM. Application of three-dimensional culture systems to study mammalian spermatogenesis, with an emphasis on the rhesus monkey (Macaca mulatta). Asian J Androl. 2015;17(6):972–80.
16. Brinster RL, Zimmermann JW. Spermatogenesis following male germ-cell transplantation. Proc Natl Acad Sci U S A. 1994;91(24):11298–302.
17. Goossens E, Frederickx V, De Block G, Van Steirteghem AC, Tournaye H. Reproductive capacity of sperm obtained after germ cell transplantation in a mouse model. Hum Reprod. 2003;18(9):1874–80.
18. Geens M, Goossens E, De block G, Ning L, Van saen D, Tournaye H. Autologous spermatogonial stem cell transplantation in man: current obstacles for a future clinical application. Hum Reprod Update. 2008;14(2):121–9.
19. Kanatsu-Shinohara M, Ogonuki N, Iwano T, Lee J, Kazuki Y, Inoue K, et al. Genetic and epigenetic properties of mouse male germline stem cells during long-term culture. Development. 2005;132(18):4155–63.
20. Weinbauer GF, Aslam H, Krishnamurthy H, Brinkworth MH, Einspanier A, Hodges JK. Quantitative analysis of spermatogenesis and apoptosis in the common marmoset (Callithrix jacchus) reveals high rates of spermatogonial turnover and high spermatogenic efficiency. Biol Reprod. 2001;64(1):120–6.
21. Wistuba J. Organization of seminiferous epithelium in primates: relationship to spermatogenic efficiency, phylogeny, and mating system. Biol Reprod. 2003;69(2):582–91.
22. Luetjens CM, Weinbauer GF, Wistuba J. Primate spermatogenesis: new insights into comparative testicular organisation, spermatogenic efficiency and endocrine control. Biol Rev Camb Philos Soc. 2005;80(3):475–88.
23. Mitchell RT, Cowan G, Morris KD, Anderson RA, Fraser HM, Mckenzie KJ, et al. Germ cell differentiation in the marmoset (Callithrix jacchus) during fetal and neonatal life closely parallels that in the human. Hum Reprod. 2008;23(12):2755–65.
24. Albert S, Ehmcke J, Wistuba J, Eildermann K, Behr R, Schlatt S, et al. Germ cell dynamics in the testis of the postnatal common marmoset monkey (Callithrix jacchus). Reproduction. 2010;140(5):733–42.

25. Langenstroth D, Kossack N, Westernströer B, Wistuba J, Behr R, Gromoll J, et al. Separation of somatic and germ cells is required to establish primate spermatogonial cultures. Hum Reprod. 2014;29(9):2018–31.
26. He Z, Kokkinaki M, Jiang J, Dobrinski I, Dym M. Isolation, characterization, and culture of human spermatogonia. Biol Reprod. 2010;82(2):363–72.
27. Sadri-Ardekani H. Propagation of human spermatogonial stem cells in vitro. Am Med Assoc. 2009;302(19):2127–34.
28. Kossack N, Terwort N, Wistuba J, Ehmcke J, Schlatt S, Schöler H, et al. A combined approach facilitates the reliable detection of human spermatogonia in vitro. Hum Reprod. 2013;28(11):3012–25.
29. Sadri-Ardekani H. In vitro propagation of human prepubertal spermatogonial stem cells. Medicine (Baltimore). 2011;305(23):2006–7.
30. Honaramooz A, Snedaker A, Boiani M, Schöler H, Dobrinski I, Schlatt S. Sperm from neonatal mammalian testes grafted in mice. Nature. 2002;418(6899):778–81.
31. Schlatt S. Progeny from sperm obtained after ectopic grafting of neonatal mouse testes. Biol Reprod. 2003;68(6):2331–5.
32. Sato Y, Nozawa S, Yoshiike M, Arai M, Sasaki C, Iwamoto T. Xenografting of testicular tissue from an infant human donor results in accelerated testicular maturation. Hum Reprod. 2010;25(5):1113–22.
33. Socie G, Salooja N, Cohen A, Rovelli A, Carreras E, Locasciulli A, et al. Nonmalignant late effects after allogeneic stem cell transplantation. Blood. 2003;101(9):3373–85.
34. Jahnukainen K, Ehmcke J, Nurmio M, Schlatt S. Autologous ectopic grafting of cryopreserved testicular tissue preserves the fertility of prepubescent monkeys which receive a sterilizing cytotoxic therapy. Cancer Res. 2012;257(5):2432–7.
35. Jahnukainen K, Hou M, Petersen C, Setchell B, Söder O. Intratesticular transplantation of testicular cells from leukemic rats causes transmission of leukemia. Cancer Res. 2001;61(2):706–10.
36. WHO. WHO laboratory manual for the examination and processing of human semen. Cambridge, UK: Cambridge University Press; 2010.
37. De Vos A, Polyzos N, Verheyen G, Tournaye H. Intracytoplasmic morphologically selected sperm injection (IMSI): a critical and evidence-based review. Basic Clin Androl. 2013;23(10):1–8.
38. Lockwood GM, Deveneau NE, Shridharani AN, Strawn EY, Sandlow JI. Isolated abnormal strict morphology is not a contraindication for intrauterine insemination. Andrology. 2015;3(6):1088–93.
39. Pereira N, Neri Q V., Lekovich JP, Spandorfer SD, Palermo GD, Rosenwaks Z. Outcomes of intracytoplasmic sperm injection cycles for complete teratozoospermia: a case-control study using paired sibling oocytes. Biomed Res Int. 2015;2015.
40. Shabtaie SA, Gerkowicz SA, Kohn TP, Ramasamy R. Role of abnormal sperm morphology in predicting pregnancy outcomes. Curr Urol Rep. 2016;17(9)
41. Tanaka A, Nagayoshi M, Takemoto Y, Tanaka I, Kusunoki H, Watanabe S, et al. Fourteen babies born after round spermatid injection into human oocytes. Proc Natl Acad Sci. 2015;(March 2014):201517466.
42. Jeyendran RS, Van der Ven HH, Perez-Pelaez M, Crabo BG, Zaneveld LJ. Development of an assay to assess the functional integrity of the human sperm membrane and its relationship to other semen characteristics. J Reprod Fertil. 1984;70(1):219–28.
43. Esteves SC, Varghese AC. Laboratory handling of epididymal and testicular spermatozoa: what can be done to improve sperm injections outcome. J Hum Reprod Sci. 2012;5(3):233–43.
44. Aktan TM, Montag M, Duman S, Gorkemli H, Rink K, Yurdakul T. Use of a laser to detect viable but immotile spermatozoa. Andrologia. 2004;36(6):366–9.
45. Nordhoff V, Schüring a N, Krallmann C, Zitzmann M, Schlatt S, Kiesel L, et al. Optimizing TESE-ICSI by laser-assisted selection of immotile spermatozoa and polarization microscopy for selection of oocytes. Andrology. 2013;1(1):67–74.

46. Nordhoff V. How to select immotile but viable spermatozoa on the day of intracytoplasmic sperm injection? An embryologist's view. Andrology. 2015;3(2):156–62.
47. Yoon SY, Eum JH, Lee JE, Lee HC, Kim YS, Han JE, et al. Recombinant human phospholipase C zeta 1 induces intracellular calcium oscillations and oocyte activation in mouse and human oocytes. Hum Reprod. 2012;27:1768–80.
48. Nomikos M, Kashir J, Swann K, Lai FA. Sperm PLCζ: from structure to Ca2+ oscillations, egg activation and therapeutic potential. FEBS Lett. 2013;587:3609–16.
49. Tesarik J, Rienzi L, Ubaldi F, Mendoza C, Greco E. Use of a modified intracytoplasmic sperm injection technique to overcome sperm-borne and oocyte-borne oocyte activation failures. Fertil Steril. 2002;78(3):619–24.
50. Ebner T, Moser M, Sommergruber M, Jesacher K, Tews G. Complete oocyte activation failure after ICSI can be overcome by a modified injection technique. Hum Reprod. 2004;19(8):1837–41.
51. Yanagida K, Katayose H, Yazawa H, Kimura Y, Sato A, Yanagimachi H, et al. Successful fertilization and pregnancy following ICSI and electrical oocyte activation. Hum Reprod. 1999;14(5):1307–11.
52. Borges E, de Almeida Ferreira Braga DP, de Sousa Bonetti TC, Iaconelli A, Franco JG. Artificial oocyte activation using calcium ionophore in ICSI cycles with spermatozoa from different sources. Reprod Biomed Online. 2009;18(1):45–52.
53. Borges E, de Almeida Ferreira Braga DP, de Sousa Bonetti TC, Iaconelli A, Franco JG. Artificial oocyte activation with calcium ionophore A23187 in intracytoplasmic sperm injection cycles using surgically retrieved spermatozoa. Fertil Steril. 2009;92(1):131–6.
54. Kyono K, Kumagai S, Nishinaka C, Nakajo Y, Uto H, Toya M, et al. Birth and follow-up of babies born following ICSI using SrCl2 oocyte activation. Reprod Biomed Online. 2008;17(1):53–8.
55. Sfontouris IA, Nastri CO, Lima MLS, Tahmasbpourmarzouni E, Raine-Fenning N, Martins WP. Artificial oocyte activation to improve reproductive outcomes in women with previous fertilization failure: a systematic review and meta-analysis of RCTs. Hum Reprod. 2015;30(8):1831–41.
56. Franken D, Oehninger S, Burkman L, Coddington C, Kruger T, Rosenwaks Z, et al. The hemizona assay (HZA): a predictor of human sperm fertilizing potential in in vitro fertilization (IVF) treatment. Vitr Fert Embryo Transf. 1989;6(1):44–50.
57. Liu D, Baker H. The proportion of human sperm with poor morphology but normal intact acrosomes detected with Pisum sativum agglutinin correlates with fertilization in vitro. Fertil Steril. 1988;50(2):288–93.
58. Franken DR, Bastiaan HS, Oehninger SC. Physiological induction of the acrosome reaction in human sperm: validation of a microassay using minimal volumes of solubilized, homologous zona pellucida. J Assist Reprod Genet. 2000;17(3):156–61.
59. Bedford J. Sperm/egg interaction: the specificity of human spermatozoa. Anat Rec. 1977;188(4):477–87.
60. Oehninger S, Mahony MC, Swanson JR, Hodgen GD. The specificity of human spermatozoa/zona pellucida interaction under hemizona assay conditions. Mol Reprod Dev. 1993;35(1):57–61.
61. Liu DY, Baker HW. Morphology of spermatozoa bound to the zona pellucida of human oocytes that failed to fertilize in vitro. J Reprod Fertil. 1992;94(1):71–84.
62. WHO. Consultation on the zona-free hamster oocyte penetration test and the diagnosis of male fertility. Int J Androl. 1986;(Suppl. 6).
63. Goossens E, De Vos P, Tournaye H. Array comparative genomic hybridization analysis does not show genetic alterations in spermatozoa and offspring generated after spermatogonial stem cell transplantation in the mouse. Hum Reprod. 2010;25(7):1836–42.
64. Goossens E, De Rycke M, Haentjens P, Tournaye H. DNA methylation patterns of spermatozoa and two generations of offspring obtained after murine spermatogonial stem cell transplantation. Hum Reprod. 2009;24(9):2255–63.

65. Carrell DT. Epigenetics of the male gamete. Fertil Steril. 2012;97(2):267–74.
66. Reik W. Epigenetic reprogramming in mammalian development. Science. 2001;1089(2001):1089–94.
67. Horsthemke B. In brief: genomic imprinting and imprinting diseases. J Pathol. 2014;232(5):485–7.
68. Kobayashi H, Sakurai T, Miura F, Imai M, Mochiduki K, Yanagisawa E, et al. High-resolution DNA methylome analysis of primordial germ cells identifies gender-specific reprogramming in mice. Genome Res. 2013;23(4):616–27.
69. Tang WWC, Dietmann S, Irie N, Leitch HG, Floros VI, Bradshaw CR, et al. A unique gene regulatory network resets the human germline epigenome for development. Cell. 2015;161(6):1453–67.
70. Laurentino S, Borgmann J, Gromoll J. On the origin of sperm epigenetic heterogeneity. Reproduction. 2016;151(5):R71–8.
71. Kobayashi H, Sato A, Otsu E, Hiura H, Tomatsu C, Utsunomiya T, et al. Aberrant DNA methylation of imprinted loci in sperm from oligospermic patients. Hum Mol Genet. 2007;16(21):2542–51.
72. Marques CJ, Costa P, Vaz B, Carvalho F, Fernandes S, Barros A, et al. Abnormal methylation of imprinted genes in human sperm is associated with oligozoospermia. Mol Hum Reprod. 2008;14(2):67–73.
73. Marques CJ, Francisco T, Sousa S, Carvalho F, Barros A, Sousa M. Methylation defects of imprinted genes in human testicular spermatozoa. Fertil Steril. 2010;94(2):585–94.
74. Hammoud SS, Purwar J, Pflueger C, Cairns BR, Carrell DT. Alterations in sperm DNA methylation patterns at imprinted loci in two classes of infertility. Fertil Steril. 2010;94(5):1728–33.
75. Poplinski A, Tüttelmann F, Kanber D, Horsthemke B, Gromoll J. Idiopathic male infertility is strongly associated with aberrant methylation of MEST and IGF2/H19 ICR1. Int J Androl. 2010;33(4):642–9.
76. Boissonnas CC, Abdalaoui HE, Haelewyn V, Fauque P, Dupont JM, Gut I, et al. Specific epigenetic alterations of IGF2-H19 locus in spermatozoa from infertile men. Eur J Hum Genet. 2010;18(1):73–80.
77. El Hajj N, Zechner U, Schneider E, Tresch A, Gromoll J, Hahn T, et al. Methylation status of imprinted genes and repetitive elements in sperm DNA from infertile males. Sex Dev. 2011;5(2):60–9.
78. Hammoud SS, Nix DA, Hammoud AO, Gibson M, Cairns BR, Carrell DT. Genome-wide analysis identifies changes in histone retention and epigenetic modifications at developmental and imprinted gene loci in the sperm of infertile men. Hum Reprod. 2011;26(9):2558–69.
79. Paradowska AS, Miller D, Spiess AN, Vieweg M, Cerna M, Dvorakova-Hortova K, et al. Genome wide identification of promoter binding sites for H4K12ac in human sperm and its relevance for early embryonic development. Epigenetics. 2012;7(9):1057–70.
80. Kläver R, Tüttelmann F, Bleiziffer A, Haaf T, Kliesch S, Gromoll J. DNA methylation in spermatozoa as a prospective marker in andrology. Andrology. 2013;1(5):731–40.
81. Kläver R, Gromoll J. Bringing epigenetics into the diagnostics of the andrology laboratory: challenges and perspectives. Asian J Androl. 2014;16(5):669–74.
82. Laurentino S, Beygo J, Nordhoff V, Kliesch S, Wistuba J, Borgmann J, et al. Epigenetic germline mosaicism in infertile men. Hum Mol Genet. 2015;24(5):1295–304.

Chapter 6
Assessment of Sperm DNA Integrity and Implications for the Outcome of ICSI Treatments

Preben Christensen and Anders Birck

6.1 Introduction

Good sperm DNA integrity is essential to preventing it from becoming damaged before fertilization of the oocyte has been completed. The nuclear genome in mature sperm is normally quite resistant to the oxidative stress caused by the cell metabolism. However, if the integrity is insufficient, the sperm DNA is likely to become damaged during the "journey" to the oocyte, or during fertilization. This is a significant problem as mature sperm has no active DNA repair mechanism [1–3].

Once the sperm DNA has become damaged, the final outcome will depend on the ability of the oocyte to repair the damage [4]. Severe damage, where the DNA has suffered double-stranded breaks (fragmentation), is highly unlikely to be repaired correctly by the oocyte. Such damage may therefore affect early embryonic development or result in poor implantation rates. If the damage to the sperm DNA is less severe, implantation and a biochemical pregnancy may occur. However, due to aberrant repair by the oocyte, a miscarriage will be the likely outcome. In some cases where non-vital genes are affected, the pregnancy continues although the embryo's genome has acquired several mutations. Under normal circumstances, an embryo may have a few mutations [5]. However, a large number of embryonic mutations are likely to result in severe implications for the offspring, such as malformations or diseases.

To avoid confusion, the term "fragmentation" in this work refers to double-stranded DNA breaks resulting in fragments. Fragmentation is perceived to be an irreversible change, where it is highly unlikely that the sperm DNA can be restored by the oocyte [6]. The term "damage" in this work refers to other types of DNA changes which are likely to be repaired by the oocyte although any such repair may result in mutations. The term "integrity" in this work refers to the robustness of the

P. Christensen (✉) • A. Birck
SPZ Lab A/S, Copenhagen OE, Denmark
e-mail: pc@spzlab.com

© Springer International Publishing AG 2018
G.D. Palermo, E.S. Sills (eds.), *Intracytoplasmic Sperm Injection*,
https://doi.org/10.1007/978-3-319-70497-5_6

DNA. The sperm DNA integrity concerns primary changes in DNA during spermatogenesis which makes it vulnerable to secondary damage. In some cases, the primary changes in the sperm DNA involve small endogenous breaks ("nicks") which make it susceptible to further damage. The secondary DNA damage occurs after the sperm has become motile in the cauda of the epididymis and is largely caused by oxidative stress [7]. Depending on the extent of secondary DNA damage, the DNA may eventually acquire double-stranded breaks and become separated into fragments ("fragmentation"). The result of a sperm DNA integrity test is expressed as a DFI value. This value describes how robust or fragile the sperm DNA is. A low DFI indicates that the sperm DNA is very robust. DFI is a continuous measurement, and the degree of DNA fragility rises with increasing DFI values. Originally, the abbreviation DFI was short for "DNA Fragmentation Index." However, in accordance with the proposed terminology, DFI stands for DNA Fragility Index.

The first clinical studies of sperm DNA integrity showed a negative impact on clinical pregnancy rates following natural intercourse [8, 9]. At the time of these studies, it was incorrectly assumed that the test detected sperm DNA fragmentation. It was therefore anticipated that different types of fertility treatments would be affected to the same extent as natural intercourse [10]. We have since learned that this assumption was incorrect. It has been shown that sperm DNA integrity affects the outcome of IVF and especially ICSI treatments to a lesser extent than IUI treatments [11–14]. Although ICSI treatment is affected to a lesser extent than other types of fertility treatment, damage of sperm DNA appears to be a factor in unsuccessful treatments for one in four couples attending fertility clinics [15]. For one in two couples receiving IUI or IVF treatments, the outcome may be negatively affected as a result of insufficient sperm DNA integrity [15]. A recent meta-analysis shows that sperm DNA damage also results in increased miscarriage rates after ICSI treatments [16].

Another concern which has been discussed since the first clinical studies of sperm DNA integrity [8–10] is the question of whether damage to the paternal genome also implies a health risk for the offspring [17, 18]. Wyrobek et al. [19] showed that advancing paternal age is correlated to a reduction in sperm DNA integrity. During the past decade, a number of studies have shown that certain diseases in the offspring appear to be linked with paternal age. The list of such diseases includes schizophrenia [20], autism [21], bipolar disorder [22], ADHD, and psychosis [23], as well as reduced learning potential (intelligence, [24]). Although these diseases occur more frequently with increasing paternal age, it has not yet been proven that the direct cause is embryonic mutations resulting from aberrant repair of sperm DNA within the oocyte after fertilization. However, this appears to be a very likely explanation as it has been shown that 94% of all mutations in children suffering from schizophrenia or autism are of paternal origin [5]. A recent study by Rahbari et al. [25] supports the observation that embryonic mutations largely appears to be of paternal origin. The incidence of mental problems diagnosed in childhood or young adulthood is currently under debate as it appears that such conditions have become more common over the past 30 years. It has been argued that the increasing prevalence of these disorders has largely been attributable to changes in reporting practice [26]. However, it has been observed that there is a likely link between mental illness and sperm DNA damage as mental illnesses appear more frequently among children of couples with reported fertility problems [27]. In addition to mental disorders, malformations occur more frequently with increasing paternal age; including Apert syndrome and achondroplasia [19], and cleft palate [28]. It should also be noted that a higher parental age appears to increase the risk of miscarriage [29, 30]. We are aware that replication errors in the spermatogonial stem cells may account for some of the mutations in the offspring and also would be linked with the age of the parent. However, it is currently perceived that this only accounts for a small proportion of the mutations.

It has been argued that sperm DNA integrity tests are of little value to the fertility clinic where most treatments are either IVF or ICSI [31, 32]. However, over the past decade, research in other fields has enhanced our understanding of DNA damage and repair and the way in which it impacts the general health of an individual. Maintenance of function in somatic cells depends on efficient repair of DNA. Cellular DNA is relatively unstable and is under constant attack due to the presence of oxygen-free radicals (oxidation), water (hydrolysis), and from self-generated by-products of metabolism such as the superoxide anion [33–35]. Oxidative DNA damage appears to be an important mechanism in the development of various diseases where cell death plays a central role [36]. Neurodegenerative disorders such as Alzheimer's and Parkinson's disease are typical examples [37, 38]. A very frequent consequence of oxidative DNA damage appears to be aberrant repair, and this may result in the mutation of genes critical for the control of cell growth. Such lesions could result in various types of cancer [39]. The link between DNA damage and different types of diseases is worth noting as it has also been shown that men with reduced fertility later in life appear to have increased mortality as a result of a wide range of diseases including cancers [40]. More recently, it has been demonstrated that DNA damage is not only a phenomenon that affects sperm, but also one which often indicates a general health problem as DNA damage also occurs simultaneously in the somatic cells [41]. It is a well-established fact that post-meiotic male germ cells are extremely sensitive to DNA damage, and that this is due to reduced DNA repair capacity in late spermatids, as compared to early spermatids and other spermatogenic cell types [3, 42–45]. When DNA becomes damaged in a cell, it may be the result of an increased rate of damage and/or a reduced rate of repair. Endogenous strand breaks ("nicks") in the late spermatids may thus be due to factors which are known to increase the rate of DNA damage such as smoking [46], or factors which appear to reduce the rate of DNA repair such as vitamin D deficiency [47]. Sperm DNA integrity may also be reduced due to poor compaction of the chromatin, initiation of apoptosis (which remains uncompleted in the mature sperm), or deficient disulfide cross-linking during the passage through the first part of the epididymis [48–51].

In light of the above information, it is clear that assessment of sperm DNA integrity is a very important step in the examination and treatment of the infertile couple. Insufficient DNA integrity may have a significant impact on treatment success rates, result in adverse outcome for the offspring, and cause implications for the general health of the man. This means that the correct and precise assessment of sperm DNA integrity is of paramount importance. Along with optimizing the chances of successful fertility treatment, fertility clinics should also aim to prevent adverse effects for the offspring, and to minimize the risk of the man acquiring serious diseases such as cancer or Alzheimer's in later life.

However, before we are able to look at the therapeutic consequences, we first need to critically review how we analyze sperm DNA integrity. During the past decade, there has been a plethora of (often contradictory) reports describing the possible impact of sperm DNA integrity on various reproductive outcomes [52–55]. A number of studies concerning IVF or ICSI treatment have focused on the impact on fertilization and embryo quality and the results have been conflicting [12, 52, 56, 57]. This is not surprising as fertilization may not depend on sperm DNA integrity and because the paternal genome is not expressed until the four- to eight-cell stage [58]. Perhaps the most important endpoint to consider in relation to sperm DNA integrity is the clinical pregnancy rate. Unfortunately, fertility studies are not easy to conduct on humans, and a number of studies have been either based on too few couples, or have been biased due to the study design. Assessment of fertility should only be based on the first treatment cycle since subsequent cycles are likely to be biased by other potential causes of subfertility or infertility in the man or woman [59]. Confusion in this field has also been caused by the fact that a number of new methods have claimed to detect sperm DNA integrity (or apoptosis) and have been made commercially available. This is despite a lack of sufficient data to demonstrate an association between the parameters measured and clinical pregnancy rates [60–63]. Another important aspect to consider is that determination of sperm DNA integrity needs to be highly precise and repeatable when used as a diagnostic tool or in experiments. A number of studies have included insufficient descriptions of the laboratory procedures, and paid little attention to measurement errors and quality control.

In this work, we will focus on the protocol described by Evenson and Jost [64]. In addition, we will describe the use of flow cytometry and discuss the quality control procedures essential to achieving results of high quality. It is our opinion that precise and accurate assessment of sperm DNA integrity is an essential diagnostic tool in the fertility clinic. This tool will allow fertility clinics to give the best possible advice to the infertile couple in relation to their choice of fertility treatment. In addition, the risk of adverse outcomes can be minimized for the offspring, and serious disease may be prevented for the male in later life.

6.2 Materials and Methods

6.2.1 Protocol for the Sperm Chromatin Structure Assay (SCSA)

The basic protocol for the sperm chromatin structure assay (SCSA) was published by Evenson et al. [65] and has been described in more detail by Evenson and Jost [64]. The principle is that sperm DNA with good integrity is robust and therefore unaffected by treatment at low pH, whereas DNA with insufficient integrity becomes denatured. After subsequent staining with acridine orange, the robust double-stranded DNA will emit a green signal, whereas the fragile, denatured, and single-stranded DNA will emit a red fluorescent signal due to the metachromatic nature of the dye. The percentage of sperm with a detectable level of red signal is identified during the analysis by a flow cytometer and is referred to as the DFI value.

One advantage of this protocol is that no washing steps are included. Washing steps may result in selective bias due to loss of sperm, and the process itself may result in damage to DNA. The first step in the process is the addition of the acid solution. After 30 s, the acridine orange staining solution is added and analysis of the sample is performed after a staining period of 2½ min.

A potential pitfall of acridine orange is that it is an equilibrium dye. This means that binding of the dye to DNA depends on the remaining concentration of dye in the solution. According to Evenson and Jost [64], an aliquot of the semen sample should be diluted to approximately 1 millon sperm/mL prior to addition of the acid solution. This will provide approximately two molecules of acridine orange per DNA phosphate group. Higher concentrations of sperm will result in insufficient staining of the DNA, and this is likely to lead to incorrect results. Another challenge when using acridine orange is that it is a very sticky dye. It therefore stains debris in the semen, which may cause problems with the analysis of some samples. The dye also adheres to the tubing and other parts of the flow cytometer. For this reason, saturation of the flow system is essential before the first analysis, and careful cleaning of the instrument is equally important after the completion of the analyses. Keeping the instrument clean is an important factor in maintaining a low level of background interference in the analyses.

6.2.2 The Semen Samples

Patients should be instructed to maintain 2–5 days of sexual abstinence before collecting a diagnostic sample. After liquefaction for 30–60 min, an aliquot of the neat semen can be analyzed directly or can be frozen for later analysis. Some semen samples become viscous after freezing and thawing so it is advisable to dilute the aliquot before freezing. The medium for dilution can be any physiological medium for sperm and does not need to contain cryoprotectants. The sample should be frozen and kept at a temperature below −80 °C until it is thawed prior to analysis.

6.2.3 Flow Cytometry and Quality Control

For a sperm test to be useful, a high degree of precision is necessary [66]. High precision means that uniform results are obtained when repeated analyses of the same sample are performed. Most semen analyses suffer from a large degree of random variation due to the fact that only a limited number of sperm are assessed [67]. A high degree of variation in a test is a significant problem as it also will result in poor accuracy [68]. For this reason, it is essential for a fertility test to be highly precise before it can have the potential to accurately predict reproductive outcome.

In contrast to microscopic assessments of a few hundred sperm, flow cytometry makes it possible to analyze 5000 sperm or more per measurement. Flow cytometry has the potential to yield highly precise results but good quality control is paramount. There are several factors in the analysis that can cause random variations in the results, and these should therefore be considered [69]. Debris in the semen sample or air bubbles in the sheath fluid of the flow cytometer (Fig. 6.1) can cause disturbances to the laminar flow and lead to incorrect results. It is only possible to detect such problems if two independent measurements are processed and analyzed separately for each semen sample. Repeating a measurement is the most essential step in the quality control of semen analysis. This enables the technician to detect any errors in sampling or processing, as well as any technical errors such as the partial blocking of a flow cytometer. The precision of any laboratory test should always be monitored on a day-to-day basis and periodic internal tests should be performed to confirm that the precision is high [59].

For the test of sperm DNA integrity, it is important to use a reference sample when setting up the instrument and to check the performance at regular intervals. Occasionally, a semen sample may provide an abnormal plot or result. In such cases, the reference sample is helpful to determine whether the plot is correct or if there is a problem with the flow cytometer.

A particular advantage of flow cytometry is that the electronic detection of fluorescence signals (Fig. 6.1) is several hundred times more sensitive than with the human eye. The flow cytometer can therefore objectively detect small changes in sperm DNA. With regard to analysis of emission signals from acridine orange, it should be noted that the green peak emission is at 520 nm and is easily detected in the 515–530 band-pass filter normally used for FL1 (Fig. 6.1). However, the red peak emission from acridine orange is at 650 nm and will not typically be easily detected by FL3, where the filter is often a 670 long-pass. Using the standard flow cytometer setup may therefore mean that sensitivity for the red signal is reduced and that DFI is underestimated. The flow cytometer needs to be equipped with a 640 or 630 nm long-pass filter for optimal detection of the red signal.

6.3   Results

During the past decade, several laboratories have taken up the Sperm Chromatin Structure Assay (SCSA) and a large number of reports have described the relationship between this test and various reproductive outcomes [8–10, 12, 14, 57, 70, 71]. Most studies have not been particularly detailed with regard to the level of internal quality assurance (IQA) in the laboratories. As a result, it has been difficult to interpret the different results that have been published. The authors of this work are

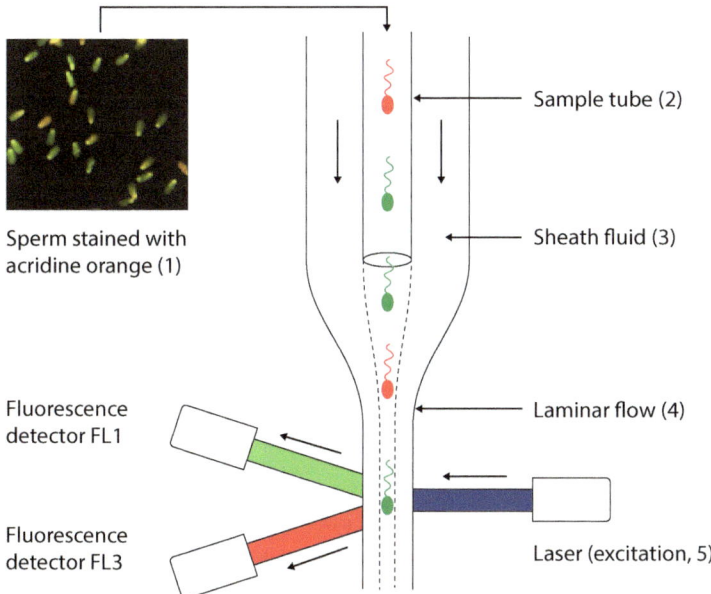

Fig. 6.1 The basic principle of flow cytometry is shown in this figure. The sperm is fluorescently stained with acridine orange (1). Stained sperm is introduced via the sample tube (2). The sheath fluid (3) surrounds the sample fluid and creates a laminar flow (4) with the sperm hydrodynamically focused in the middle of the stream. Disturbances in the sheath fluid (typically air bubbles) or sample tube (typically debris) may cause turbulence in the laminar flow and result in incorrect analyses. Dilution of the semen sample during the processing ensures that sperm pass through the flow cytometer individually at a rate of 100–200 per second. A beam of laser light (488 nm, 5) is directed at the stream of fluid for excitation of the fluorescently stained sperm. Emission light is separated and collected by fluorescent detectors. Green fluorescence (FL1) is collected through a 515–530 band-pass filter. Red fluorescence (FL3) is collected through a 630 or 640 long-pass filter

aware that a number of laboratories do not routinely perform repeated measurements, despite the fact that this is essential when carrying out quality control. To omit repeated measurements poses a significant problem as it is possible that the data produced also contains some outliers. In the clinical setting, a diagnosis could be incorrect and lead to wrong advice and treatment being given to a couple. In research projects, the true biological relationships may remain concealed [72].

6.3.1   Variation Between Measurements (Measurement Error)

The theoretical standard deviation (SD) for a result is 1.4% when 5000 sperm are analyzed. With appropriate quality control procedures, outliers can be identified and the respective samples can be re-analyzed. It is therefore possible to achieve a smaller variation, i.e., below 1% [69]. To achieve a high degree of precision, it is essential to assess the variation between the repeated measurements, and to perform a re-analysis when the level of variation exceeds a predetermined threshold. This is a time-consuming procedure as 5–10 % of the samples may need to be re-analyzed.

6.3.2 Periodic Internal Test

Due to small differences in the daily setup and adjustment of a flow cytometer, a small day-to-day variation in results should be expected [69]. Although laboratory technicians are well trained, small differences between technicians may also contribute to random variation in results [69]. As several factors can affect the results, it is important that periodic internal tests are performed to assess its repeatability. Figure 6.2 shows the results of a periodic internal test performed blinded by two laboratory technicians. The results show a diagram of the measurements and only a minor scattering of the points around the regression line is seen. The standard deviation for the spreading of the points around the regression line ($SD_{y,x}$) is 1.8% and the coefficient of correlation r is 0.99. The average standard deviation between the repeated measurements (SD_r) was 0.57%.

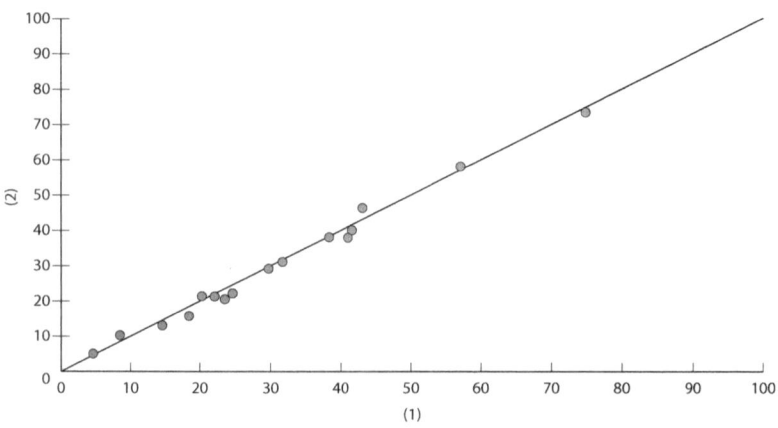

Fig. 6.2 The diagram shows the result of a periodic internal test. The flow cytometric assessment of sperm DNA integrity was performed on two different days by two blinded laboratory technicians. The values on the x-axis represent the measurements made by one technician (1) against the measurements performed by the other technician (y-axis, 2). The black line indicates a slope of 1.0. Each point represents the results of a semen sample analyzed by the two technicians. There is only a minor scattering of the points around the line indicating a good agreement between the measurements. Standard deviation ($SD_{y,x}$ = 1.8%)

6.3.3   Intra-individual Variation

Although a test is very precise, the results may not be repeatable over time due to differences between semen samples from the same male. Standard seminal parameters such as sperm concentration, motility, and morphology can be highly variable over time within individuals [59, 73, 74]. Evenson et al. [75] demonstrated that sperm DNA integrity is a very stable parameter with a standard deviation between measurements in the same individuals (standard deviation within donor, SD_w) of 5.0%. Zini et al. [76, 77] confirmed the low variation in the assessment of sperm DNA integrity, but a couple of studies have since reported a higher degree of variation [78, 79]. Differences in methodology or quality control procedures may be responsible for the conflicting results. Recently, we were involved in a double-blinded and randomized controlled trial (RCT), where the analysis of sperm DNA integrity of the control-group individuals ($N = 28$) were found to be highly repeatable over time with a SD_w of 3.3% [80].

6.3.4   Comparison of Results Between Different Laboratories

Use of flow cytometry enables measurements to be objective. When good quality control is performed in different laboratories using the same method, a high correlation between results can be achieved [81]. For assessment of sperm DNA integrity, a very high correlation between results obtained by different laboratories (coefficient of correlation $r = 0.98$) was reported by Evenson [82]. Such high agreement between the results will obviously depend on good internal quality control in the laboratories.

6.3.5   Relationship Between Sperm DNA Integrity and Fertility

Accuracy defines the relationship between the result of a test and the "true" value. To assess the accuracy of a fertility test, we will have to compare the results of the test against reproductive outcome.

Assessment of fertility is not an easy task when working with humans [59]. To detect small differences in male fertility, the ideal study should only include females with high fertility and each male should be "tested" on several females [59]. Obviously, such a study is not possible on humans for ethical and biological reasons. Often the only possibility is to use data from the fertility clinic. However, couples attending a clinic may have a number of issues affecting fertility in the male, in the woman or both. To avoid bias and to achieve the best possible data, we should therefore only use data from the first cycle of treatment. Using subsequent cycles will result in the data being biased from the other factors.

The next point to consider is how many couples need to be enrolled in a study to see a difference in fertility. It may be more convenient to look at only a few couples, but a small number of observations will make the outcome as random as "flipping a coin" [83]. If we want to perform a study, we will need to calculate the statistical power based on the proportion of couples with a defined reduction in pregnancy rate. The number of couples that need to be enrolled is likely to be 200 or above and estimates should be based on the expected outcome.

If we want to study the impact on IUI, IVF, and ICSI treatments, we need to perform separate studies for each type of treatment. The amount of secondary damage to the sperm DNA depends on the length of the "journey" that the sperm has to travel to reach the oocyte, and also on whether it has to penetrate the zona pellucida or not (Fig. 6.3). Obviously, the impact on outcome will be different for IUI, IVF, and ICSI treatments.

For IVF and ICSI treatments, it is tempting to study endpoints such as fertilization, cleavage rates or embryo development and morphology. However, when we study the impact of sperm DNA integrity the more significant events occur after embryo transfer and include implantation and miscarriage. The most important endpoint is clinical pregnancy rate, preferably confirmed as a positive scan at 12 weeks of pregnancy.

The relationship between sperm DNA integrity (as assessed using the SCSA protocol and flow cytometry) and clinical pregnancy rates are described below. The results are only described for studies which included more than 100 couples, and where there were no obvious deficiencies with regard to design, statistical analysis, or endpoints. It should be noted that insufficient sperm DNA integrity is a very frequent problem among couples attending the fertility clinic. For approximately 1 in 2 of the men, the sperm DNA integrity is insufficient (a DFI value above 15). For approximately 1 in 4 of the men, the integrity is suboptimal (DFI is between 15 and 25). For approximately 1 in 4 of the men, the integrity is poor (DFI is above 25).

6.3.6 Natural Intercourse

The first large-scale study to demonstrate the relationship between sperm DNA integrity and the outcome of natural intercourse was published by Evenson et al. [8]. In brief, this study showed that the time taken to achieve pregnancy was increased significantly if the DFI value was between 15 and 30 and that almost no couples achieved pregnancy with a DFI value of over 30. Additionally, Evenson et al. [8] observed that the incidence of miscarriage was higher with increased DFI values. Evenson's results were confirmed by Spano et al. [9], who had followed a group of 215 "first-pregnancy-planners" for a period up to 2 years or until they achieved pregnancy.

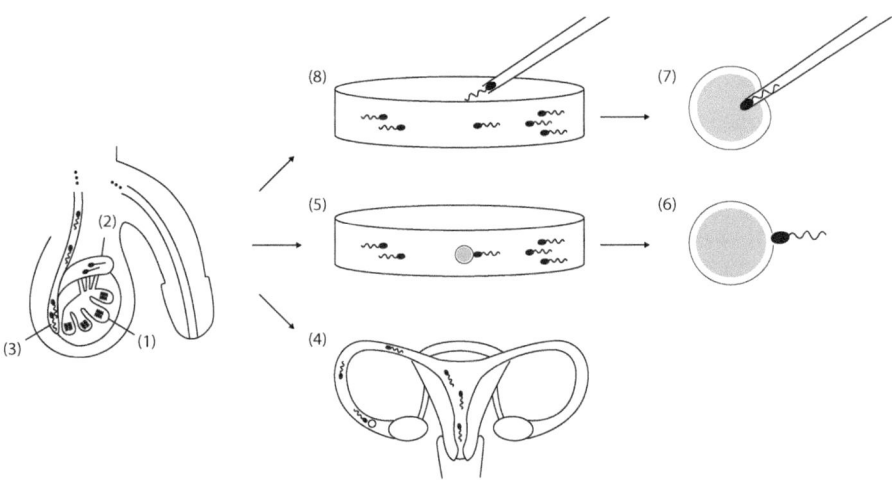

Fig. 6.3 The "two-step" hypothesis of sperm DNA damage is shown in this figure. The primary changes in the sperm DNA occur in the testicle and result in insufficient DNA integrity (1). The primary changes may be due to reduced DNA repair capacity in the late spermatids causing endogenous "nicks." The primary changes may also result from incomplete apoptosis, poor protamination, or by deficient disulfide cross-linking during the passage through the first part of the epididymis (2). Insufficient integrity makes the sperm DNA vulnerable to secondary damage. This is largely caused by oxidative stress as a result of metabolism once the sperm becomes motile in the cauda of the epididymis (3). Secondary DNA damage is most pronounced in connection with natural intercourse or after IUI treatment. In these cases, the sperm has a long "journey" to the oocyte and needs to perform fertilization (4). In IVF, the "journey" is made shorter as the sperm is placed with the oocyte in the fertilization medium (5). Washing procedures, incubation in the laboratory, as well as the process of fertilization (6) may result in DNA damage when IVF is performed. In ICSI treatments, the sperm is placed directly into the oocyte and bypasses fertilization (7). However, if the sperm DNA integrity is poor (DFI value above 25), the DNA may become damaged already in the cauda of the epididymis (3) or as a result of washing procedures or incubation in the laboratory (8)

6.3.7 Intrauterine Insemination (IUI)

The relationship between DFI and the outcome of IUI treatments was explored in a study of 387 cycles (first or second treatment cycle, [14]). Of the 66 IUI cycles performed with semen samples where the DFI value was above 30, only 2 resulted in a clinical pregnancy (3% per cycle). One pregnancy led to a miscarriage and the delivery rate was therefore only 1.5% per cycle. In contrast, IUI treatments performed with semen where the DFI value was below 30 resulted in an average delivery rate of 19%. Results for IUI have since been confirmed by Yang et al. [71] who analyzed sperm DNA integrity in a study of 482 first or second IUI treatments. A DFI value of 25 was used as the threshold. Of the 95 IUI treatments performed with semen where the DFI value was above 25, only 5.3% achieved a clinical pregnancy. When the DFI value was below 25, the clinical pregnancy rate was 15.3%.

6.3.8   *In Vitro Fertilization (IVF) and Intracytoplasmic Sperm Injection (ICSI)*

Bungum et al. [14] also studied the impact of sperm DNA integrity on the outcome of IVF ($N = 388$) and ICSI treatments ($N = 223$). When the outcome of ICSI versus IVF was compared, no significant difference was observed when the DFI value was below 30. However, if the DFI value was above 30, the results were significantly better for ICSI versus IVF, with an odds ratio of 2.25 for clinical pregnancy (95% CI 1.10–4.60), and 2.17 for delivery (95% CI 1.04–4.51).

A retrospective analysis of the relationship between sperm DNA integrity and the outcome of 210 IVF cycles was reported by Christensen et al. [84]. It was the first IVF treatment for the couples involved. IVF treatment was only recommended to the couple if the men had a DFI value below 25. Clinical pregnancy was confirmed by ultrasound in the 12th week of gestation and the outcome was assessed for groups with a DFI value below or above 15 (Fig. 6.4a). The clinical pregnancy rate was 45.1% when the DFI value was below 15 and diminished to 24.6% when the DFI value was between 15 and 25. The odds ratio for low versus high DFI group (adjusted for female age, sperm motility, and concentration) was 2.45 ($P = 0.01$, 95% CI 1.25–5.18). Christensen et al. [84] also reported results for 196 ICSI cycles. For ICSI cycles, the DFI value varied from 2.4% to 61.2% and treatment outcome was assessed for groups with a DFI value below or above 25. The clinical pregnancy rate was 48.7% when the DFI value was below 25. Above this threshold, the clinical pregnancy rate was only 29.6% (Fig. 6.4b). The odds ratio for the low versus high DFI group (adjusted for female age, sperm motility, and concentration) was 1.97 ($P < 0.05$, 95% CI 1.02–3.84).

6.4   Discussion

The most significant impact of insufficient sperm DNA integrity is seen on the clinical pregnancy rates after natural intercourse and IUI treatments [8, 9, 14, 71, 85]. The reduction in pregnancy rates results from secondary damage to the DNA, largely caused by oxidative stress due to metabolism in the sperm on its long "journey" to the oocyte and also during fertilization. In addition to human studies, several studies in animal species have demonstrated a clear relationship between insufficient sperm DNA integrity and reduced fertility after insemination [86–88].

According to the "two-step" hypothesis [7], the degree of secondary damage to sperm DNA can be reduced if the journey of the sperm to the oocyte is shortened. This is the case with IVF treatments, where clinical pregnancy rates are affected to a lesser extent than for IUI treatments [14, 84]. However, in IVF the sperm still needs to become hyperactivated and penetrate the oocyte investments including the zona pellucida (Fig. 6.3). This is an energy-demanding task and the sperm DNA may therefore become damaged due to oxidative stress caused by its own

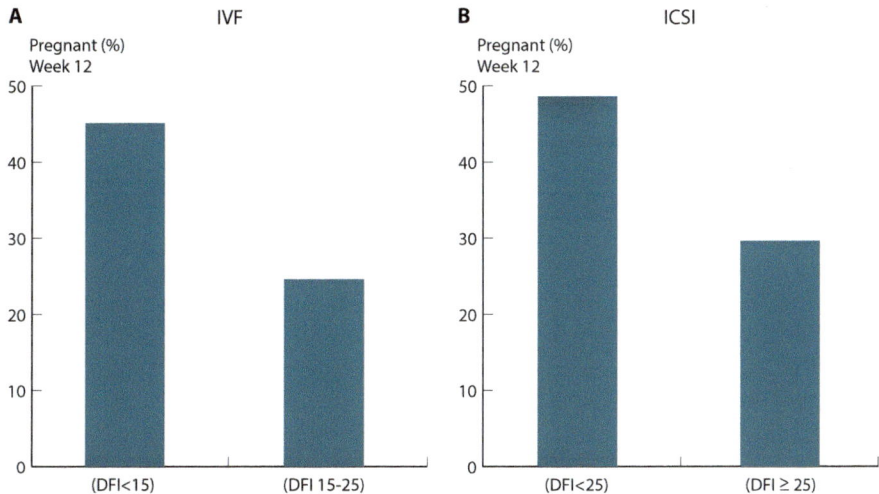

Fig. 6.4 (**a**) The diagram shows the percentage of ongoing pregnancies after first cycle IVF treatments for 210 couples. Pregnancy was confirmed by ultrasound at 12-week gestation. When the DFI value was below 15, the pregnancy rate was 45.1%. The pregnancy rate diminished to 24.6% when the DFI value was between 15 and 25. The odds ratio adjusted for female age, sperm concentration, and motility was 2.45 ($P = 0.01$, 95% CI 1.25–5.18, [84]). (**b**) This diagram shows the results of 196 first cycle ICSI treatments. When the DFI value was below 25, the pregnancy rate was 48.6%. When the DFI was above 25, the pregnancy rate was only 29.6%. The odds ratio adjusted for female age, sperm concentration, and motility was 1.97 ($P < 0.05$, 95% CI 1.02–3.84, [84])

metabolism. It is thus not surprising that clinical pregnancy rates are higher for ICSI treatments in comparison to IVF treatments [14, 84]. ICSI appears to protect the sperm DNA from becoming damaged before fertilization is completed. However, when the DNA integrity is poor (DFI value above 25) clinical pregnancy rates also appear to be affected negatively for ICSI treatments [84]. Poor integrity seems to make the sperm DNA so vulnerable that it already becomes damaged in the cauda of the epididymis or during incubation in the laboratory (Fig. 6.3). A new meta-analysis and review have confirmed that outcome of ICSI treatments are affected negatively by poor DNA integrity [89].

The "two-step" hypothesis helps us to understand why the various types of fertility treatments are affected to a different extent by insufficient sperm DNA integrity. In addition, this hypothesis can help us to develop a strategy for the most optimal treatment of a couple in the fertility clinic. An obvious part of such a strategy is the reduction of the secondary oxidative damage to the DNA that occurs after the sperm has become motile. When the sperm DNA integrity is poor (DFI value above 25), ICSI treatments may be combined with the use of sperm aspirated from the testicle (TESA) or epididymis (PESA) [90, 91]. Aspirated sperm will not have suffered any secondary damage at this stage, but may do so if incubated after retrieval [86, 92–94].

A number of methods have claimed to provide a selection of "the best sperm" in connection with ICSI treatments. IMSI (intracytoplasmic morphological selected sperm injection) has been recommended [95], but results of this technology are still controversial [96]. It should be noted that sperm DNA integrity may be insufficient, even though the sperm morphology is normal [97, 98]. Another reported method is the selection of "non-apoptotic" sperm by use of annexin V [61, 99]. So far, use of this technology has not resulted in trials demonstrating a positive effect on clinical pregnancy rates. Other reports concerning annexin V have shown that labeling with this marker may be a result of phosphatidylserine externalization occurring during capacitation [100]. It has also been shown that apoptotic markers, such as Fas, can only be demonstrated on a small proportion of the sperm in a semen sample [51, 101]. It therefore seems that endogenous strand breaks ("nicks") in the sperm DNA may be caused by mechanisms which do not involve an apoptotic pathway [3]. The hyaluronic acid-binding technique has also been recommended for sperm selection but does not appear to result in increased clinical pregnancy rates [102, 103].

The selection of the best embryos for transfer is important in order to ensure high treatment success rates for IVF and ICSI [104, 105]. However, it should be kept in mind that the paternal genome is not expressed until the four- to eight-cell stage [58]. Impact on development and morphology of the embryo may not be obvious unless the sperm DNA integrity is very poor or if the transfer of blastocysts is performed [106, 107]. Despite good embryo or blastocyst development, we may not be able to identify the embryos or blastocysts which later result in a miscarriage or adverse outcome for the offspring [16, 108, 109].

The treatment strategy should also consider the possible etiologic factors that cause insufficient DNA integrity. Factors known to impact sperm DNA integrity should be considered, identified, and treated before fertility treatment is initiated. By improving the DNA integrity, the sperm DNA becomes more robust and less likely to be damaged by secondary oxidative stress. The overall aim is to increase treatment success rates and minimize possible risks of adverse outcomes for the offspring. In addition, improving the DNA integrity in the male is also likely to have a positive effect on the somatic cells and hence improve his general health [36, 39–41]. One very obvious recommendation to men with insufficient sperm DNA integrity is to stop smoking [46, 110]. Smoking appears to cause a general increase in the oxidative stress and has recently been demonstrated to be a direct cause of de novo mutations in the offspring [111]. However, smoking and other factors causing DNA damage may affect individuals differently. This means that some male smokers may not suffer from sperm DNA damage [112]. The impact of smoking may be more pronounced in individuals who are also insufficient with regard to antioxidants [113]. A number of studies have shown that men with an increased body mass index (BMI) are more likely to have insufficient sperm DNA integrity [114, 115]. Another study has shown that weight loss is likely to improve sperm DNA integrity [116]. However, one recent study has not confirmed a link between BMI and insufficient sperm DNA integrity [117]. It is possible that this may be due to epigenetic differences [118] or because insufficient DNA integrity is not caused by high BMI, but results from accompanying insulin resistance [119, 120]. With regard to obesity and insulin resistance, it seems that the pro-inflammatory cytokine tumor necrosis factor α (TNF-α) is involved in DNA alterations [121–123]. It is therefore important to keep in mind that insufficient DNA integrity may have an etiology which does not involve oxidative stress.

Treatment with antioxidants has been reported frequently, but a number of reports have failed to demonstrate a positive effect on pregnancy rates [124–128]. A lack of certain micronutrients may result in oxidative DNA damage and has been associated with increased risk of various types of cancer [129]. However, treatment with antioxidants is not recommended for all men with insufficient sperm DNA integrity. Treatment with large doses of antioxidants is only recommended if the deficiency of a particular vitamin or mineral has been diagnosed. Several vitamins and minerals exhibit pro-oxidant properties when their concentration exceeds the required physiological level [130–132]. The pro-oxidant effect may then cause an oxidative effect and lead to serious adverse outcome for the patient [133].

Treatment of etiological factors responsible for insufficient sperm DNA integrity may result in sperm with more robust DNA. Treatment of factors such as smoking, insulin resistance, or an underlying inflammatory condition is essential and should be combined with sufficient doses of vitamins or minerals when a deficiency has been diagnosed. In some cases, this intervention may not result in improvement of sperm DNA integrity. It should be kept in mind that the underlying cause could be due to other factors such as the knockout of genes important for DNA repair or protamination [134]. Retesting of the sperm DNA integrity after a minimum period of 3 months can confirm if the intervention has been successful and the new DFI value can be utilized to recommend the most optimal type of fertility treatment to the couple. If the DFI value is below 15 (normal DNA integrity), IUI or IVF treatment is recommended. When the DFI value is between 15 and 25 (suboptimal DNA integrity), ICSI treatment is more likely to result in a successful outcome than IVF. ICSI treatment provides better protection of the sperm DNA and is thus less likely to result in a miscarriage or adverse outcome for the offspring. If the DFI value is above 25 (poor DNA integrity), combining ICSI treatment with sperm aspirated from the epididymis or testicle should be considered. The purpose of this invasive approach is to prevent the sperm DNA from becoming damaged. For the male with insufficient DNA integrity, the increased risk of acquiring various diseases later in life also needs to be addressed. Therapy to reduce oxidative stress or improve DNA repair should be considered in order to maintain good health, and new antioxidant formulations which are not based on micronutrients may be an option [135, 136].

It is our hope that further research into this field will lead to an increased number of products and methods aimed at treating insufficient DNA integrity in the future. This could lead to more optimal treatment of couples in the fertility clinics and may also help to reduce possible adverse outcomes for the offspring as well as lead to improved male health.

References

1. Sega GA, Sotomayor RE, Owens JG. A study of unscheduled DNA synthesis induced by X-rays in the germ cells of male mice. Mutat Res. 1978;49:239–57.
2. Olsen AK, Duale N, Bjoras M, Larsen CT, Wiger R, Holme JA, et al. Limited repair of 8-hydroxy-7,8-dihydroguanine residues in human testicular cells. Nucleic Acids Res. 2003;423:1351–63.
3. Marchetti F, Wyrobek AJ. DNA repair decline during mouse spermiogenesis results in the accumulation of heritable DNA damage. DNA Repair (Amst). 2008;7:572–81.
4. Genesca A, Caballin MR, Miro R, Benet J, Germa JR, Egozcue J. Repair of human sperm chromosome aberrations in the hamster egg. Hum Genet. 1992;89:181–6.
5. Kong A, Frigge ML, Masson G, Besenbacher S, Sulem P, Magnusson G, et al. Rate of de novo mutations and the importance of father's age to disease risk. Nature. 2012;488:471–5.
6. Sakkas D, Alvarez JG. Sperm DNA fragmentation: mechanisms of origin impact on reproductive outcome, and analysis. Fertil Steril. 2010;93:1027–36.
7. Aitken RJ, Bronson R, Smith TB, De Iuliis GN. The source and significance of DNA damage in human spermatozoa; a commentary on diagnostic strategies and straw man fallacies. Mol Hum Reprod. 2013;19:475–85.
8. Evenson DP, Jost LK, Marshall D, Zinaman MJ, Clegg E, Purvis K, et al. Utility of the sperm chromatin structure assay as a diagnostic and prognostic tool in the human fertility clinic. Hum Reprod. 1999;14:1039–49.
9. Spano M, Bonde JP, Hjøllund HI, Kolstad HA, Cordelli E, Leter G, et al. Sperm chromatin damage impairs human fertility. The Danish First Pregnancy Planer Study. Fertil Steril. 2000;73:43–50.
10. Larson KL, De Jonge CJ, Barnes AM, Jost LK, Evenson DP. Sperm chromatin structure assay parameters as predictors of failed pregnancy following assisted reproductive techniques. Hum Reprod. 2000;15:1717–22.
11. Gandini L, Lombardo F, Paoli D, Caruso F, Eleuteri P, Leter G, et al. Full-term pregnancies achieved with ICSI despite high levels of sperm chromatin damage. Hum Reprod. 2004;19:1409–17.
12. Virro MR, Larson-Cook KL, Evenson DP. Sperm chromatin structure assay (SCSA®) parameters are related to fertilization, blastocyst development, and ongoing pregnancy in in vitro fertilization and intracytoplasmic sperm injection cycles. Fertil Steril. 2004;81:1289–95.
13. Payne JF, Raburn DJ, Couchman GM, Price TM, Jamison MG, Walmer DK. Redefining the relationship between sperm deoxyribonucleic acid fragmentation as measured by the sperm chromatin structure assay and outcomes of assisted reproductive techniques. Fertil Steril. 2005;84:356–64.
14. Bungum M, Humaidan P, Axmon A, Spano M, Bungum L, Erenpreiss J, et al. Sperm DNA integrity assessment in prediction of assisted reproduction technology outcome. Hum Reprod. 2007;22:174–9.
15. Christensen P, Birck A. Comparison of methods for assessment of sperm DNA damage (fragmentation) and implications for the assisted reproductive technologies. In: Scott Sills E, editor. Screening the single euploid embryo, molecular genetics in reproductive medicine. New York: Springer; 2015.
16. Zhao J, Zhang Q, Wang Y, Li Y. Whether sperm deoxyribonucleic acid fragmentation has an effect on pregnancy and miscarriage after in vitro fertilization/intracytoplasmic sperm injection: a systematic review and meta-analysis. Fertil Steril. 2014;102:998–1005.
17. Hansen M, Kurinczuk JJ, Bower C, Webb S. The risk of major birth defects after intracytoplasmic sperm injection and in vitro fertilization. N Engl J Med. 2002;346:725–30.
18. Olson CK, Keppler-Noreuil KM, Romitti PA, Budelier WT, Ryan G, Sparks AE, et al. In vitro fertilization is associated with an increase in major birth defects. Fertil Steril. 2005;84:1308–15.
19. Wyrobek AJ, Eskenazi B, Young S, Arnheim N, Tiemann-Boege I, Jabs EW, et al. Advancing age has differential effects on DNA damage, chromatin integrity, gene mutations, and aneuploidies in sperm. PNAS. 2006;103:9601–6.

20. Sipos A, Rasmussen F, Harrison G, Tynelius P, Lewis G, Leon DA, et al. Paternal age and schizophrenia: a population based cohort study. BMJ. 2004;329:1070.
21. Reichenberg A, Gross R, Weiser M, Bresnahan M, Silverman J, Harlap S, et al. Advancing paternal age and autism. Arch Gen Psychiatry. 2006;63:1026–32.
22. Frans EM, Sandin S, Reichenberg A, Lichtenstein P, Långström N, Hultman CM. Advancing paternal age and bipolar disorder. Arch Gen Psychiatry. 2008;65:1034–40.
23. D'Onofrio BM, Rickert ME, Frans E, Kuja-Halkola R, Almqvist C, Sjölander A, et al. Paternal age at childbearing and offspring psychiatric and academic morbidity. JAMA Psychiat. 2014;71:432–8.
24. Malaspina D, Gilman C, Kranz TM. Paternal age and mental health of offspring. Fertil Steril. 2015;103:1392–6.
25. Rahbari R, Wuster A, Lindsay SJ, Hardwick RJ, Alexandrov LB, Turki SA, et al. Timing, rates and spectra of human germline mutation. Nat Genet. 2016;48:126–36.
26. Hansen SN, Schendel DE, Parner ET. Explaining the increase in the prevalence of autism spectrum disorders. The proportion attributable to changes in reporting practices. JAMA Pediatr. 2015;169:56–62.
27. Svahn MF, Hargreave M, Nielsen TSS, Plessen KJ, Jensen SM, Kjaer SK, et al. Mental disorders in childhood and young adulthood among children born to women with fertility problems. Hum Reprod. 2015;30:2129–37.
28. Bille C, Skytthe A, Vach W, Knudsen LB, Nybo Andersen AM, Murray JC, et al. Parent's age and the risk of oral clefts. Epidemiology. 2005;16:311–6.
29. de La Rochebrochard E, Thonneau P. Paternal age and maternal age are risk factors for miscarriage; results of a multicentre European study. Hum Reprod. 2002;17:1649–56.
30. Kleinhaus K, Perrin M, Friedlander Y, Paltiel O, Malaspina D, Harlap S. Paternal age and spontaneous abortion. Obstet Gynaecol. 2006;108:369–77.
31. Collins JA, Barnhart KT, Schlegel PN. Do sperm DNA integrity tests predict pregnancy with in vitro fertilization? Fertil Steril. 2008;89:823–31.
32. ASRM Practice Committee. The clinical utility of sperm DNA integrity testing: a guideline. Fertil Steril. 2013;99:673–7.
33. Crine P, Verly WG. A study of DNA spontaneous degradation. BBA. 1976;442:50–7.
34. Lindahl T. Instability and decay of the primary structure of DNA. Nature. 1993;362:709–15.
35. Kanduc D, Mittelman A, Serpico R, Sinigaglia E, Sinha AA, Natale C, et al. Cell death: apoptosis versus necrosis (review). Int J Oncol. 2002;21:165–70.
36. Cooke MS, Evans MD, Dizdaroglu M, Lunec J. Oxidative DNA damage: mechanisms, mutation, and disease. FASEB. 2003;17:1195–214.
37. Alam ZI, Jenner A, Daniel SE, Lees AJ, Cairns N, Marsden CD, et al. Oxidative DNA damage in the parkinsonian brain: an apparent selective increase in 8-hydroxyguanine levels in substantia nigra. J Neurochem. 1997;69:1196–203.
38. Lovell MA, Gabbita SP, Markesbery WR. Increased DNA oxidation and decreased levels of repair products in Alzheimer's disease ventricular CSF. J Neurochem. 1999;72:771–6.
39. Hoeijmakers JAJ. Genome maintenance mechanisms for preventing cancer. Nature. 2001;411:366–74.
40. Jensen TK, Jacobsen R, Christensen K, Nielsen NC, Bostofte E. Good semen quality and life expectancy: a cohort study of 43,277 men. Am J Epidemiol. 2009;170:559–65.
41. Baumgartner A, Kurzawa-Zegota M, Laubenthal J, Cemeli E, Anderson D. Comet-assay parameters as rapid biomarkers of exposure to dietary/environmental compounds—an in vitro feasibility study on spermatozoa and lymphocytes. Mutat Res. 2012;743:25–35.
42. Shelby MD. Selecting chemicals and assays for assessing mammalian germ cell mutagenicity. Mutat Res. 1996;325:159–67.
43. Sotomayor RE, Sega GA. Unscheduled DNA synthesis assay in mammalian spermatogenic cells: an update. Environ Mol Mutagen. 2000;36:255–65.
44. Baarends WM, van der Laan R, Grootegoed JA. DNA repair mechanisms and gametogenesis. Reproduction. 2001;121:31–9.

45. Olsen AK, Lindeman B, Wiger R, Duale N, Brunborg G. How do male germ cells handle DNA damage? Toxicol Appl Pharmacol. 2005;207:521–31.
46. Potts RJ, Newbury CJ, Smith G, Notarianni LJ, Jefferies TM. Sperm chromatin damage associated with male smoking. Mutat Res. 1999;423:103–11.
47. Nair-Shalliker V, Armstrong BK, Fenech M. Does vitamin D protect against DNA damage? Mutat Res. 2012;733:50–7.
48. McPherson S, Longo FJ. Chromatin structure-function alterations during mammalian spermatogenesis: DNA nicking and repair in elongating spermatids. Eur J Histochem. 1993;37:109–28.
49. Manicardi GC, Bianchi PG, Pantano S, Azzoni P, Bizzaro D, Bianchi U, et al. Presence of endogenous nicks in DNA of ejaculated spermatozoa and its relationship to chromomycin A_3 accessibility. Biol Reprod. 1995;52:864–7.
50. Rodriguez I, Ody C, Araki K, Garcia I, Vassalli P. An early and massive wave of germinal cell apoptosis is required for the development of functional spermatogenesis. EMBO J. 1997;16:2262–70.
51. McVicar CM, McClure N, Williamson K, Dalzell LH, Lewis SE. Incidence of Fas positivity and deoxyribonucleic acid double-stranded breaks in human ejaculated sperm. Fertil Steril. 2004;81(Suppl 1):767–74.
52. Morris ID, Ilott S, Dixon L, Brison DR. The spectrum of DNA damage in human sperm assessed by single cell gel electrophoresis (Comet assay) and its relationship to fertilization and embryo development. Hum Reprod. 2002;17:990–8.
53. Henkel R, Hajimohammad M, Stalf T, Hoogendijk C, Mehnert C, Menkveld R, et al. Influence of deoxyribonucleic acid damage on fertilization and pregnancy. Fertil Steril. 2004;81:965–72.
54. Schlegel PN, Paduch DA. Yet another test of sperm chromatin structure. Fertil Steril. 2005;84:854–9.
55. Li Z, Wang L, Cai J, Huang H. Correlation of sperm DNA damage with IVF and ICSI outcomes: a systematic review and meta-analysis. J Assist Reprod Genet. 2006;23:367–76.
56. Lopes S, Sun JG, Jurisicova A, Meriano J, Casper RF. Sperm deoxyribonucleic acid fragmentation is increased in poor-quality semen samples and correlates with failed fertilization in intracytoplasmic sperm injection. Fertil Steril. 1998;69:528–32.
57. Larson-Cook KL, Brannian JD, Hansen KA, Kasperson KM, Aamold ET, Evenson DP. Relationship between the outcomes of assisted reproductive techniques and sperm DNA fragmentation as measured by the sperm chromatin structure assay. Fertil Steril. 2003;80:895–902.
58. Braude P, Bolton V, Moore S. Human gene expression first occurs between the four- and eight-cell stages of preimplantation development. Nature. 1988;332:459–61.
59. Amann RP. Can the fertility potential of a seminal sample be predicted accurately? J Androl. 1989;10:89–98.
60. Barroso G, Morshedi M, Oehninger S. Analysis of DNA fragmentation, plasma membrane translocation of phosphatidylserine and oxidative stress in human spermatozoa. Hum Reprod. 2000;15:1338–44.
61. Grunewald S, Paasch U, Glander HJ. Enrichment of non-apoptotic human spermatozoa after cryopreservation by immunomagnetic cell sorting. Cell Tissue Bank. 2001;2:127–33.
62. Muriel L, Meseguer M, Fernandez JL, Alvarez J, Jose R, Pellicer A, et al. Value of the sperm chromatin dispersion test in predicting pregnancy outcome in intrauterine insemination: a blind prospective study. Hum Reprod. 2006;21:738–44.
63. Muriel L, Garrido N, Fernández JL, Remohí J, Pellicer A, de los Santos MJ, et al. Value of the sperm deoxyribonucleic acid fragmentation level, as measured by the sperm chromatin dispersion test, in the outcome of in vitro fertilization and intracytoplasmic sperm injection. Fertil Steril. 2006;85:371–83.
64. Evenson DP, Jost LK. Sperm chromatin structure assay for fertility assessment. Curr Protoc Flow Cytom. 2000;7.13.1–7.13.27.
65. Evenson DP, Darzynkiewicz Z, Melamed MR. Relation of mammalian sperm chromatin heterogeneity to fertility. Science. 1980;240:1131–3.

66. Matson PL. Clinical value of tests for assessing male infertility. Bal Clin Obstet Gynaecol. 1997;11:641–54.
67. WHO. WHO laboratory manual for the examination and processing of human semen. 5th ed. Geneva: World Health Organization; 2010.
68. Christensen P, Stryhn H, Hansen C. Discrepancies in the determination of sperm concentration using Bürker-Türk, Thoma and Makler counting chambers. Theriogenology. 2005;63:992–1003.
69. Boe-Hansen GB, Ersbøll AK, Christensen P. Variability and laboratory factors affecting the sperm chromatin structure assay in human semen. J Androl. 2005;26:360–8.
70. Brandt Boe-Hansen GB, Fedder J, Ersbøll AK, Christensen P. The sperm chromatin structure assay as a diagnostic tool in the human fertility clinic. Hum Reprod. 2006;21:1576–82.
71. Yang XY, Zhang Y, Sun XP, Cui YG, Qian XQ, Liao A. Sperm chromatin structure assay predicts the outcome of intrauterine insemination. Zhonghua Nan Ke Xue. 2011;17:977–83.
72. Björndahl L, Barratt CLR, Mortimer D, Jouannet P. 'How to count sperm properly': checklist for acceptability of studies based on human semen analysis. Hum Reprod. 2016;31:227–32.
73. Mallidis C, Howard EJ, Baker HW. Variation of semen quality in normal men. Int J Androl. 1991;14:99–107.
74. Alvarez C, Castilla JA, Martinez L, Ramirez JP, Vergara F, Gaforio JJ. Biological variation of seminal parameters in healthy subjects. Hum Reprod. 2003;18:2082–8.
75. Evenson DP, Jost LK, Baer RK, Turner TW, Schrader SM. Individuality of DNA denaturation patterns in human sperm as measured by the sperm chromatin structure assay. Reprod Toxicol. 1991;5:115–25.
76. Zini A, Kamal K, Phang D, Willis J, Jarvi K. Biologic variability of sperm DNA denaturation in infertile men. Urology. 2001;58:258–61.
77. Zini A, Bielecki R, Phang D, Zenzes M. Correlations between two markers of sperm DNA integrity. DNA denaturation and DNA fragmentation in fertile and infertile men. Fertil Steril. 2001;75:674–7.
78. Erenpreiss J, Bungum M, Spano M, Elzanaty S, Orbidans J, Giwercman A. Intra-individual variation in sperm chromatin structure assay parameters in men from infertile couples: clinical implications. Hum Reprod. 2006;21:2061–4.
79. Oleszczuk K, Giwercman A, Bungum M. Intra-individual variation of the sperm chromatin structure assay DNA fragmentation index in men from infertile couples. Hum Reprod. 2011;26:3244–8.
80. Blomberg Jensen M, Lawaetz JG, Pedersen JH, Juul A, Joergensen N. Effects of vitamin D and calcium supplementation on semen quality, reproductive hormones and live birth rate: a randomized clinical trial. JECM. 2017 Accepted.
81. Christensen P, Hansen C, Liboriussen T, Lehn-Jensen H. Implementation of flow cytometry for quality control in four Danish bull studs. Anim Reprod Sci. 2005;85:201–8.
82. Evenson DP. Sperm chromatin structure assay: 30 years of experience with the SCSA. In: Zini A, Agarwal A, editors. Sperm chromatin biological and clinical applications in male infertility and assisted reproduction. New York: Springer; 2011. p. 125–50.
83. Jeyendran RS, Zaneveld LJ. Controversies in the development and validation of new sperm assays. Fertil Steril. 1993;59:726–8.
84. Christensen P, Sills ES, Fischer R, Naether OGJ, Walsh D, Rudolf K, et al. Impact of sperm DNA fragmentation on reproductive outcome following IVF and ICSI: a retrospective analysis of 406 cases. Hum Reprod. 2013;28:i128:P-026.
85. Duran EH, Morshedi M, Taylor S, Oehninger S. Sperm DNA quality predicts intrauterine insemination outcome: a prospective cohort study. Hum Reprod. 2002;17:3122–8.
86. Love CC, Thompson JA, Lowry VK, Varner DD. Effect of storage time and temperature on stallion sperm DNA and fertility. Theriogenology. 2002;57:1135–42.
87. Boe-Hansen GB, Christensen P, Vibjerg D, Nielsen MBF, Hedeboe AM. Sperm chromatin structure integrity in liquid stored boar semen and its relationships with field fertility. Theriogenology. 2008;69:728–36.

88. Christensen P, Labouriau R, Birck A, Boe-Hansen GB, Pedersen J, Borchersen S. Relationship among seminal quality measures and field fertility of young dairy bulls using low-dose inseminations. J Dairy Sci. 2011;94:1744–54.

89. Simon L, Zini A, Dyachenko A, Ciampi A, Carrell DT. A systematic review and meta-analysis to determine the effect of sperm DNA damage on in vitro fertilization and intracytoplasmic sperm injection outcome. Asian J Androl. 2017;19:80–90.

90. Ollero M, Gil-Guzman E, Lopez MC, Sharma RK, Agarwal A, Larson K, et al. Characterization of subsets of human spermatozoa at different stages of maturation: implications in the diagnosis and treatment of male infertility. Hum Reprod. 2001;16:1912–21.

91. Greco E, Scarselli F, Iacobelli M, Rienzi L, Ubaldi F, Ferrero S, et al. Efficient treatment of infertility due to sperm DNA damage by ICSI with testicular spermatozoa. Hum Reprod. 2005;20:226–30.

92. Dalzell LH, McVicar CM, McClure N, Lutton D, Lewis SE. Effects of short and long incubations on DNA fragmentation of testicular sperm. Fertil Steril. 2004;82:1443–5.

93. Boe-Hansen GB, Ersbøll AK, Greve T, Christensen P. Increasing storage time of extended boar semen reduces sperm DNA integrity. Theriogenology. 2005;63:2006–19.

94. Matsuura R, Takeuchi T, Yoshida A. Preparation and incubation conditions affect the DNA integrity of ejaculated human spermatozoa. Asian J Androl. 2010;12:753–9.

95. Antinori M. Intracytoplasmic morphologically selected sperm injection: a prospective randomized trial. RBM Online. 2008;16:835–41.

96. Setti AS, Paes de Almeida Ferreira Braga D, Iaconelli A Jr, Aoki T, Borges E Jr. Twelve years of MSOME and IMSI: a review. Reprod Biomed Online. 2013;27:338–52.

97. Avendaño C, Franchi A, Taylor S, Morshedi M, Bocca S, Oehninger S. Fragmentation of DNA in morphologically normal human spermatozoa. Fertil Steril. 2009;91:1077–84.

98. Oleszczuk K, Augustinsson L, Bayat N, Giwercman A, Bungum M. Prevalence of high DNA fragmentation index in male partners of unexplained infertile couples. Andrology. 2013;1:357–60.

99. Said TM, Grunewald S, Paasch U, Glander HJ, Baumann T, Kriegel C, et al. Advantage of combining magnetic cell separation with sperm preparation techniques. Reprod Biomed Online. 2005;10:740–6.

100. Gadella BM, Harrison RA. The capacitating agent bicarbonate induces protein kinase A-dependent changes in phospholipid transbilayer behavior in the sperm plasma membrane. Development. 2000;127:2407–20.

101. Weng SL, Taylor SL, Morshedi M, Schuffner A, Duran EH, Beebe S, et al. Caspase activity and apoptotic markers in ejaculated human sperm. Mol Hum Reprod. 2002;8:984–91.

102. Worrilow KC, Eid S, Woodhouse D, Perloe M, Smith S, Witmyer J, et al. Use of hyaluronan in the selection of sperm for intracytoplasmic sperm injection (ICSI): significant improvement in clinical outcomes—multicenter, doubleblinded and randomized controlled trial. Hum Reprod. 2013;28:306–14.

103. Beck-Fruchter R, Shalev E, Weiss A. Clinical benefit using sperm hyaluronic acid binding technique in ICSI cycles: a systematic review and meta-analysis. RBM Online. 2016;32:286–98.

104. Ramsing NB, Callesen H. Detecting timing and duration of cell division by automated image analysis may improve selection of viable embryos. Fertil Steril. 2006;86:S189.

105. Kirkegaard K, Kesmodel US, Hindkjær JJ, Ingerslev HJ. Time-lapse parameters as predictors of blastocyst development and pregnancy outcome in embryos from good prognosis patients: a prospective cohort study. Hum Reprod. 2013;28:2643–51.

106. Seli E, Gardner DK, Schoolcraft WB, Moffatt O, Sakkas D. Extent of nuclear DNA damage in ejaculated spermatozoa impacts on blastocyst development after in vitro fertilization. Fertil Steril. 2004;82:378–83.

107. Tesarik J, Greco E, Mendoza C. Late, but not early, paternal effect on human embryo development is related to sperm DNA fragmentation. Hum Reprod. 2004;19:611–5.

108. Carrell DT, Liu L, Peterson CM, Jones KP, Hatasaka HH, Erickson L, et al. Sperm DNA fragmentation is increased in couples with unexplained recurrent pregnancy loss. Arch Androl. 2003;49:49–55.
109. Robinson L, Gallos ID, Conner SJ, Rajkhowa M, Miller D, Lewis S, et al. The effect of sperm DNA fragmentation on miscarriage rates: a systematic review and meta-analysis. Hum Reprod. 2012;27:2908–17.
110. Sepaniak S, Forges T, Gerard H, Foliguet B, Bene MC, Monnier-Barbarino P. The influence of cigarette smoking on human sperm quality and DNA fragmentation. Toxicology. 2006;223:54–60.
111. Laubenthal J, Zlobinskaya O, Poterlowicz K, Baumgartner A, Gdula MR, Fthenou E, et al. Cigarette smoke-induced transgenerational alterations in genome stability in cord blood of human F1 offspring. FASEB J. 2012;26:3946–56.
112. Sergerie M, Ouhilal S, Bissonnette F, Brodeur J, Bleau G. Lack of association between smoking and DNA fragmentation in the spermatozoa of normal men. Hum Reprod. 2000;15:1314–21.
113. Fraga CG, Motchnik PA, Wyrobek AJ, Rempel DM, Ames BN. Smoking and low antioxidant levels increase oxidative damage to sperm DNA. Mutat Res. 1996;35:199–203.
114. Chavarro JE, Toth TL, Wright DL Meeker JD, Hauser R. Body mass index in relation to semen quality, sperm DNA integrity, and serum reproductive hormone levels among men attending an infertility clinic. Fertil Steril. 2010;93:2222–31.
115. Dupont C, Faure C, Sermondade N, Boubaya M, Eustache F, Clément P, et al. Obesity leads to higher risk of sperm DNA damage in infertile patients. Asian J Androl. 2013;15:622–5.
116. Håkonsen LB, Thulstrup AM, Aggerholm AS, Olsen J, Bonde JP, Andersen CY, et al. Does weight loss improve semen quality and reproductive hormones? Results from a cohort of severely obese men. Reprod Health. 2011;8:24.
117. Bandel I, Bungum M, Richtoff J, Malm J, Axelsson J, Pedersen HS, et al. No association between body mass index and sperm DNA integrity. Hum Reprod. 2015;30:1704–13.
118. Arcidiacono B, Iiritano S, Nocera A, Possidente K, Nevolo MT, Ventura V, et al. Insulin resistance and cancer risk: an overview of the pathogenetic mechanisms. Exp Diabetes Res. 2012;2012:789174. https://doi.org/10.1155/2012/789174.
119. Duale N, Steffensen IL, Andersen J, Brevik A, Brunborg G, Lindeman B. Impaired sperm chromatin integrity in obese mice. Andrology. 2014;2:234–43.
120. Leisegang K, Bouic PJ, Henkel RR. Metabolic syndrome is associated with increased seminal inflammatory cytokines and reproductive dysfunction in a case-controlled male cohort. Am J Reprod Immunol. 2016;76:155–63.
121. Koçak I, Yenisey C, Dündar M, Okyay P, Serter M. Relationship between seminal plasma interleukin-6 and tumor necrosis factor alpha levels with semen parameters in fertile and infertile men. Urol Res. 2002;30:263–7.
122. Nordström EA, Rydén M, Backlund EC, Dahlman I, Kaaman M, Blomqvist L, et al. A human-specific role of cell death-inducing DFFA (DNA fragmentation factor-alpha)-like effector A (CIDEA) in adipocyte lipolysis and obesity. Diabetes. 2005;54:1726–34.
123. Perdichizzi A, Nicoletti F, La Vignera S, Barone N, D'Agata R, Vicari E, et al. Effects of tumour necrosis factor-alpha on human sperm motility and apoptosis. J Clin Immunol. 2007;27:152–62.
124. Suleiman SA, Ali ME, Zaki ZM, el-Malik EM, Nasr MA. Lipid peroxidation and human sperm motility: protective role of vitamin. J Androl. 1996;17:530–7.
125. Kodama H, Yamaguchi R, Fukuda J, Kasai H, Tanaka T. Increased oxidative deoxyribonucleic acid damage in the spermatozoa of infertile male patients. Fertil Steril. 1997;68:519–24.
126. Geva E, Lessing JB, Lerner-Geva L, Amit A. Free radicals, antioxidants and human spermatozoa: clinical implications. Hum Reprod. 1998;13:1422–4.
127. Comhaire FH, Christophe AB, Zalata AA, Dhooge WS, Mahmoud AM, Depuydt CE. The effects of combined conventional treatment, oral antioxidants and essential fatty acids on sperm biology in subfertile men. Prostaglandins Leukot Essent Fatty Acids. 2000;63:159–65.
128. Greco E, Romano S, Iacobelli M, Ferrero S, Baroni E, Minasi MG, et al. ICSI in cases of sperm DNA damage: beneficial effect of oral antioxydant treatment. Hum Reprod. 2005;20:2590–4.

129. Ames BN. Micronutrients prevent cancer and delay aging. Toxicol Lett. 1998;102–103:5–18.
130. Bowry VW, Ingold KU, Stocker R. Vitamin E in human low-density lipoprotein. When and how this antioxidant becomes a pro-oxidant. Biochem J. 1992;288:341–4.
131. Podmore ID, Griffiths HR, Herbert KE, Mistry N, Mistry P, Lunec J. Vitamin C exhibits pro-oxidant properties. Nature. 1998;392:559.
132. Tvrda E, Peer R, Sikka SC, Agarwal A. Iron and copper in male reproduction: a double-edged sword. J Assist Reprod Genet. 2015;32:3–16.
133. Durup D, Jørgensen HL, Christensen J, Tjønneland A, Olsen A, Halkjær J, et al. A reverse J-shaped association between serum 25-hydroxyvitamin D and cardiovascular disease mortality: the CopD study. J Clin Endocrinol Metab. 2015;100:2339–46.
134. Balhorn R, Corzett M, Mazrimas J, Watkins B. Identification of bull protamine disulfides. Biochemistry. 1991;30:175–81.
135. Fedder MD, Jakobsen HB, Giversen I, Christensen LP, Parner ET, Fedder J. An extract of pomegranate fruit and galangal rhizome increases the numbers of motile sperm: a prospective, randomized, controlled, double-blinded trial. PLoS One. 2014;9(9):e108532. https://doi.org/10.1371/journal.pone.0108532.
136. Gharagozloo P, Gutiérrez-Adán A, Champroux A, Noblanc A, Kocer A, Calle A, et al. A novel antioxidant formulation designed to treat male infertility associated with oxidative stress: promising preclinical evidence from animal models. Hum Reprod. 2016;31:252–62.

Chapter 7
Sperm Evaluation Using the Comet Assay

Océane Albert and Bernard Robaire

7.1 Introduction

Since 1980, the World Health Organization (WHO) has developed and updated standard semen reference values and operating procedures to assess human semen quality based on six essential parameters: semen volume, sperm concentration, total sperm number, total progressive motility, morphologically normal sperm, and sperm vitality [1]. While fundamental to establish an initial diagnosis, the standard semen analysis has been shown to be a poor predictor of fertility, in part because of the seasonal, geographical, and intra-individual heterogeneity of human semen [2]. More importantly, none of these parameters assess the quality of sperm nuclear material, which has been proven to be sensitive to a wide range of physical, chemical, and environmental agents [3]. There is growing evidence that sperm chromatin quality plays a crucial role in the success of assisted reproductive technologies (ART). Recent studies show associations between sperm DNA integrity and fertility, success of in vitro fertilization (IVF) or intracytoplasmic sperm injection (ICSI), embryo quality, and pregnancy rates and outcomes [4], suggesting the prognostic value of sperm chromatin quality assays.

Available sperm DNA quality assays include detection of chromosomal aberrations, DNA fragmentation and compaction, and protamination defects [3, 5]. Among those, the single-cell gel electrophoresis, or comet assay, gives a comprehensive measure of DNA integrity by revealing single- and double-strand DNA breaks and alkali-labile sites under specific treatment conditions. The comet assay offers the unique feature of collecting data at the level of the single cell; the assessment of 50 individual cells is enough to deliver accurate information on sperm quality [6, 7], opening the possibility of analysis to severely oligozoospermic patients. However,

O. Albert • B. Robaire (✉)
Department of Pharmacology and Therapeutics and of Obstetrics and Gynecology,
McGill University, Montreal, QC, Canada
e-mail: oceane.albert@mcgill.ca; bernard.robaire@mcgill.ca

© Springer International Publishing AG 2018
G.D. Palermo, E.S. Sills (eds.), *Intracytoplasmic Sperm Injection*,
https://doi.org/10.1007/978-3-319-70497-5_7

this feature, together with the single-slide classic output of the assay, makes comet assessment a low throughput procedure that renders large cohort analysis extremely challenging. Furthermore, the sensitivity of unwound sperm DNA and the multiple steps of the assay make it inherently variable and call for a standardization of the procedure [4, 8, 9].

In this chapter, we present the basic aspects of the comet assay and discuss its advantages and disadvantages as well as recent improvements of the procedure. Studies associating sperm DNA damage, as assessed by the comet assay, with the success of ICSI procedures are also reviewed.

7.2 The Human Sperm Comet Assay

7.2.1 Principle

The concept of a microgel electrophoresis to reveal DNA damage in somatic cells was first introduced by Ostling and Johanson [10]. In 1988, Singh and collaborators modified the original protocol and introduced alkaline conditions in order to improve assay sensitivity [11]. However, to reveal DNA damage in spermatozoa, additional steps were required to induce chromatin decondensation and DNA migration. Indeed, sperm chromatin has a highly organized, compact heterogeneous structure. This condensed nature is believed to allow for the preservation of the paternal genome integrity during transportation through the male and female reproductive tracts. Sperm chromatin compaction results from complex topological and protein-aceous rearrangements during spermiogenesis: a large proportion of histone-based nucleosomes are first replaced by transition proteins, and then by small arginine-rich proteins called protamines that allow the DNA to fold into highly condensed toroids [12]. As a consequence, Singh and collaborators developed a specific comet procedure for human and mouse spermatozoa [13].

The principle of the assay is to embed spermatozoa in low melting-point agarose and spread the mix on a glass slide, followed by several treatments designed to induce cell lysis and DNA unwinding (see Fig. 7.1a). In the initial description of the assay, these treatments were: (a) a high concentration aqueous salt, detergent, and reducing agent dithiothreitol (DTT) mix to induce cell lysis; (b) a proteinase K treatment at 37 °C to remove residual proteins; (c) a neutral to alkaline solution to induce DNA unwinding. After a brief electrophoresis, each cell is stained with a DNA-specific fluorescent dye resulting in a structure resembling a comet, consisting of a round-shaped head made of high molecular weight undamaged DNA, and a tail containing the leading ends and lower heterogeneous molecular weight fragments of damaged DNA. Each comet is given a score that reflects its length and the amount of DNA present in the tail: the longer and brighter the comet tail, the more damaged the spermatozoon.

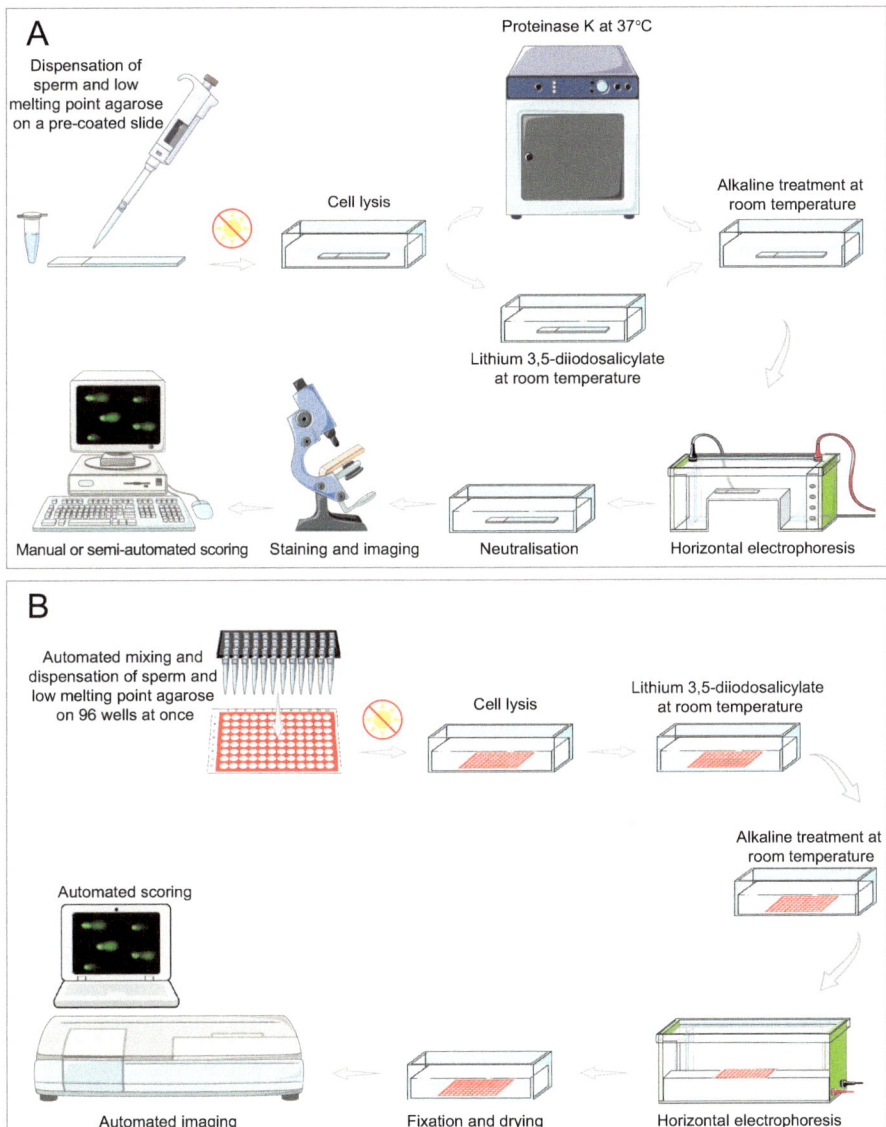

Fig. 7.1 The classical comet assay versus HT-COMET. The classic comet assay (**a**) is a procedure comprising manual mixing of sperm and agarose, distribution on a single glass slide, various cell lysis and DNA unwinding treatments, electrophoresis, time-consuming manual imaging, and laborious manual or semi-automated scoring of the comets. Due to numerous protocol variations, the procedure is also often described as inherently variable. To circumvent these effects, we developed HT-COMET (**b**), comprising automated mixing, distribution, imaging, and scoring of 96-well slides, and a simpler treatment procedure. Individual illustrations of laboratory equipment were used and modified from Servier Medical Arts

Using this approach, it was soon discovered that spermatozoa exhibit a higher baseline level of DNA migration than somatic cells [13]. Because such migration was not described after a neutral treatment, the larger comets were attributed to alkali-sensitive sites rather than preexisting strand breaks. However, this particularity, together with the largely described sensitivity of the assay to protocol modifications [8], confers an inherent degree of variability to the comet assay that has been depicted as a weakness of this method. Next, we discuss the protocol variations that have been described in the literature, and the steps that have been taken towards minimizing these confounders leading to greater standardization.

7.2.1.1 Variation in Agarose Distribution

Although treatment with different enzymes or at different pH is often identified as a major factor in comet assay variability, one technical variable is often overlooked. Indeed, agarose evenness across and between the slides is a sine qua non-condition to reach reproducibility and accuracy. Heterogeneous agarose levels and textures can lead to artifactual trends in DNA damage [14]. Homogeneous distribution of agarose is ensured by a strict control of agarose temperature when mixed with sperm and pipetted onto the slide, and a quick dispensation of the mix across conditions. In the original protocol [13], a thin layer of low melting-point agarose was spread on a glass slide. The cell suspension in agarose was pipetted onto this first layer and immediately overlaid with a coverslip. The slides were then kept at 4 °C for 5 min to allow solidification of the agarose. After gently removing the coverslip, the slides were covered with a third layer of low melting agarose by using a coverslip and then placed horizontally in a steel tray and returned to 4 °C. Some protocol emphasize that these slides should be fully frosted for greater surface adhesion [6, 15]. More recently, commercial options for 2, 24, and 96-well slides specifically developed for the comet assay have been made available, reducing the number of technical steps and thereby decreasing the variability attributable to agarose distribution.

7.2.1.2 Lysis Buffer

Depending on the protocol, cell lysis can be done first as a separate step in an aqueous salt solution without supplements, or combined with DNA unwinding steps in a buffer supplemented with DTT, Proteinase K, and/or 3,5-diiodosalicylate (LIS). There is a general consensus on the basic composition of the lysis buffer (2.5 mM NaCl, 100 mM EDTA, and 10 mM Tris) [16]. Alternative protocols include the addition of 10% DMSO to scavenge radicals and 1% Triton to increase membrane permeability [17], or, more rarely for spermatozoa, 1% of the surfactant sodium sarcosinate [7, 13].

7.2.1.3 Enzymatic Treatment

The original protocol, as well as most currently used protocols, include an exposure to the broad-spectrum serine protease Proteinase K to remove protamines, thereby allowing sperm DNA to decondense and migrate [13]. However, there are discrepancies in this technique: incubation with Proteinase K can be done directly in the lysis solution or as an additional step after lysis, performed at different concentrations, either at room temperature or 37 °C, and for durations varying from 3 to 18 h [8]. Prolonged incubations with high concentrations of Proteinase K have been reported to increase the baseline DNA damage observed with sperm [17]. Whether this is attributable to de novo DNA damage or further supercoil relaxation is still unclear. Other protocols include two enzymatic digestion steps with RNAse and Proteinase K [18]. Such variations in the procedure can greatly affect the sensitivity of the assay and aggravate the inability to compare data between laboratories. More recently, protocol modifications introduced incubation with the chaotropic agent LIS instead of Proteinase K [14, 15, 19]. This permitted reduction of both experimental time and background DNA damage [15]. Hence, LIS appears to be the better option as it shortens and simplifies the process and prevents agarose softening as, unlike Proteinase K, it is active at room temperature.

7.2.1.4 pH Conditions

One of the most critical and debated parameters in the comet procedure is the pH of the third and final treatment of the cells. Two versions of the sperm comet assay have been described: one done under neutral conditions where protein removal is immediately followed by electrophoresis in a neutral buffer, and the other where electrophoresis is preceded by treatment with an alkaline solution. Authors often erroneously attempt to associate the pH conditions with the nature of DNA breaks detected; there is a common belief that alkaline conditions are required to reveal single-strand DNA breaks, and consequently that neutral conditions would only pick up double-strand DNA breaks. These incorrect statements are believed to arise from comparisons with historical procedures to detect DNA damage, such as alkaline sucrose gradient sedimentation, alkaline elution, or alkaline unwinding [20]. It has been demonstrated that while decreasing the sensitivity of the assay, neutral conditions still mainly detect single-strand DNA breaks [13, 20, 21]. The increased sensitivity of the alkaline assay is well documented in the literature and believed to be due to the unravelling of alkali-labile sites (such as apurinic and apyrimidinic sites which arise from the loss of a damaged base) [22] and further detachment of DNA strand breaks from the nuclear matrix [20].

While drastic alkaline conditions (pH > 13) [23, 24] were recommended by international experts for genotoxicity testing to maximize the expression of alkali-labile sites, there are nearly as many different protocols for human sperm comet as there are laboratories. Electrophoresis is done in different buffers, with pH conditions varying from 8.2 to 13.5 [8]. This contributes to the large variability in baseline

DNA migration observed between procedures [8], and further emphasizes the need for a standardized assay.

7.2.2   Staining and Imaging

After electrophoresis, slides can either be immediately neutralized, stained and imaged, or fixed and dehydrated in ethanol and dried for 48–72 h before staining and imaging [7]. The original protocol included staining with the intercalating agent ethidium bromide [11], but, primarily because of the toxicity of this chemical, other DNA-specific fluorescent dyes have been used since, including propidium iodide [7], 4,6-diamidino-2-phenylindole (DAPI), SYBR Green I and YOYO-1 (benzoxazolium-4-quinolinum oxazole yellow homodimer) [20] or, more recently, SYBR® Gold [14]. Analysis of traditional comets is a tedious process involving manual selection, focusing, imaging, and semi-automated scoring. This substantial task accounts for a significant part of the classical comet low throughput.

7.3   Analysis and Scoring

There are four ways by which comet images can be analyzed [20]:

- Visual inspection and classification, typically into five categories (0 representing undamaged cells, and 1–4 representing increasing tail intensities). A sum of the individual scores from 100 comets will give a total score ranging from 0 to 400. This qualitative method is not only extremely tedious but is also subjective and creates intra- and inter-individual variability.
- Comet tail measurement using a graticule. While quantitative, this laborious method gives limited information on the extent of the damage in DNA: the tail length has been reported to be the most variable characteristic of the comet, and to plateau quickly to a maximum length [20], reducing the useful range of the assay.
- Semi-automated image analysis using commercially available software. Comets are individually selected by the operator, automatically analyzed and given a score (see scoring options below).
- Fully automated image analysis using commercially available software [14] or freeware [25]. Comets are picked and scored automatically with minimal experimenter intervention.

Of all these methods, the last two are the most currently used, reliable, and widely accepted. Comet measurements include the percentage DNA in the tail (accounting for the proportion of damaged DNA) and the tail length (determined by the relative size of DNA fragments). The product of the latter two gives a score called the tail extent moment (TEM). While theoretically more informative, the

TEM is poorly standardized across laboratories because it has no generally accepted units. As a consequence, the percentage of DNA in the tail is believed to be the most accurate and least variable measure of DNA damage. The Olive tail moment (OTM), a product of the percentage of DNA in the tail and the displacement between the means of the head and tail distribution [26], is equally used.

7.4 Towards a Standardized High Throughput Comet Assay

Of all sperm chromatin quality assays, the comet offers the unique feature of collecting data at the level of the single cell. However, this very feature, together with the classical single-well slide output of the assay, makes comet laborious and renders large cohort analysis extremely challenging.

Since the early 2000s, multiple attempts have been made to circumvent the inherent low throughput and laboriousness of the comet assay, mostly within the frame of genotoxicity screening of drug compounds in somatic cells. These endeavors started with the concept of a multigel assay [27] for somatic cells to avoid cell trypsinization: cells were cultured in multichamber plates with removable walls followed by agarose coating [28]. Other attempts included manually dispensed minigels on GelBond® sheets [29] and homemade micropatterned arrays dubbed CometChip arrays [30–32]. The later involved single-cell trapping and automatic detection and scoring using a suite of custom analyses in MATLAB®. However, all the above-mentioned methods require intensive manual handling of both the cells and the agarose gels, which can be compounding factors for variability. More importantly, none of these methods were specifically developed for human sperm chromatin, the condensed and insoluble nature of which requires a specific treatment.

To fill in this experimental gap, we developed a novel automated approach for high throughput assessment of human sperm chromatin quality called HT-COMET [14]. This method circumvents the major technical and data extraction disadvantages of the classical comet assay as it includes (Fig. 7.1b): (a) the automated mixing and distribution of sperm in low melting-point agarose on a 96-well slide with an automated liquid handling system to ensure evenness across the plate and avoid artifactual DNA damage trends; (b) optimized cell lysis and DNA decondensation conditions for human sperm; (c) a fully automated detection of SYBR® Gold stained comets using a high content imaging system; (d) a fully automated scoring of comets by the Columbus™ image analysis software that includes assessment of typical comet criteria (% DNA in the tail, tail length, and tail extent moment), and that compares well with a commonly used commercial software. HT-COMET was shown to reduce agarose handling, mixing, and distribution time by nearly 80%, treatment procedure time by over 90% and imaging and scoring time by 95%, reducing overall experimental time by more than 90%, while ensuring more accuracy and reproducibility through automation.

7.5   Human Sperm Comet and ICSI

7.5.1   Comet Assay Applicability to the Fertility Clinic

The human sperm comet assay is unique in its ability to give a direct measure of DNA damage at the level of the single cell. However, like many other sperm chromatin quality assays, it is a destructive procedure that does not allow for the selection of an undamaged spermatozoon to perform ICSI. As a consequence, the prognostic value of the assay lies in the characterization of DNA damage in a single or several ejaculates.

7.5.1.1   Novel Output Measures

For many years, the mean DNA damage, tail extent moment or Olive tail moment have been used as output measures and prognostic factors for ART outcome. Researchers have been trying to rethink these criteria to adapt comet assay data better for personalized clinical use. Hence, the DNA damage profile was first introduced by exploiting the high throughput single-cell data produced by the HT-COMET [14]. By plotting the percentage of DNA in the tail against the tail length for each comet, we can visualize a patient's sperm chromatin damage profile (see Fig. 7.2). In each graph, a black curve showing the arbitrary threshold of a tail extent moment of 10 allows to determine the proportions of highly damaged cells. The shape of each scatter plot can also provides essential information regarding the overall nature of DNA damage within a sample: a trend towards a horizontal cloud suggests longer comets, i.e., multiple smaller pieces of DNA migrating further, while a convergence towards the vertical axis reveals the presence of short DNA rich comet tails, i.e., of longer fragments of DNA (Fig. 7.2a). For example, using these profiles, comparison between fertility groups revealed that a severely oligozoospermic patient (see Fig. 7.2b) displayed only 15% of highly damaged cells, whereas a normozoospermic patient had as much as 35% (see Fig. 7.2c) [14], exemplifying the absence of correlation between sperm count and sperm chromatin quality [2].

Soon after, another team proposed to use a comet distribution plot to discriminate fertile vs. infertile men by classifying sperm comet data into three main categories: type A plots (high proportion of undamaged cells), type B plots (Gaussian distribution), and type C plots (high proportion of damaged cells) [19]. Of 132 couples undergoing ART, 66% of couples with type A plots achieved clinical pregnancy, while couples with type C plots achieved 33% pregnancies. Both these methods could be of use in guiding patients' options when considering assisted reproductive technologies provided scientists reach an international consensus on a DNA damage threshold for human sperm.

These novel output measures are of particular importance when comparing comet data with Sperm Chromatin Structure Assay (SCSA) or Terminal

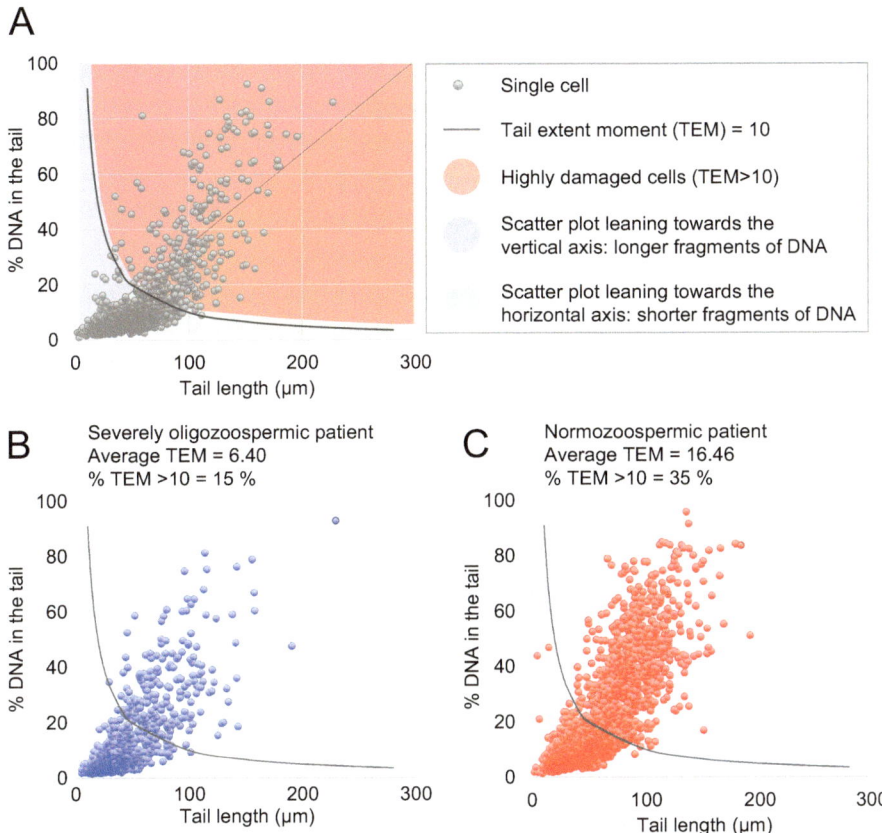

Fig. 7.2 DNA damage profiling using the automated alkaline HT-COMET [14]. A guide to reading the HT-COMET DNA damage profile is presented (**a**). The dark curve identifies the limit of a tail extent moment (TEM) equal to 10 as an arbitrary threshold for high damage: every dot above the curve represents a highly damaged cell (red area). A scatter-plot leaning towards the horizontal axis (green area) suggests longer comets, i.e., multiple smaller pieces of DNA migrating further, while a convergence towards the vertical axis (blue area) reveals the presence of short DNA rich comet tails, i.e., of longer fragments of DNA. Comet data from individual spermatozoa from a selected severe oligozoospermic (**b**) and a normozoospermic (**c**) patient were used to produce individual DNA damage profiles as a proposed tool for fertility prognosis. The fertility group, average TEM and percentage of highly damaged cells within the total population of comets (% TEM >10) are indicated above each profile; $n = 6$ wells from one 96-well slide were plotted for each patient. In this example, a patient categorized as normozoospermic per WHO criteria displays more damaged sperm than a severely oligozoospermic patient

deoxynucleotidyl transferase (TdT) dUTP Nick-End Labeling (TUNEL) data. Indeed, contrary to the comet measurements, the two latter assessments describe the proportion of highly damaged cells within a population. In TUNEL, terminal deoxynucleotidyl transferase catalyzes the addition of labeled nucleotides to 3′-OH ends at single- and double-strand DNA breaks to create a signal. Each scored sperm is determined as positively or negatively labeled, and the proportion of labeled sperm is considered. SCSA determines the susceptibility of sperm chromatin to in situ denaturation in acid. Based on the differential staining of chromatin single- and double-strand breaks by the dichromatic dye acridine orange [33, 34], SCSA allows the indirect measurement of the extent of sperm DNA fragmentation by determining the proportion of cells fluorescing in red (damaged) over those fluorescing in green (undamaged). Comet is more informative as it can provide a direct measure of both the extent of DNA damage in individual cells and the proportion of highly damaged cells in a population. Importantly, only the comparison of the proportion of highly damaged spermatozoa among comet, SCSA, and TUNEL experiments is valid.

7.5.1.2   DNA Damage Threshold for Human Sperm

No internationally accepted clinical threshold has been defined for the human comet assay, either in its neutral or alkaline form [2, 35]. So far, the very few epidemiological studies using the comet assay on human sperm vary in procedure and analysis and have defined study-dependent thresholds. For instance, in 2010, Simon et al. reported two threshold values to calculate odds ratios for IVF using the comet assay: 56% for unprocessed sperm and 48% for sperm selected by density gradient centrifugation. In another study using the same protocol but a different analysis, this threshold was brought up to 82% [36]. A valid threshold would have to be determined using a large population of proven fathers using a standardized protocol.

7.5.2   Comet Sperm DNA Damage and ICSI Outcome: Epidemiological Studies

Although still debated, the robustness of sperm DNA damage as a biomarker for ART outcome is supported by a large number of studies using SCSA, TUNEL, or the Sperm Chromatin Dispersion assay (SCD) [9]. There are very few studies, however, looking at the associations between ICSI outcome and DNA damage as assessed by the comet assay.

In 2002, Morris et al. first showed that sperm DNA damage assessed by the neutral comet assay is positively associated with impairment of post-fertilization embryo cleavage following ICSI [37]. Because it has been shown to be more sensitive, the alkaline comet assay has since then been presented as the better option. A large cohort study of infertile couples showed no significant association between alkaline comet DNA fragmentation and fertilization rate, embryo cumulative scores, and clinical pregnancy after ICSI treatment [38]. However, the predictive power of the assay was significantly increased by adding a step to convert oxidized purines into measureable strand breaks through exposure to formamidopyrimidine DNA glycosylase (FPG); there was significantly more damage in the group of patients that did not achieve clinical pregnancy after ICSI. The same group published a small cohort study showing no correlation between comet DNA fragmentation and fertilization rates or embryo quality after ICSI, including only 24 infertile men [39]. Another study on 149 men from infertile couples undergoing ICSI treatment showed no direct association between fertilization rate and comet DNA damage [36]. However, when the fertilization rate was categorized into normal and abnormal DNA damage groups (based on an 82% abnormal comet threshold value established specifically from the odds ratio of this study), sperm DNA damage above the threshold value resulted in significantly reduced fertilization rates after ICSI. Sperm DNA damage measured by comet was also negatively correlated with embryo quality measured on day 2, 3, and 5 post-injection, and positively correlated with percentage of blastocyst arrested. The mean implantation rate was higher when sperm DNA damage was below the threshold value, and there was a decrease in sperm DNA damage when more than one embryo was implanted. Finally, the mean percentage of sperm with DNA damage in the native semen was significantly higher in semen from non-pregnant couples compared to pregnant couples, confirming the prognostic value of the alkaline comet assay on ICSI outcome. In this study, the alkaline comet assay was shown to be more sensitive and predictive than SCSA. Both of these studies present the major drawback of not excluding female factor infertility, potentially reducing the prognostic value of sperm DNA tests. In an attempt to circumvent this flaw, the same research group analyzed semen from a cohort of 115 men from couples undergoing ICSI treatment and classified the causes of infertility into male, female, or unexplained categories [40]. Using the alkaline comet assay, and based on the presence or absence of a tail in 50–100 cells, their sperm were categorized into low, intermediate, or high damage. In the male infertility group, after ICSI treatment, DNA damage was positively associated with peri-fertilization defect and the percentage of poor quality embryos, and negatively associated with the percentage of good quality embryos.

7.6   Comet Sperm DNA Damage and ICSI Outcome: Meta-Analysis

Extant literature on the predictive value of sperm DNA damage on ART outcome remains controversial. Given the scarcity of comet-based studies on human sperm, the inclusion of comet data in systematic meta-analyses regarding associations between DNA damage and ICSI outcome is only recently possible.

One meta-analysis showed no significant association between DNA damage assessed by comet and miscarriage rates after IVF and ICSI [41]. This study comprised only one peer-reviewed comet study and one set of unpublished comet data, which considerably limited the statistical power of the work. Another report found no significant association between DNA damage assessed by comet and pregnancy or miscarriage rates after IVF or ICSI [42], but only took two comet-based studies into account within a comet- and acridine orange-based pool of four studies without a valid experimental rationale. In 2016, a study showed the predictive accuracy of the comet assay for pregnancy following ART was found to be fair compared to the poor predictive capacity of SCSA and SCD [43]. A meta-regression showed no significant difference in predictive value between IVF and ICSI for the comet assay, showing that the fertility treatment did not affect the estimated effect of sperm DNA damage; however, there was significant heterogeneity across studies in the sensitivity and specificity of the assay [43]. The most recent systematic review and meta-analysis examining the effects of sperm DNA damage on IVF and ICSI outcome showed that there is a statistically significant adverse effect of sperm DNA damage as assessed by the comet assay on clinical pregnancy [44]. Using a random effects model, the combined odds ratio estimates from seven independent comet-based studies revealed a statistically significant effect of DNA damage on IVF outcome.

7.7   Conclusion

Despite the numerous advantages of the comet assay, its prognostic value for ICSI outcome is still debated. To circumvent the scarcity of comparable human studies using the comet assay, the following steps should be undertaken: (a) reach an international consensus on an alkaline comet assay procedure to limit intra- and interlaboratory variability; (b) develop an international standard for criteria used to describe comets (number of damaged cells vs. percentage of DNA in the tail or tail extent moment); (c) define a threshold for the latter on a large population of proven fathers; (d) design large-scale epidemiological studies in couples with identified male factor infertility undergoing ICSI treatment. By standardizing the comet assay procedure and making it high throughput, the HT-COMET renders those aims possible in the short term.

References

1. World Health Organization. Examination and processing of human semen. Geneva: World Health Organization; 2010. p. 1–287.
2. Lewis SEM. Is sperm evaluation useful in predicting human fertility? Reproduction. 2007;134(1):31–40.
3. Delbes G, Hales BF, Robaire B. Toxicants and human sperm chromatin integrity. Mol Hum Reprod. 2009;16(1):14–22.
4. Zini A, Albert O, Robaire B. Assessing sperm chromatin and DNA damage: clinical importance and development of standards. Andrology. 2014;2(3):322–5.
5. Shamsi MB, Imam SN, Dada R. Sperm DNA integrity assays: diagnostic and prognostic challenges and implications in management of infertility. J Assist Reprod Genet. 2011;28(11):1073–85.

6. Hughes CM, Lewis S, McKelveyMartin VJ, Thompson W. Reproducibility of human sperm DNA measurements using the alkaline single cell gel electrophoresis assay. Mutat Res. 1997;374(2):261–8.
7. Olive PL, Banáth JP. The comet assay: a method to measure DNA damage in individual cells. Nat Protoc. 2006;1(1):23–9.
8. Speit G, Vasquez M, Hartmann A. The comet assay as an indicator test for germ cell genotoxicity. Mutat Res. 2009;681(1):3–12.
9. Bach PV, Schlegel PN, Sperm DNA. Damage and its role in IVF and ICSI. Basic Clin Androl. 2016;26(1):15.
10. Ostling O, Johanson KJ. Microelectrophoretic study of radiation-induced DNA damages in individual mammalian cells. Biochem Biophys Res Commun. 1984;123(1):291–8.
11. Singh NP, McCoy MT, Tice RR, Schneider EL. A simple technique for quantitation of low levels of DNA damage in individual cells. Exp Cell Res. 1988;175(1):184–91.
12. Ward WS. The structure of the sleeping genome: implications of sperm DNA organization for somatic cells. J Cell Biochem. 1994;55(1):77–82.
13. Singh NP, Danner DB, Tice RR, McCoy MT, Collins GD, Schneider EL. Abundant alkali-sensitive sites in DNA of human and mouse sperm. Exp Cell Res. 1989;184(2):461–70.
14. Albert O, Reintsch WE, Chan P, Robaire B. HT-COMET: a novel automated approach for high throughput assessment of human sperm chromatin quality. Hum Reprod. 2016;31(5):938–46.
15. Donnelly ET, McClure N, Lewis SE. The effect of ascorbate and alpha-tocopherol supplementation in vitro on DNA integrity and hydrogen peroxide-induced DNA damage in human spermatozoa. Mutagenesis. 1999;14(5):505–12.
16. Simon L, Carrell DT. Sperm DNA damage measured by comet assay. Methods Mol Biol. 2013;927(Chapter 13):137–46.
17. Hughes CM, Lewis SEM, McKelvey-Martin VJ, Thompson W. A comparison of baseline and induced DNA damage in human spermatozoa from fertile and infertile men, using a modified comet assay. Mol Hum Reprod. 1996;2(8):613–9.
18. Duty SM, Singh NP, Ryan L, Chen Z, Lewis C, Huang T, et al. Reliability of the comet assay in cryopreserved human sperm. Hum Reprod. 2002;17(5):1274–80.
19. Simon L, Aston KI, Emery BR, Hotaling J, Carrell DT. Sperm DNA damage output parameters measured by the alkaline comet assay and their importance. Andrologia. 2017;49(2).
20. Collins AR, Oscoz AA, Brunborg G, Gaivão I, Giovannelli L, Kruszewski M, et al. The comet assay: topical issues. Mutagenesis. 2008;23(3):143–51.
21. Angelis KJ, Dusinská M, Collins AR. Single cell gel electrophoresis: detection of DNA damage at different levels of sensitivity. Electrophoresis. 1999;20(10):2133–8.
22. Karlsson HL. The comet assay in nanotoxicology research. Anal Bioanal Chem. 2010;398(2):651–66.
23. Tice RR. Single cell gel/comet assay: guidelines for in vitro and in vivo genetic toxicology testing. Environ Mol Mutagen. 2000;35(3):6–21.
24. Hartmann A, Agurell E, Beevers C, Brendler-Schwaab S, Burlinson B, Clay P, et al. Recommendations for conducting the in vivo alkaline comet assay. 4th International Comet Assay Workshop. Mutagenesis. 2003;18:45–51.
25. Gyori BM, Venkatachalam G, Thiagarajan PS, Hsu D, Clement M-V. OpenComet: an automated tool for comet assay image analysis. Redox Biol. 2014;2:457–65.
26. Olive PL, Banáth JP, Durand RE. Heterogeneity in radiation-induced DNA damage and repair in tumor and normal cells measured using the "comet" assay. Radiat Res. 1990;122(1):86–94.
27. Witte I, Plappert U, de Wall H, Hartmann A. Genetic toxicity assessment: employing the best science for human safety evaluation part III: the comet assay as an alternative to in vitro clastogenicity tests for early drug candidate selection. Toxicol Sci. 2007;97(1):21–6.
28. Stang A, Witte I. Performance of the comet assay in a high-throughput version. Mutat Res. 2009;675(1–2):5–10.
29. Gutzkow KB, Langleite TM, Meier S, Graupner A, Collins AR, Brunborg G. High-throughput comet assay using 96 minigels. Mutagenesis. 2013;28(3):333–40.

30. Wood DK. Single cell trapping and DNA damage analysis using microwell arrays. PNAS. 2010;107:10008–13.
31. Weingeist DM, Ge J, Wood DK, Mutamba JT, Huang Q, Rowland EA, et al. Single-cell micro-array enables high-throughput evaluation of DNA double-strand breaks and DNA repair inhibitors. Cell Cycle. 2013;12(6):907–15.
32. Ge J, Chow DN, Fessler JL, Weingeist DM, Wood DK, Engelward BP. Micropatterned comet assay enables high throughput and sensitive DNA damage quantification. Mutagenesis. 2015;30(1):11–9.
33. Neville DM, Bradley DF. Anomalous rotatory dispersion of acridine orange-native deoxyribo-nucleic acid complexes. Biochim Biophys Acta. 1961;50:397–9.
34. Evenson DP. Sperm chromatin structure assay (SCSA®). Methods Mol Biol. 2013;927(Chapter 14):147–64.
35. Lewis SEM, Simon L. Clinical implications of sperm DNA damage. Hum Fertil (Camb). 2010;13(4):201–7.
36. Simon L, Liu L, Murphy K, Ge S, Hotaling J, Aston KI, et al. Comparative analysis of three sperm DNA damage assays and sperm nuclear protein content in couples undergoing assisted reproduction treatment. Hum Reprod. 2014;29(5):904–17.
37. Morris ID, Ilott S, Dixon L, Brison DR. The spectrum of DNA damage in human sperm assessed by single cell gel electrophoresis (comet assay) and its relationship to fertilization and embryo development. Hum Reprod. 2002;17(4):990–8.
38. Simon L, Brunborg G, Stevenson M, Lutton D, McManus J, Lewis SEM. Clinical significance of sperm DNA damage in assisted reproduction outcome. Hum Reprod. 2010;25(7):1594–608.
39. Simon L, Castillo J, Oliva R, Lewis SEM. Relationships between human sperm protamines, DNA damage and assisted reproduction outcomes. Reprod Biomed Online. 2011;23(6):724–34.
40. Simon L, Murphy K, Shamsi MB, Liu L, Emery B, Aston KI, et al. Paternal influence of sperm DNA integrity on early embryonic development. Hum Reprod. 2014;29(11):2402–12.
41. Robinson L, Gallos ID, Conner SJ, Rajkhowa M, Miller D, Lewis S, et al. The effect of sperm DNA fragmentation on miscarriage rates: a systematic review and meta-analysis. Hum Reprod. 2012;27(10):2908–17.
42. Zhao J, Zhang Q, Wang Y, Li Y. Whether sperm deoxyribonucleic acid fragmentation has an effect on pregnancy and miscarriage after in vitro fertilization/intracytoplasmic sperm injection: a systematic review and meta-analysis. Fertil Steril. 2014;102(4):998–1005.e8.
43. Cissen M, Wely MV, Scholten I, Mansell S, de Bruin JP, Mol BW, et al. Measuring sperm DNA fragmentation and clinical outcomes of medically assisted reproduction: a systematic review and meta-analysis. PLoS One. 2016;11(11):e0165125.
44. Simon L, Zini A, Dyachenko A, Ciampi A, Carrell DTA. Systematic review and meta-analysis to determine the effect of sperm DNA damage on in vitro fertilization and intracytoplasmic sperm injection outcome. Asian J Androl. 2017;19(1):80–90.

Chapter 8
Automated Morphology Detection from Human Sperm Images

Seyed Abolghasem Mirroshandel and Fatemeh Ghasemian

8.1 Introduction

The inability to conceive after 12 months of unprotected intercourse is generally defined as infertility. Almost 15% of reproductive age couples experience infertility and at least 30–40% are attributed to male factor infertility [1, 2]. Several factors modulate male fertility potential, and one of the most important of these is sperm morphology—considered to be a chief feature [3]. Types of abnormalities in sperm morphology (teratozoospermia) is head defects (e.g., tapered, pyriform, round, pin and amorphous head, two head, head with small acrosome or without acrosome, and vacuolated head), neck and midpiece defects (e.g., bent or asymmetrical neck, and thin or thick midpiece), tail defects (e.g., short, bent, and coiled tail and two tail), and excess residual cytoplasm more than one-third head.

Defective sperm morphology is likely to affect male fertility potential and may also be associated with abnormal DNA fragmentation [4, 5]. Indeed, a close correlation between sperm morphology abnormalities and embryo quality as observed in vitro at later developmental stages has been reported [6]. Defects in sperm maturation can manifest as abnormal sperm morphology and also cause problems during oocyte fertilization [7]. Several factors of seminal plasma and sperm parameters can reflect male infertility, such as semen viscosity, volume, pH and sperm morphology, vitality, motility, and concentration [4]. Morphology defects include abnormality of head (nucleus), neck, midpiece, tail, and the presence of residual cytoplasm.

S.A. Mirroshandel (✉)
Department of Computer Engineering, University of Guilan, Rasht, Guilan, Iran
e-mail: mirroshandel@guilan.ac.ir

F. Ghasemian
Department of Biology, University of Guilan, Rasht, Guilan, Iran
e-mail: ghasemian@guilan.ac.ir

© Springer International Publishing AG 2018
G.D. Palermo, E.S. Sills (eds.), *Intracytoplasmic Sperm Injection*,
https://doi.org/10.1007/978-3-319-70497-5_8

Following semen analysis, samples are classified as normal or abnormal [8]. Identifying atypical morphological patterns of sperm heads specially could have clinical utility as infertility treatment strategies are developed. Therefore, a complete and real-time analysis of different sperm components as normal vs. abnormal could be critical during intracytoplasmic sperm injection (ICSI).

As discussed elsewhere in this book, the first ICSI offspring live-birth was achieved in 1992 [9]. In recent years, various infertile couples with normal, mildly, or severely abnormal semen forms have undergone treatment incorporating ICSI [10]. The positive correlation between normal sperm morphology and favorable ICSI outcomes has been established from many studies; low fertilization, implantation, and conception (pregnancy) rates in cases with severe abnormality of the sperm head have likewise been reported [11].

Normal sperm morphology as defined by Menkveld et al. [12] includes the following characteristics: the sperm head is oval, and length and width of the sperm head are 3–5 and 2–3 µm, respectively (between three-fifths and two-thirds of the head length). The acrosome is well defined in the anterior aspect of the sperm head and comprises 40–70% of the sperm head (by volume). The width and size of midpiece are <1 µm and 1.5× the sperm head dimension, oriented axially. Cytoplasmic residue may be observed as less than half of the sperm's head size. The normal sperm tail was defined as uniformly thinner than the midpiece, uncoiled, and with a total length of 45 µm [12].

Different efforts have been proposed to facilitate sperm morphology evaluation during ICSI, including intracytoplasmic morphologically selected sperm injection (IMSI). In this procedure, sperm selection is performed at high magnification (usually ×6000) [11]. However, laboratories are commonly equipped with lower magnification (400–600×) microscopes, thus selection and injection of sperm are routinely performed at these magnifications. Such subjective manual methods are subjective, inexact, non-repeatable, and unteachable, leading to widely varying results.

Computer-assisted sperm (CASA) morphology assessment has been introduced to supply standardization and objectivity in the assessment of sperm morphology during injection to control methods and standards among laboratories and technicians [13]. Even methods of CASA reflect some variation [14–17], and identical and standard methods are absent across existing studies. Thus, the need persists among researcher to develop a new methodology and knowledge enrichment for analysis, classification, and selection the best sperm morphology, in real-time, during ICSI [15]. Given this background, automated methods to select the best sperm morphology without staining will be more suitable for embryologists and technicians.

This chapter is organized as follows: In Sect. 13.2, data assessing human sperm morphology are reviewed. In Sect. 13.3, detection and analysis of unstained human sperm using a sperm morphology analysis (SMA) algorithm are described. The results of applying the suggested algorithm are presented in Sect. 13.4. In Sect. 13.5, advantages and benefits of the SMA algorithm are discussed. In many studies, sperm was fixed, stained, and photographed although such sperm is not useful for ICSI in real-time. In contrast, a different method has been proposed where fresh human sperm is selected for injection in real-time at low magnification (×400 and ×600) [18]. It has an appropriate level of stability to evaluate sperm in the provided image. The key contribution of this research is the ability to work on noisy, low quality, and unstained images. Furthermore, the proposed algorithm reduces noise without the loss of any information in the image. Another advantage of this method is that sperm defects can be detected by low computation cost [18].

8.2 Related Works

Sanchez et al. described computer-assisted analyzed a fraction of boar spermatozoa heads and defined normal as a pattern of intracellular density distribution [15, 16]. They first described a deviation measure from this model, and computed the deviation from the model for each of sperm's head image. Then, they selected an optimal value for each classification of sperm cells. They were performed on the sperm tail removal and hole filling in the contours of the head using morphological closing. In the next stage, separation of the sperm's head from the background was done using Otsu's method [17].

An automated screening method for detecting stained spermatozoa was described by Vandewoestyne et al. [19]. All steps of processing, analysis, and evaluation were stored in an Axio Vision Commander Script, which could be run automatically using stored images to distinguish sperm heads from epithelial cells. This algorithm splits the image into disjoint regions containing only one nucleus and is based on the topology of the image.

Sperm components (i.e., acrosome, nucleus, midpiece, tail) were identified and discriminated as fully automatic by Bijar et al. [14]. In this study, microscopic images were captured from stained human semen smears. Using a Bayesian classifier, sperm parts were segmented using an entropy-based algorithm of expectation maximization (EM) and Markov random field (MRF) model. It is necessary to mention that in this study, stained sperm were used and analysis was performed at a high magnification (×1000). It has been reported that the different staining methods change morphometric dimensions of frozen human sperm in comparison to fresh ones [20]. Therefore, it is better that unstained and fresh sperm cells are used to analyze its morphometric dimensions. Thus, both cell dimensions will be unaffected by staining methods and also sperm can be used in real-time ICSI.

In another study, Alegre et al. [21] used digital image processing and learning vector quantization (LVQ) to classify boar sperm (acrosome) automatically. They captured sperm head images using a phase-contrast microscope, and evaluation of the acrosome status was performed according to staining features. The rate of overall test error of this sperm classification technique was reported 6.8%.

In other research, extraction of image features and normal sperm diagnosis were performed using the principal component analysis (PCA) and K-nearest neighbor (KNN), respectively. Assay performance (approximately 87%) was reported in this study derived from a small dataset [22]. A gold-standard assay was proposed by

Chang et al. [23] to improve framework for detection and segmentation of human sperm with attention to acrosome and nucleus components. They deployed a clustering and histogram approach to segment sperm head parameters with a combination of different color spaces. In this study, an improved result of >98% was reported to detect the sperm head. However, in this study, stained sperm images were also used for automatic detection and analysis [23].

Abbiramy and Shanthi [7] analyzed typical and atypical forms of sperm cells using a four-stage process. (1) Image preprocessing, (2) detection and extraction of individual sperm, (3) spermatozoa segmentation, and (4) statistical measurement of sperm. In the first stage, the RGB images were converted to a gray-scale images and noise removal was completed using a median filter, while Sobel edge detection algorithm was used in the stage II. The segmentation of each sperm element into head, midpiece, and tail was performed in stage III, and in the end, classification of sperm cells was done as normal and abnormal forms in the final stage.

The morphometric dimensions of sperm nuclei were compared for species of sheep, cattle, goat, and pig by Vicente-Fie et al. [24] and sperm processing was done using ImageJ [25]. The analysis and identification of sperm cells was also performed using open-access software and clustering procedures, respectively. In this study, they used a combination of computer-assisted sperm morphology analysis-fluorescence (CASMA-F) technology and multivariate cluster analyses [24]. Sperm cells obtained from the epididymis were stained with DNA-specific stain (Feulgen) and evaluated by Ramos et al. [26] using a system of computerized karyometric image analysis (CKIA) at a high magnification (×1000). A computerized assessment of ram sperm morphology was performed by Yaniz et al. using stained images from fluorescence microscopy, and the ImageJ program was used to analyze sperm nuclei [27]. Bellastella et al. [28] used a semi-automated Integrated Sperm Analysis System (ISAS) computer-aided system to quantify sperm head parameters, including length, width, area, perimeter, and acrosomal area.

8.3 Patient Recruitment and Sample Processing

Sperm samples were obtained from infertile couples who visited the IVF center of Alzahra hospital. Written informed consent was obtained from all study participants and the investigation was approved by the ethics committee of Guilan University of Medical Sciences (GUMS). Human sperm images were captured at low magnification (×400 and ×600) where image resolution is known to be low. Therefore, the SMA algorithm was used to enable effective sperm analysis by analyzing different sperm components. As the sperm has three main elements (head, neck/midpiece, and tail), any abnormality identified resulted in the designation of abnormal sperm; generally, low fertility has been reported for such abnormal sperm cases [4].

Initially, noise reduction of images was performed. Then, detection and analysis of different sperm components were completed as summarized in Fig. 8.1. Because

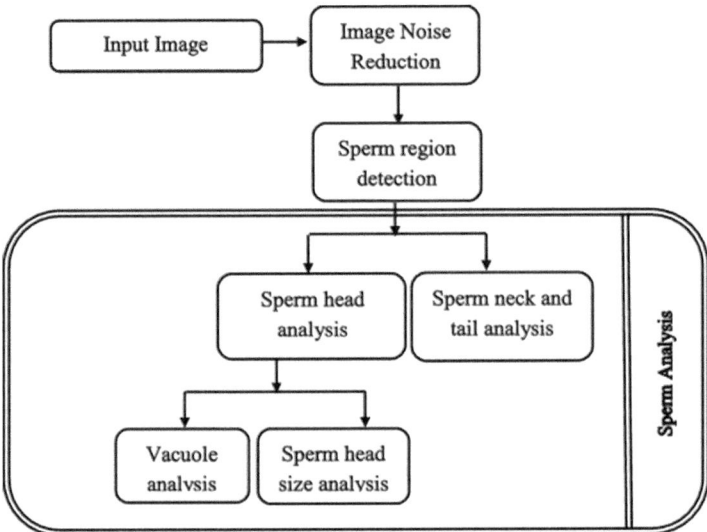

Fig. 8.1 The proposed algorithm

Fig. 8.2 Noise reduction algorithm

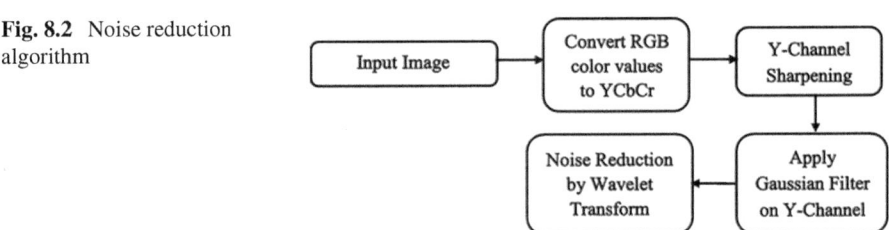

of the poor image quality captured at low magnification, the important pre-processing step is considered as "noise reduction" (see Fig. 8.2).

At the first step of noise reduction, RGB color images were converted into YCbCr, where color components could be discriminated as red, green, and blue [29]. A color space is formed from these three components and a multidimensional space. Each dimension of a color space is one color component. During the digital image processing, several color spaces are seen such as RGB, YCbCr, HSV, CMY, and CMYK. Moreover, YCbCr has three components: Y (luminance), Cb (Chromatic blue), and Cr (Chromatic red). YCbCr is often abbreviated as YCC. There are three components in the HSV color space: Hue, Saturation, and Value. The components of the CMY and CMYK color space are: C (cyan), M (magenta), Y (yellow), and K (black) [30].

The RGB image can be stored in a three-dimensional array. There are three values of red, green, and blue in each pixel. However, Y shows luminance, Cb and Cr are the different components of blue and red, respectively, in the YCbCr color space.

The color space of YCbCr is derived from the RGB color space and can be expressed as follows [31]:

$$
\begin{bmatrix} Y \\ Cb \\ Cr \end{bmatrix} = \begin{bmatrix} 16 \\ 128 \\ 128 \end{bmatrix} + \begin{bmatrix} 65.481 & 128.553 & 24.966 \\ -37.797 & -74.203 & 112.000 \\ 112.000 & -93.786 & -18.214 \end{bmatrix} \begin{bmatrix} R \\ G \\ B \end{bmatrix}.
$$

In the first step of the noise reduction algorithm, RGB color values are converted to YcbCr. In the next steps of the algorithm, the Y dimension is used. The noise of the original image in a gray-scale image comes from the Y dimension. There is a uniform distribution of noise in all parts of the images. Thus, the sharpening of the noise to separate this from the texture of image is proposed as the first step in this algorithm. After performance of this sharpening step, noise appears as image edges. A Gaussian filter is used to smooth these images and the noise shape is changed. At this time, the applying of wavelet transformation would be appropriate for the resulting image. In this study, a two-dimensional wavelet analysis function was used to remove noise of images. Wavelet decomposition of the matrix X at level N was returned by this algorithm. There are different types of wavelet families. By using different wavelet families, there are different trade-offs between the smoothness of the basic functions and how compactly they are localized in space. There are wavelet subclasses in each of wavelet family. Using of the iteration level and the coefficients number could distinguish these subclasses, and assignment of wavelets to a particular family is often done on the basis of number of vanishing moments. Indeed, the number of vanishing moments is an extra mathematical relationship set for coefficients that is directly correlated to the coefficient number and must be satisfied [32].

In the suggested algorithm, Coiflet 2 is used and the performance of decomposition is shown at level 4. After applying the aforesaid wavelet transformation, noise removal of input images can be performed at an acceptable rate.

8.3.1   Sperm Region Detection

Signal noise reduction enables image quality to be of suitable quality to apply the algorithm for edge detection to detect sperm components. In other words, noise has been smoothed during the pre-processing step, and there is minimal noise in the format of sharpened edges. Therefore, the noises will not be considered as edges during the phase of edge detection. In Fig. 8.3, the algorithm of sperm part detection has been shown.

Image segmentation can be performed by applying the edge detection algorithm of Sobel, which measures a 2D spatial gradient [33]. For each point from a gray-scale image, the approximate absolute gradient magnitude was determined. A pair

Fig. 8.3 Sperm compartment detection algorithm

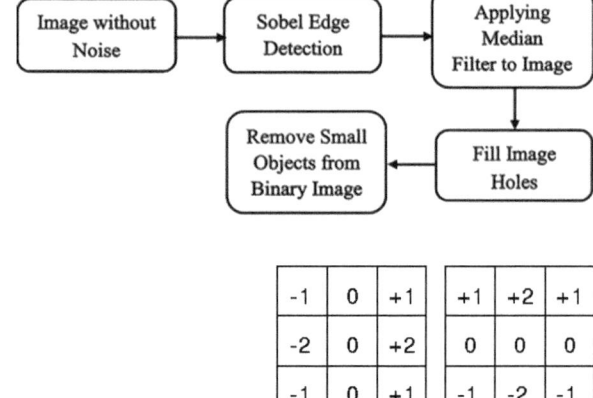

Fig. 8.4 Sobel operator matrices used for human sperm image processing and analysis

-1	0	+1
-2	0	+2
-1	0	+1

Gx

+1	+2	+1
0	0	0
-1	-2	-1

Gy

3 × 3 kernels was then used (see Fig. 8.4), which are convolved with gray-scale image to estimate gradients in both x and y axes.

To calculate gradient magnitude, the following formula was used:

$$|G| = \sqrt{Gx^2 + Gy^2}$$

Also, an approximate magnitude can be calculated using this approach:

$$|G| = |Gx| + |Gy|$$

After application of the Sobel edge detection method, some divergence in detected edges may be seen, or non-sperm parts of the input image could be incorrectly classified as edges. Thus, a second step to detect this situation in the proposed algorithm is the applying of a median filter. In this step, tiny regions are deleted without destructing the proposed edge. The last steps in sperm region detection are filling of image holes and small object subtraction, respectively. After edge detection, the small input image holes were filled to make a uniform image followed by removal of small extraneous image objects. In this way, the algorithm with a threshold value was applied, while debris and image noise are eliminated.

8.3.2 Sperm Analysis

After detection of the different sperm parts, each component was analyzed. Each part (i.e., head, neck/midpiece, and tail) was detected and analyzed. The first aspect of sperm is the head (nucleus), which undergoes additional analysis including the presence of vacuoles. After calculation of total sperm head size, measured values

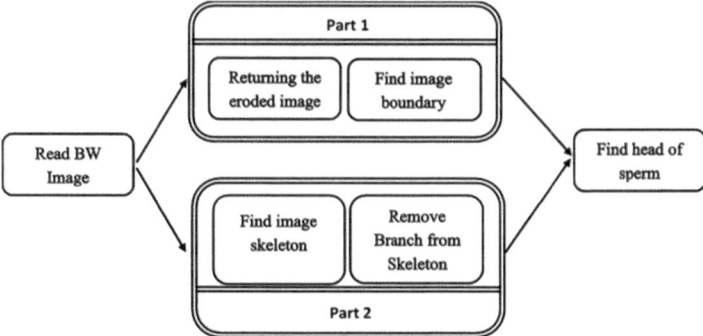

Fig. 8.5 Sperm head phase recognition

were compared to a standard range. If the value is not within this expected range, then that particular sperm is considered unsuitable and is not injected.

As shown in Fig. 8.5, the phase of the sperm head is also assessed. There are two main parts in phase of sperm head recognition, boundary recognition, and skeleton finding. To achieve this, images are converted to black and white (BW) space. Next, the erosion morphology operator is used on the BW images. It should be noted that during morphological image processing, all operations are based on two fundamental elements: erosion and dilation.

The binary erosion of A by B, denoted $A \ominus B$, is defined as the set operation $A \ominus B = \{z | B_z \subseteq A\}$. In other words, $A \ominus B$ is the set of pixel locations z, where the structuring element translated to location z overlaps only with foreground pixels in A. The detection of the image boundary can be done via subtracting the eroded image from the main image. The analysis of sperm head is attained using this boundary.

As summarized in Fig. 8.5, BW image skeletons are found in Part 2 and an operator of morphology is applied to input images. Recognition of the skeleton was performed with removal of pixels on the object boundaries using this algorithm. On the other hand, breaking apart of objects should not happen. Therefore, the image skeleton is determined by the remaining pixels. By this option the Euler number is preserved. Then, branch removal is performed behind the skeleton detection of an image. In this way, the remaining skeleton now is the same sperm backbone. Subsequently, there are two images: (1) boundary and (2) skeleton. A composite image can be produced via overlaying the two images that include only a boundary of sperm and its backbone, and analysis of the sperm head can now be performed based on standard criteria. As sperm head shape is oval, its center is considered to be along a line with maximum transverse width. The algorithm initially recognizes the nearest point between skeleton and boundary. By measuring line lengths and the connection between the backbone line and longest line, the center of the head is determined. After calculating of the head center, the head boundary can easily be recognized. In the section of experimental results of this chapter, the complete analysis is explained. The recognition of the sperm head also facilitates detection of large vacuoles and sperm head size. The vacuole (seen as a dark element within the

Fig. 8.6 Absolute length of each pixel by microscope at ×400 (**a**) and ×600 (**b**) magnification

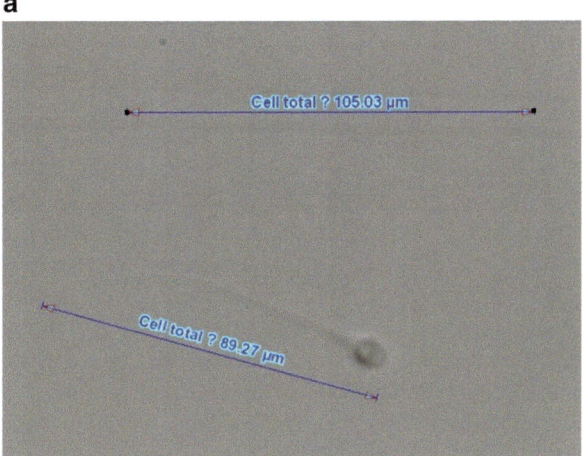

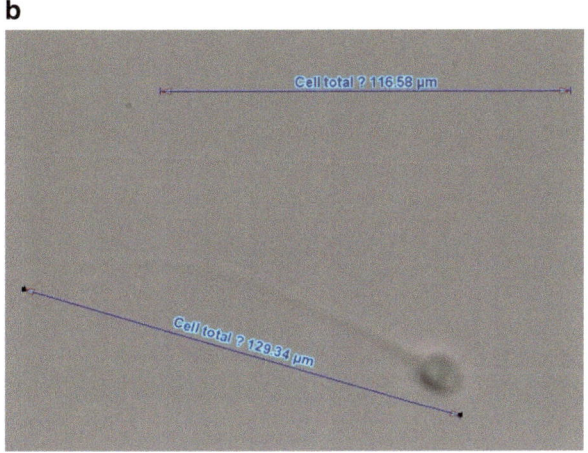

head of sperm) is associated with chromatin abnormality, DNA fragmentation, and aneuploidy [34]. In other words, sperm quality is impacted by vacuole presence, especially the presence of large vacuoles and the formation of vacuoles in the nucleus. Indeed, poor reproductive outcomes have been reported after use of sperm with large vacuoles with ICSI [34]. The algorithm identifies any gray region which represents vacuoles, from two conditions: (1) the area should be smaller than the threshold, and (2) the area should be dark. By determining sperm head area, the threshold is calculated. When the darkness of the vacuole is more than 70, this value is consistent with the presence of a large vacuole. It should be mentioned that this value was obtained from experimental studies. Proper measurement of various sperm components is an important factor in sperm selection during ICSI. If a sperm has a head that deviates from normal, the algorithm recognizes this abnormality. This algorithm requires an absolute length of each pixel (imicrometers) as captured by a calibration microscope and camera. In Fig. 8.6, this is shown at two magnification levels, ×400 and ×600, where 7.7875 pixels equal 1 μm.

Two criteria were used to validate the proposed algorithm: First, the length and width of the sperm head should be between 3–5 and 2–3 μm, respectively. Second, the width ratio of the sperm should be between three-fifths and two-thirds of the height, and sperm suitable for injection should meet both criteria. According to previous calculations, the skeleton length of the head should be equivalent to the longitude of the sperm head. Optimal tail features are as follows: uncoiled, uniform, and thinner than the midpiece. The presence of any observed abnormality in the sperm tail will change the length of the tail which must be 45 μm. Based on the equivalent micrometer in pixels, the length of the sperm was calculated as shown in Fig. 8.6. The sperm with any tail anomaly is unsuitable for injection (the presence of sperm with double tail is easily detected by the proposed SMA algorithm after the skeleton recognition, where two lines are seen as their skeleton).

The algorithm can also calculate the shape and size of the midpiece, and the presence of thin or thick midpiece was recognized in this evaluation. Another frequently encountered abnormality in sperm is a bent neck. The key element to identify the malformed midpiece (bent neck) is considered during defining the sperm skeleton. Based on previous findings, the skeleton angle on the conjunction of head border and tail should be between 150–210°. This angle can be easily calculated by comparing the slope of two lines of the corresponding angle. In this way, another anatomical abnormality in sperm (deformed neck) can be identified.

8.4 Methods and Results

Washed sperm samples were incubated at 37 °C in preparation for ICSI. During the injection process, one drop of the processed sperm was placed in 10% polyvinylpyrrolidone (PVP, Vitrolife; Sweden) and one sperm was selected for provisional injection. At the time of sperm injection, images of each sperm cell were captured at ×400 and ×600 magnification (IX70, Olympus; Japan) fitted with a CCD camera (DP71, Olympus; Japan). All images were captured using a chromatic infinity objective lenses with resolution of 576×764 pixels in RGB color space.

For sperm morphology assessment, a total of 1457 sperm images were studied; different sperm morphologies were captured first with low resolution. The diverse morphologies of sperm from different patients were entered into this dataset as human sperm morphology analysis dataset (HSMA-DS), which included both normal and abnormal sperm morphologies. Expert embryologists annotated all dataset images according to the criteria of Menkveld et al. [12]. The different sperm features including head morphology, presence of vacuoles, neck dimensions, and tail morphology were tagged as binary (0 vs. 1; where 1 = problem/abnormal and 0 = normal). Examples of normal and abnormal findings tabulated using this method are presented in Fig. 8.7.

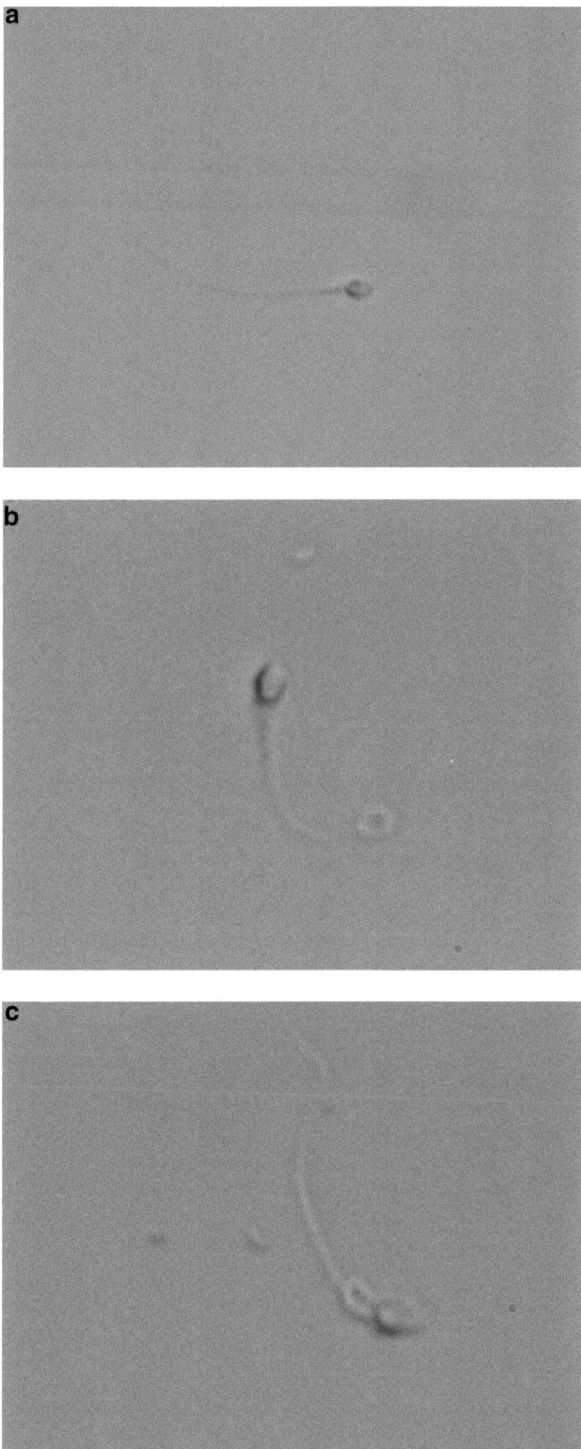

Fig. 8.7 Different sperm images: (**a**) normal, (**b**) coiled tail, (**c**) debris in image, (**d**) vacuole, (**e**) enlarged head, (**f**) amorphous head, (**g**) excess residual cytoplasm, and (**h**) abnormal midpiece (×600)

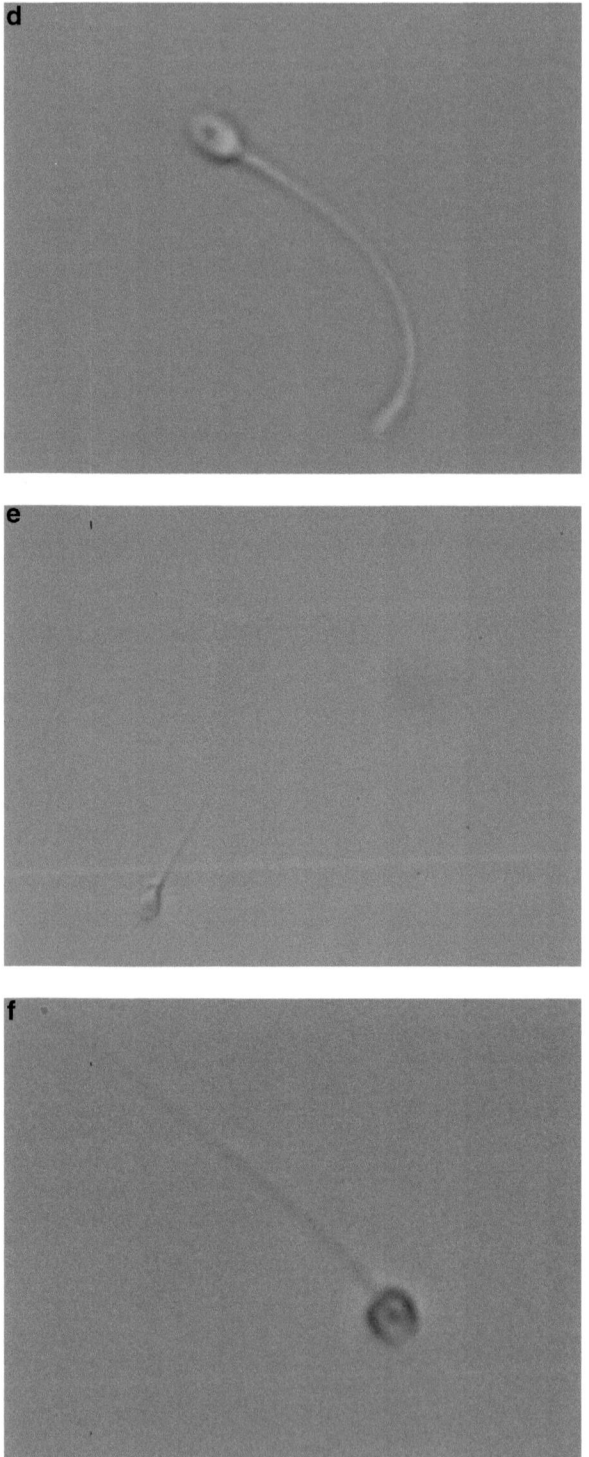

Fig. 8.7 (continued)

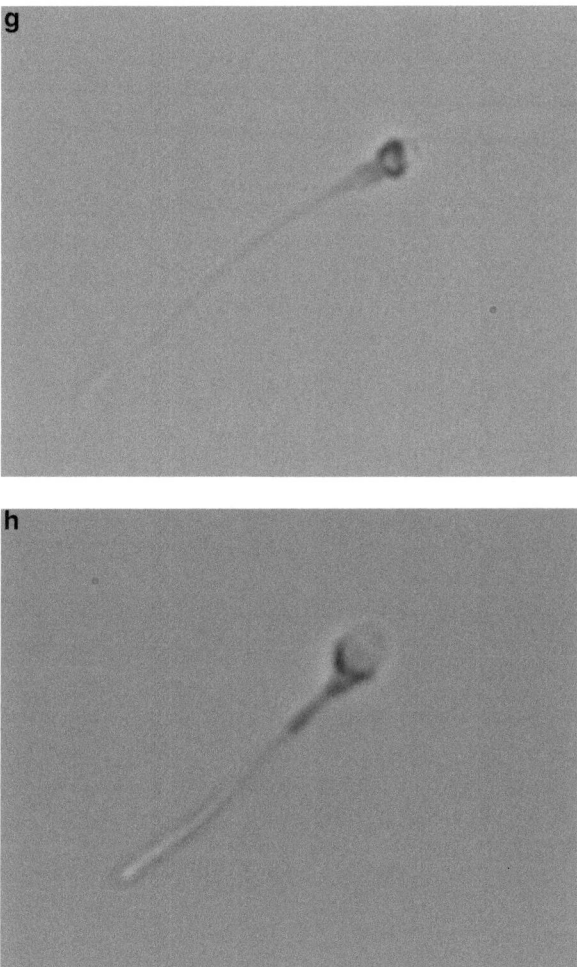

Fig. 8.7 (continued)

Each sperm image was classified based on information obtained from each patient ($n = 235$); this classification also permits comparison of sperm images among different patients. The sperm abnormalities in 1457 images from this study's dataset consist of 358 images with a large vacuole, 16 images with abnormal tails, and 502 with head/nuclear abnormalities. Overall, 750 images of normal sperm and 707 images of abnormal sperm were captured and used for ICSI performance (see Table 8.1). Note that the full dataset is freely available for academic purposes at: http://nlp.guilan.ac.ir/dataset.aspx.

Table 8.1 Distribution of sperm morphology characteristics (n) in HSMA-DS

Normal sperm	Abnormal head	Abnormal neck/tail	Total
707	502	358	1457

8.5   Evaluation Metrics

Four metrics were used to assess the SMA algorithm which include true negative (TN), true positive (TP), false negative (FN), and false positive (FP). In this study, the samples without problem are characterized as positive (P) and any problem is shown as negative (N). Therefore, aforesaid metrics can be considered as:

- TN indicatives the number of negative samples that the suggested algorithm correctly recognized.
- TP indicatives the number of positive samples that the proposed algorithm correctly recognized as positive.
- FN indicatives the number of positive samples. This means that expert embryologists tagged the samples as positive and the suggested algorithm are incorrectly also recognized as negative.
- FP indicatives the number of negative samples. This means that expert embryologists tagged the samples as negative and the suggested algorithm are incorrectly recognized as positive.

Thus, each image in the dataset was tagged as either positive or negative for different parts of sperm such as head, large vacuole, midpiece, and tail. Accuracy was also used in this study [35], which is a standard value and evaluated the suggested method. This value is computed as follows:

$$\text{Accuracy} = \frac{\text{TP} + \text{TN}}{\text{TP} + \text{FP} + \text{FN} + \text{TN}}$$

8.5.1   Noise Reduction

As noted in the dataset section, image quality, due to the low resolution microscope, is poor. The sperm identification is not easy given the considerable noise in the images. Figure 8.8 shows the steps of noise reduction. An input sperm image is shown in Fig. 8.8a, which in the RGB images is converted to YCbCr space and in Fig. 8.8b seen as Y component. Due to the high noise level in this figure, the sharpening step was performed to convert noises to edges (see Fig. 8.8c). These noises are clearly evident in this figure. To smooth the noises of the sharpened image, a Gaussian filter is applied. After applying this filter, the noise level of this image is reduced (see Fig. 8.8d). However, the residual amount of signal noise is still not acceptable for further processing.

Next, a wavelet transformation (Coiflet 2 type) can be applied on the image obtained from the Gaussian filter output. In this way, a Level 4 filter was selected and used based on the quality of sperm images. Using a lower level than 4 for filtering led to some noise remaining in the image, while there is no sensible change for filters at higher level than 4. A sample input image and the output of wavelet transform are shown in Fig. 8.9a,b, respectively. Therefore, the images without noises were produced to detect the sperm parts (see Fig. 8.9).

8.5.2 Detection of Sperm Elements

The final steps to remove noise are shown in Fig. 8.10, where images without noise include only sperm and/or debris. The Sobel algorithm is used next to define image edges (see Fig. 8.10a). The median filter is applied to remove any extraneous signals, fill in small holes, and delete small regions. Figure 8.10b shows the output image resulting from application of the median filter. These images are shown to correctly recognize different sperm components. Among the various steps of the algorithm, the aspect of successful noise reduction is perhaps the most crucial for sperm component detection.

8.6 Sperm Nucleus/Head Detection

Image analysis sequence for recognition of the sperm head are depicted in Fig. 8.11. As mentioned previously, the algorithm defines the sperm head after recognition of the cellular boundary (see Fig. 8.11b); in this way, its skeleton can be computed (see Fig. 8.11c). The output of overlaid images of boundary and skeleton (see Fig. 8.11d) allows computation of skeleton distance from each boundary point (i.e., nearest point on the skeleton); these distances appear as red lines in Fig. 8.11e. The sperm nuclear center is defined as the maximum distance between the point of skeleton and boundary. It should be noted that the skeleton size and the head length are equal, and the width of head is equal to twice the shortest line length from the head's center to the head boundary (this line is shown as green in Fig. 8.11e). To find any vacuoles, small nuclear regions are searched which have a value less than threshold value of 70.

8.7 Algorithm Performance

The ability of the algorithm to identify morphological abnormalities in sperm head, midpiece, tail, and the presence of large vacuoles was estimated using TP, TN, FP, and FN (see Table 8.2). High values for TN and TP in this study indicate the algorithm yields a satisfactory ability to achieve the diagnostic objective, in an accurate and efficient manner facilitating real-time assessment for ICSI (see Tables 8.3 and 8.4).

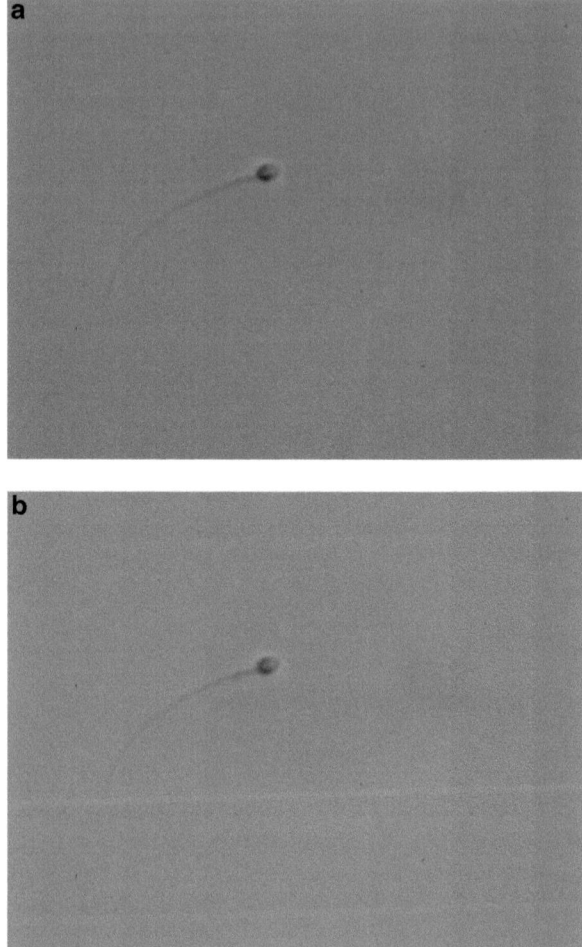

Fig. 8.8 The steps of noise reduction. (**a**) Raw input image. (**b**) Y component of image in YCbCr. (**c**) Sharpened image. (**d**) After applying Gaussian Filter

8.8 Discussion

One important characteristic of this algorithm is its ability to evaluate low resolution images. Previous investigations have assessed the utility of automated or semi-automated processes to evaluate sperm images; however, those algorithms required stained and/or high resolution images as inputs. Indeed, the algorithm described here may be applied under difficult or less than ideal conditions (i.e., unstained images with low resolution) and is thus not comparable to other existing methods.

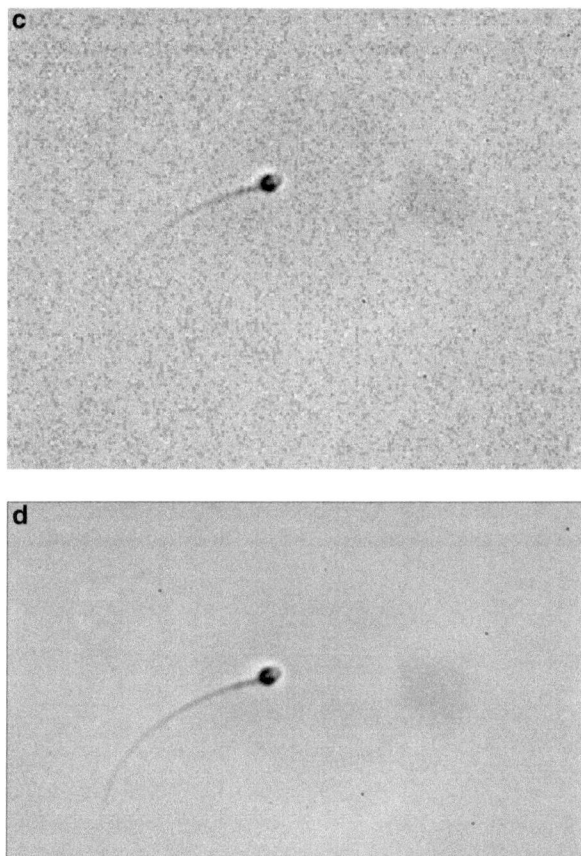

Fig. 8.8 (continued)

It should be mentioned that the TN rate to detect various sperm components is desirable, and the rate for tail abnormality recognition can easily reach 100%. The small FN rate observed with this algorithm could be ascribed to a high noise rate. For example, in the noise removal step of this algorithm, a tail section might be incorrectly deleted and thus impact the FN rate. Likewise, using the aforementioned threshold value to identify vacuoles of some blurred images was not possible and such cells were wrongly considered as normal.

On the other hand, a microscope's light reflection could itself generate some artifact which interferes in the determination of sperm size. However, the algorithm

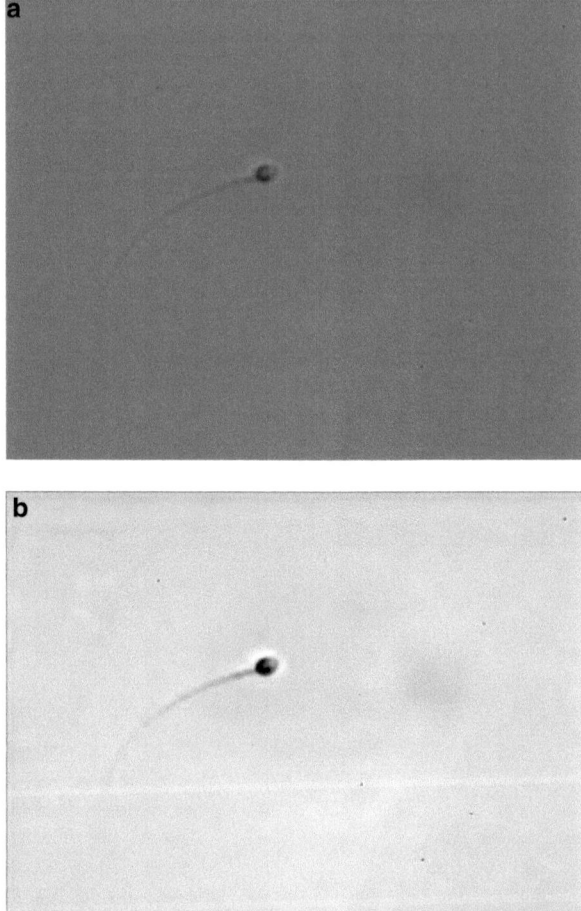

Fig. 8.9 Applying wavelet transformation. (**a**) The output of Gaussian filter, (**b**) output of the wavelet transformation

under study could successfully overcome this problem and help embryologists to measure the sperm size.

However, to the best of our knowledge, there have not been any reports describing automated detection of sperm morphology from unstained images in real-time for ICSI. In most studies, the images of stained and/or high resolution were used; stained sperm will of course not be useful for therapeutic injection for ICSI. In this way, the current algorithm aims to satisfy two requirements: desirable accuracy and speed, and also maintaining the sperm in an unaltered state for safe use in ICSI.

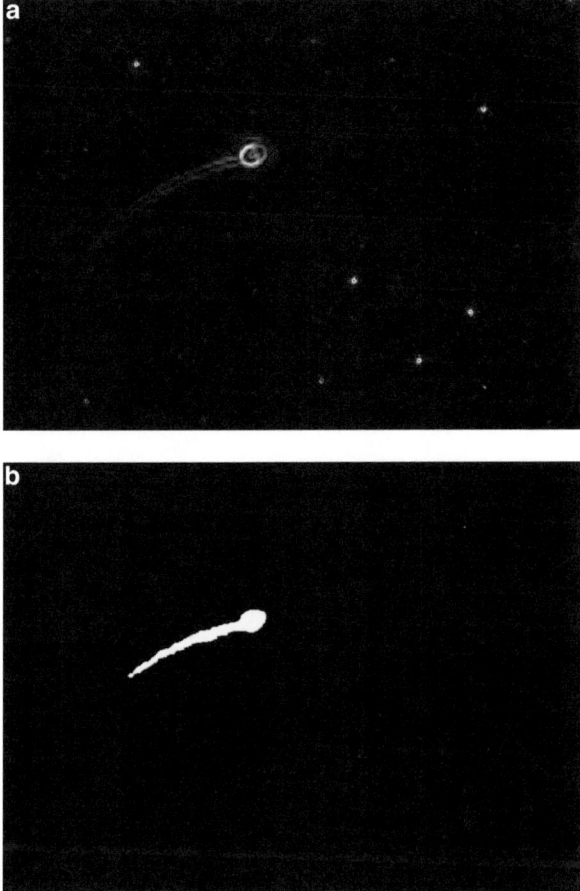

Fig. 8.10 Final stages of algorithm to remove noise. (**a**) Applying Sobel algorithm. (**b**) Applying median filter

Recognition of sperm parts requires determination of the image size automatically. In spite of the fact that this algorithm could certainly work on fixed/stained sperm images more rapidly, such staining of sperm may also modify its dimensions and are in any case would not be suitable for clinical use. In addition, the recognition of human sperm in real-time during ICSI can help to predict reproductive outcomes in other intelligent systems. The output of this method was used in a data mining system for prediction of pregnancy using each sperm [36]. Thus, the current algorithm not only could directly help during ICSI process for injection of the best sperm, but it may also be useful in other applications.

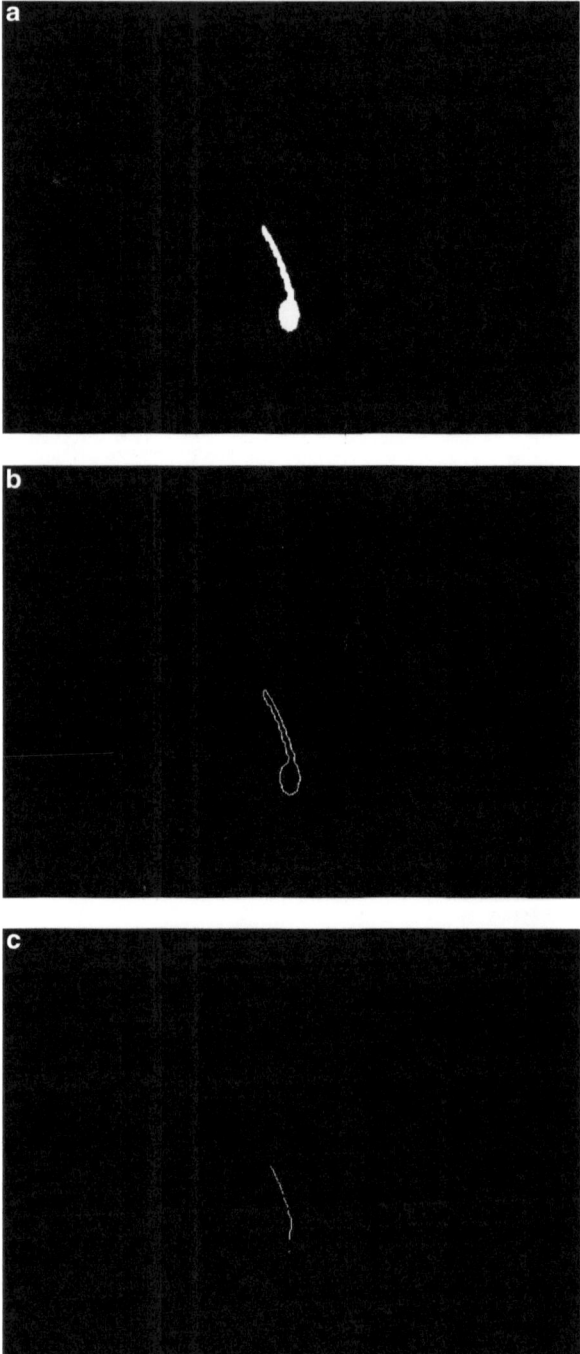

Fig. 8.11 Sperm head recognition by image analysis. (**a**) Input sperm image after noise removal, (**b**) input sperm boundary, (**c**) sperm skeleton, (**d**) overlaying of boundary and skeleton, (**e**) processed image, and (**f**) recognized sperm head/nucleus

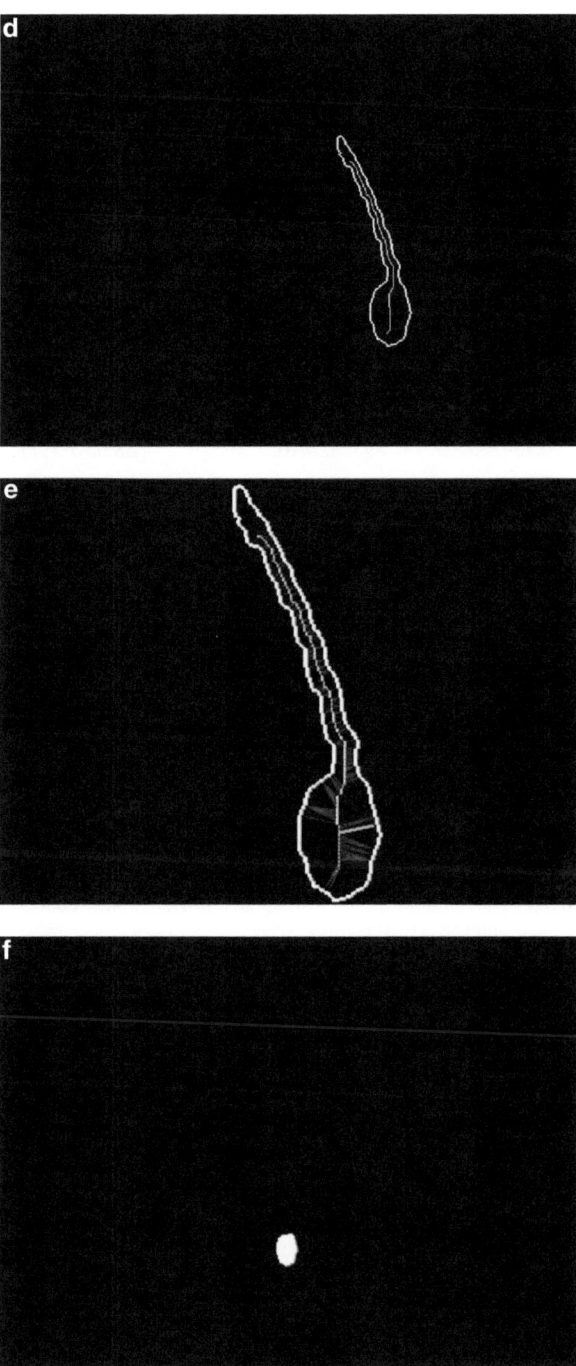

Fig. 8.11 (continued)

Table 8.2 Observed values for TP, TN, FP, and FN

	Large vacuole (*n*)		Tail and neck (*n*)		Head (*n*)	
Images analyzed (*n*)	–	+	–	+	–	+
	358	1099	16	1441	502	955
TP	309		1342		831	
TN	1013		16		452	
FP	86		0		50	
FN	49		99		124	

Table 8.3 Algorithm accuracy as observed from experimental data

	Vacuole (*n*/TN)	Tail and neck (*n*/TN)	Head (*n*/TN)	Overall (TN)
Images (*n*)	1099/1457	16/1457	502/1457	1457
Accuracy	90.73438572	93.2052162	88.05765271	90.19275145

n number, *TN* total

Table 8.4 Algorithm efficiency as a function of component steps (in seconds)

	Image noise reduction	Sperm region detection	Sperm head analysis	Sperm tail analysis	Overall process
Average time (in second)	4.793046	4.234021	0.842012	0.0000312	8.96911

Acknowledgements The authors of this study acknowledge the cooperation of the Guilan University of Medical Sciences (Rasht, Iran).

References

1. Isidori A, Latini M, Romanelli F. Treatment of male infertility. Contraception. 2005;72:314–8.
2. Stouffs K, Tournaye H, Van der Elst J, Liebaers I, Lissens W. Is there a role for the nuclear export factor 2 gene in male infertility? Fertil Steril. 2008;90:1787–91.
3. Katz D, Overstreet J, Samuels S, Niswander P, Bloom T, Lewis E. Morphometric analysis of spermatozoa in the assessment of human male fertility. J Androl. 1986;7(4):203–10.
4. WHO. World Health Organization—laboratory manual for the examination and processing of human semen. 5th ed. Geneva: World Health Organization; 2010.
5. Kobayashi T, Jinno M, Sugimura K, Nozawa S, Sugiyama T, Iida E. Sperm morphological assessment based on strict criteria and in-vitro fertilization outcome. Hum Reprod. 1991;6(7):983–6.

6. Blahova E, Machal J, Machal L, Milakovic I, Hanulakova S. Eliminating the effect of patho-morphologically formed sperm on resulting gravidity using the intracytoplasmic sperm injection method. Exp Ther Med. 2014;7:1000–4.
7. Abbiramy VS, Shanthi V. Spermatozoa segmentation and morphological parameter analysis based detection of teratozoospermia. Int J Comput Appl. 2010;3:19–23.
8. Auger J. Assessing human sperm morphology: top models, underdogs or biometrics? Asian J Androl. 2010;12(1):36–46.
9. Palermo G, Joris H, Devroey P, Van Steirteghem AC. Pregnancies after intracytoplasmic injection of single spermatozoon into an oocyte. Lancet. 1992;340:17–8.
10. Babayev SN, Park CW, Bukulmez O. Intracytoplasmic sperm injection indications: how rigorous? Semin Reprod Med. 2014;32:283–90.
11. Lo Monte G, Murisier F, Piva I, Germond M, Marci R. Focus on intracytoplasmic morphologically selected sperm injection (IMSI): a mini-review. Asian J Androl. 2013;15:608–15.
12. Menkveld R, Stander FS, Kotze TJ, Kruger TF, van Zyl JA. The evaluation of morphological characteristics of human spermatozoa according to stricter criteria. Hum Reprod. 1990;5:586–92.
13. Soler C, de Monserrat J, Gutiérrez R, Nuñez J, Nuñez M, Sancho M, et al. Use of the sperm-class analyzer for objective assessment of human sperm morphology. Int J Androl. 2003;26(5):262–70.
14. Bijar A, Benavent AP, Mikaeili M, Khayati R. Fully automatic identification and discrimination of sperm's parts in microscopic images of stained human semen smear. JBiSE. 2012;5:384–95.
15. Sánchez L, Petkov N, Alegre E. Statistical approach to boar semen evaluation using intracellular intensity distribution of head images. Cell Mol Biol. 2007;52:38–43.
16. Sánchez L, Petkov N, Alegre E. Statistical approach to boar semen head classification based on intracellular intensity distribution. In: Proceedings of the international conference on computer analysis of images and patterns, CAIP, LNCS, vol 3691. 2005. p. 88–95.
17. Otsu NA. Threshold selection method from gray-level histograms. IEEE Trans Syst Man Cybernet. 1979;9:62–6.
18. Ghasemian F, Mirroshandel SA, Monji-Azad S, Azarnia M, Zahiri Z. An efficient method for automatic morphological abnormality detection from human sperm images. Comput Methods Prog Biomed. 2015;122(3):409–20.
19. Vandewoestyne M, Van Hoofstat D, Van Nieuwerburgh F, Deforce D. Automatic detection of spermatozoa for laser capture microdissection. Int J Legal Med. 2009;123:169–75.
20. Maree L, du Plessis SS, Menkveld R, van der Horst G. Morphometric dimensions of the human sperm head depend on the staining method used. Hum Reprod. 2010;25:1369–82.
21. Alegrea E, Biehl M, Petkov N, Sanchez L. Automatic classification of the acrosome status of boar spermatozoa using digital image processing and LVQ. Comput Biol Med. 2008;38:461–8.
22. Li J, Tseng KK, Dong H, Li Y, Zhao M, Ding M. Human sperm health diagnosis with principal component analysis and K-nearest neighbor algorithm. In: IEEE in medical biometrics (ICMB), 2014 international conference on medical biometrics. 2014. p. 108–13.
23. Chang V, Saavedra JM, Castañeda V, Sarabia L, Hitschfeld N, Härtel S. Gold-standard and improved framework for sperm head segmentation. Comput Methods Prog Biomed. 2014;117(2):225–37.
24. Vicente-Fiel S, Palacín I, Santolaria P, Yániz JL. A comparative study of sperm morphometric subpopulations in cattle, goat, sheep and pigs using a computer-assisted fluorescence method (CASMA-F). Anim Reprod Sci. 2013;139:182–9.
25. Schneider CA, Rasband WS, Eliceiri KW. NIH image to ImageJ: 25 years of image analysis. Nat Methods. 2012;9:671–5.
26. Ramos L, De Boer P, Meuleman EJ, Braat DD, Wetzels AM. Evaluation of ICSI-selected epididymal sperm samples of obstructive Azoospermic males by the CKIA system. J Androl. 2004;25:406–11.

27. Yániz JL, Vicente-Fiel S, Capistrós S, Palacín I, Santolaria P. Automatic evaluation of ram sperm morphometry. Theriogenology. 2012;77:1343–50.
28. Bellastella G, Cooper TG, Battaglia M, Ströse A, Torres I, Hellenkemper B, Soler C, Sinisi AA. Dimensions of human ejaculated spermatozoa in Papanicolaou-stained seminal and swim-upsmears obtained from the integrated semen analysis system (ISAS(®)). Asian J Androl. 2010;12:871–9.
29. Rogowitz B, Pappas T, Daly S. Human vision and electronic imaging XII. In: SPIE. 2007.
30. Ibraheem NA, Hasan MM, Khan RZ, Mishra PK. Understanding color models: a review. ARPN J Sci Technol. 2012;2:265–75.
31. Hamilton E. JPEG file interchange format. C-cube microsystems; 1992.
32. Graps A. An introduction to wavelets. In: Computational science engineering, IEEE. 1995. p. 50–61.
33. Vincent OR, Folorunso O. A descriptive algorithm for sobel image edge detection. In: Proceedings of informing science & IT education conference (InSITE), vol 40. 2009. p. 97–107.
34. Park YS, Park S, Ko DS, Park DW, Seo JT, Yang KM. Observation of sperm-head vacuoles and sperm morphology under light microscope. Clin Exp Reprod Med. 2014;41:132–6.
35. Han J, Kamber M, Pei J. Data mining: concepts and techniques: concepts and techniques. 3rd ed. Burlington: Morgan Kaufmann Publisher; 2011.
36. Mirroshandel SA, Ghasemian F, Monji-Azad S. Applying data mining techniques for increasing implantation rate by selecting best sperms for intra-cytoplasmic sperm injection treatment. Comput Methods Prog Biomed. 2016;137:215–29.

Chapter 9
Clinical Approaches to Male Factor Infertility

Omer A. Raheem and Tung-Chin Hsieh

Abbreviations

ASA	Antisperm antibodies
AUA	American Urological Association
CASA	Computer-aided sperm analysis
CBAVD	Congenital bilateral absence of the vasa deferentia
CFTR	Cystic fibrosis transmembrane conductance regulator
CLIA	Clinical laboratory improvement amendments
FSH	Follicle-stimulating-hormone
HOS	Hypoosmotic swelling
ICSI	Intracytoplasmic sperm injection
IUI	Intrauterine insemination
IVF	In vitro fertilization
LH	Luteinizing hormone
MicroTESE	Microscopic testicular sperm extraction
RCTs	Randomized controlled trials
ROS	Reactive oxygen species
SA	Semen analysis
SPA	Sperm penetration assay
TRUS	Transrectal Ultrasonography
WHO	World Health Organization

O.A. Raheem
Department of Urology, University of Washington, Seattle, WA, USA
e-mail: oraheem@uw.edu

T.-C. Hsieh (✉)
Department of Urology, University of California San Diego Health, San Diego, CA, USA
e-mail: t7hsieh@ucsd.edu

© Springer International Publishing AG 2018   123
G.D. Palermo, E.S. Sills (eds.), *Intracytoplasmic Sperm Injection*,
https://doi.org/10.1007/978-3-319-70497-5_9

9.1   Introduction

Infertility is a condition with psychological, economic, and medical implications that can be difficult and stressful for both clinicians and patients alike. According to the World Health Organization (WHO), infertility is a disease of the reproductive system defined by failure to achieve clinical pregnancy after 12 months or more of regular unprotected sexual intercourse [1]. It can also be defined as failure of couple to conceive after 12 months of regular intercourse without the use of contraception in women <35 years, and after 6 months of regular intercourse without contraception in women ≥35 years [2]. After 1 year of unprotected intercourse, approximately 15% of couples of unknown fertility status are unable to conceive [3]. A male factor is solely responsible in ~30% of such couples, whereas combined male and female factors are present in an additional 20% [4]. Hence, male factor contributes to approximately 50% of infertility presentations. Nonetheless, male factor infertility is often defined by abnormal semen parameters but may be present even when the semen analysis is normal. Male infertility can be due to a variety of identifiable and reversible conditions, such as ductal obstruction and hypogonadotropic hypogonadism. Other factors are identifiable but not reversible, such as bilateral testicular atrophy secondary to gonadal insult (e.g., viral orchitis). When identification of the etiology of an abnormal semen analysis is not possible (as is the case for many patients), the condition is termed idiopathic. When the reason for infertility is unclear with a normal semen analysis and partner evaluation, the infertility is termed unexplained.

   In recent decades, the incidence of male factor infertility has been increasing as highlighted in various published studies supporting a decline in sperm quality and fertility outcomes worldwide over time [5–7]. Although analysis of retrospective data indicates that sperm counts may have declined in some parts of the world, there seems to be some geographical variation in semen quality [8]. The reason for such variance in semen characteristics is not clear, but it was postulated to be due to environmental, nutritional, socioeconomic, or other causes. The decline in semen quality coincides with an increasing incidence of abnormalities of the male genital tract including testicular cancer and cryptorchidism in various countries [7, 8]. Thus a new emphasis on evidence-based clinical practice guidelines and on consensus/expert opinion has emerged in the face of lacking adequate scientific studies. This has prompted the American Urological Association (AUA) and the American Society for Reproductive Medicine (ASRM) to produce a joint guideline covering several aspects of the evaluation and management of male infertility aiming to guide clinicians in counseling and treatment for infertile men.

9.2   Research Design and Method

Data analysis was performed via the MEDLINE, Cochrane Library Central Search, Web of Science, and Google Scholar. Initial search terms were evaluation and male factor infertility. Search results were screened for appropriate studies with particular emphasis placed on clinical and experimental studies as well as review articles. Referenced articles were screened to maximize review and inclusion of pertinent data. We utilized peer reviewed publications, review articles, and text-books discussing clinical evaluation and male factor infertility including the 2010 American Urological Association (AUA) "Best Practice" statement, optimal eval-uation of the infertile male, as part of an updated series on male infertility [9]. Additionally, data from the 2015 ASRM practice committee statement and the infertility in the male were included [10, 11]. While English language text was not a specific search parameter, only English language publications were considered.

Although inability to conceive pregnancy within 1 year of regular unprotected intercourse should trigger comprehensive infertility evaluation for the couple, an ear-lier evaluation may be warranted if (1) male infertility risk factors such as a history of bilateral cryptorchidism are known to be present; (2) female infertility risk factors, including advanced female age (over 35 years), are suspected; or (3) the couple ques-tions the male partner's fertility potential. Men who question their fertility status despite the absence of a current partner should be offered an evaluation of their fertil-ity potential. Moreover, a man may have a history of previous fertility, this does not exclude the possibility that he has acquired a new, or secondary, male infertility fac-tor. Hence, men with secondary infertility should also be evaluated in the same way as men who have never initiated a pregnancy (primary infertility) [9].

The primary goals of the evaluation of the infertile male are to identify: (1) revers-ible etiologic conditions; (2) irreversible conditions that may require the use of the assisted reproductive technique (ART) using the male partner's sperm; (3) irrevers-ible conditions not amenable to ART such that donor insemination or adoption is more advisable; (4) significant medical pathologies underlying the male's infertility; and (5) genetic etiologies that may have implications for the patient and/or his offspring.

9.3   Comprehensive Male Infertility Evaluation

9.3.1   Medical History

A careful history should be obtained including detailed and complete medical, surgi-cal, and reproductive history, including (1) coital frequency and timing; (2) duration of infertility and prior fertility; (3) childhood illnesses (e.g., bilateral cryptorchidism and developmental history); (4) systemic medical illnesses (e.g., diabetes mellitus and upper respiratory diseases) and prior surgeries; (5) sexual history including sex-ually transmitted infections; and (6) gonadal toxin exposure including heat.

9.3.2   Clinical Examination

A thorough clinical examination should be performed by a urologist or other spe-cialist in male reproduction with particular emphasis on the external genitalia including (1) examination of the penis, including the location of the urethral meatus;

(2) palpation of the testes and measurement of their size; (3) presence and consistency of both the vasa and epididymides; (4) presence of a varicocele; (5) secondary sex characteristics including body habitus, hair distribution, and breast development; and (6) digital rectal exam. The diagnosis of congenital bilateral absence of the vasa deferentia (CBAVD) is established by palpating the spermatic cord structures and vasa bilaterally. Patient should be also examined in standing position for the presence of a varicocele within the spermatic cord and the surrounding testicle. If scrotal examination is difficult or ambiguous, then scrotal ultrasound can be obtained.

9.3.3 *Endocrine Evaluation*

Hormonal profile and/or endocrine referral may be considered in some patients undergoing evaluation for male factor infertility focusing primarily on the hypothalamic-pituitary testicular axis. Endocrine disorders are uncommon in men with normal semen parameters. Despite the lack of established guidelines, advocates have suggested that infertile men should have an endocrine evaluation with hormonal profile and subsequent endocrine referral as appropriate. As per the 2010 AUA best practice statement on the optimal evaluation of the infertile male, an endocrine evaluation is indicated for men having: (1) abnormal semen parameters, particularly when the sperm concentration is <10 million/mL; (2) impaired sexual function; or (3) other clinical findings that suggest specific endocrine-related abnormalities. Moreover, it is recommended that the minimum initial hormonal evaluation should include early morning measurement of serum follicle-stimulating hormone (FSH) and total testosterone (T) levels. When the total T level is low (<300 ng/mL), further evaluation is indicated and should include a second early morning measurement of total T, free T, luteinizing hormone (LH), and prolactin (PRL) [9]. The relationships among serum T, FSH, LH, and PRL levels help delineate any endocrinopathy (see Table 9.1). For example, markedly elevated serum FSH level clearly points out to underlying defective spermatogenesis. Additional tests may include measurement of the thyroid-stimulating hormone (TSH) level obtained in men who require a more thorough endocrine evaluation. Serum inhibin B level secreted by the testicular Sertoli cells has been proposed as a marker for spermatogenesis and exerts its function to downregulate FSH synthesis and inhibits FSH secretion. Inhibin B levels are significantly lower in infertile men than in fertile men and correlate better than FSH levels with sperm parameters [12]. Owing to the higher cost of the inhibin B assay, FSH currently remains the preferred test for screening purposes.

In azoospermic men, obstructive azoospermia (OA) results in normal hormonal levels, whereas pre-testicular and some testicular abnormalities may have abnormal levels in non-obstructive azoospermia (NOA) (see Table 9.2). Furthermore, low T with elevated FSH and LH may be found in primary testicular failure (hypergonadotropic hypogonadism) such as Klinefelter's syndrome [13]. Conversely, if low T with normal to low FSH and LH levels are present, then secondary testicular failure

Table 9.1 Hormonal profile levels for various clinical conditions

Conditions	Follicle-stimulating hormone	Luteinizing hormone	Testosterone	Prolactin
Normal spermatogenesis	Normal	Normal	Normal	Normal
Hypogonadotropic hypogonadism	Low	Low	Low	Normal
Abnormal spermatogenesis	High/normal	Normal	Normal	Normal
Primary testicular failure/ hypergonadotropic hypogonadism	High	High	Normal/low	Normal
Prolactin-secreting pituitary tumor	Normal/low	Normal/low	Low	High

Adapted from Practice Committee of the American Society for Reproductive Medicine. Diagnostic evaluation of the infertile male: a committee opinion. Fertil Steril. 2015 [10]

Table 9.2 Typical hormone levels profiles observed in azoospermic men

Etiology	Follicle-stimulating hormone	Luteinizing hormone	Testosterone
Obstructive azoospermia	Normal	Normal	Normal
Non-obstructive azoospermia (NOA); pre-testicular	Low	Low	Low
NOA; exogenous testosterone	Low	Low	High
NOA; testicular	High	±High	±Low

(hypogonadotropic hypogonadism) such as Kallmann's syndrome should be considered. In addition, PRL level should be assessed to differentiate between hypogonadotropic hypogonadism (normal PRL) vs. prolactin-secreting pituitary tumor (elevated PRL). Endocrine referral may also be considered for further evaluation when indicated.

9.3.4 Semen Analysis

After completing the medical history and clinical examination, appropriate laboratory testing should be performed including semen analysis (SA). SA represents the cornerstone of the evaluation of the infertile male and defines the severity of the male factor. At least two semen samples should be evaluated, separated by at least a 1-month interval. Standard instructions for semen collection should be provided to patients including an abstinence period of 2–5 days, masturbation or coitus interruptus (not ideal as initial portion of ejaculate may be lost), or with a special seminal collection condom devoid of spermicidal agents. These condoms may be used to obtain semen at home, keeping the sample at room (or body) temperature during transport, and examined within 1 h of collection.

Table 9.3 Common reference ranges for human semen parameters by WHO, 1999 [12]

Parameters	Reference range
Volume	$\geq$2.0 mL
pH	$\geq$7.2
Sperm concentration	$\geq$20 million sperm/mL
Total sperm count per ejaculate	40 million sperm
Motility	$\geq$50% with grade A+B motility or $\geq$25% with grade A motility
Morphology	$\geq$15% by strict criteria
Viability	$\geq$75% of sperm viable
WBC (white blood cell)	< million/mL

While there are no universally accepted semen analysis reference ranges, the 1999 WHO reference values have been utilized increasingly, and for scoring sperm morphology, are in contrast to the Kruger (Tygerberg) strict morphological criteria [14, 15]. Table 9.3 summarizes the 1999 WHO reference values of semen parameters. Values that fall outside these ranges suggest male factor infertility and indicate the need for additional clinical and/or laboratory evaluation. It must be stressed that while the WHO values for semen parameters may be adequate for pregnancy by ART (including intrauterine insemination (IUI)), this should not be confused with the semen parameters necessarily for unassisted conception. Additionally, men with semen variables outside the reference ranges may still be fertile, while patients with values within the reference range may still be infertile.

In an effort to improve and standardize the semen analysis, the computer-aided sperm analysis (CASA) has been developed as a sophisticated instrument utilizing microscopic or video imaging to determine specific semen parameters. Computer-aided sperm analysis (CASA) is most useful for assessing sperm motility and motion parameters, such as velocity or speed and head movement, which may be important factors in determining sperm fertility potential [16]. While CASA remains a valuable research tool, it has not proven to be superior clinically or more cost-effective than manual assessment [17].

9.4 Semen Abnormalities

A complete semen analysis should provide accurate information on sample volume, sperm concentration, motility, and morphology. If no specific sperm abnormalities are found during this evaluation, then a female factor, inappropriate coitus habits, erectile dysfunction, defective sperm function, or antisperm antibodies should be considered. If defective sperm function is identified, then the couple should be offered in vitro fertilization (IVF) with intracytoplasmic sperm injection (ICSI). If no defective sperm function is present, IUI combined with controlled ovarian hyperstimulation or IVF may be considered.

9.4.1   Azoospermia

Azoospermia implies the absence of sperm from the semen. It should be differentiated from anejaculation in which no antegrade semen is produced. Azoospermia should not be diagnosed until the semen specimen is centrifuged at maximum speed (preferably $3000 \times g$) for 15 min, and the pellet is examined [18]. The goals of managing the azoospermic male are to determine the etiology and subsequently either treat the cause when possible, or retrieve sperm to enable IVF ICSI. Azoospermia is believed to be present in 1% of all men and accounts for 10–20% of male factor infertility [19]. Etiology of azoospermia is commonly categorized into either obstructive or post-testicular (adequate sperm production in the presence of ductal obstruction), or nonobstructive or testicular azoospermia (absence of sperm production).

Obstructive azoospermia accounts for 40% of azoospermia [19] and can result from several causes which may be due to a structural (e.g., vasectomy, prior inguinal hernia repair with mesh, prior hydrocele repair, orchiopexy), congenital bilateral absence of the vasa deferentia (CBAVD), chlamydial or gonococcal infection, or a functional problem (e.g., drug-induced anejaculation, spinal injury, neurological disease, prior retroperitoneal surgery). Men with obstructive azoospermia classically have normal FSH and normal testes on clinical examination and ultrasound. Patients with CBAVD can also have absent or atretic mullerian duct structures. CBAVD is usually associated with a mutation in cystic fibrosis transmembrane conductance regulator (CFTR) and is often seen with renal agenesis requiring renal sonographic evaluation [20, 21].

Nonobstructive azoospermia may also be classified into pre-testicular causes (hypogonadotropic hypogonadism) such as Kallmann's syndrome (anosmia, delayed puberty), post pituitary surgery, or exogenous testosterone. Testicular NOA (hypergonadotropic hypogonadism) is associated with impaired spermatogenesis such as Klinefelter's syndrome (47,XXY), maldescended testes/torsion, varicocele, testicular cancer, drugs, steroid abuse, chemotherapy, gonadotoxins, as well as mumps orchitis. Pre-testicular and post-testicular azoospermia are often treatable, whereas testicular causes (except azoospermia associated with varicocele) are generally uncorrectable [15].

In addition to the semen analysis and endocrinologic evaluation, genetic testing is also indicated in the setting of azoospermia, particularly karyotyping, Y-chromosome microdeletion analysis, and cystic fibrosis transmembrane conductance regulator (CFTR) mutation. For example, in Y-chromosome abnormalities, three microdeletions (AZFa, AZFb, and AZFc) on the long arm of the Y-chromosome (Yq) account for about 7% of severely oligospermic/azoospermic males [22]. AZFa (associated with Sertoli cell only syndrome) and AZFb (associated with maturation arrest) patients are azoospermic [23]. AZFc has a variable phenotype ranging from azoospermia to oligospermia [24]. Men with nonobstructive azoospermia should be tested for Y-chromosome microdeletions—if ICSI is utilized, these aberrations will be passed onto male children [25]. If AZFa or AZFb microdeletions are detected, it is highly unlikely that any sperm will be found and thus microscopic testicular sperm extraction (microTESE) is not indicated [26]. However, there is up to 70% sperm retrieval rate with AZFc with microTESE [23]. Cystic fibrosis (CF) is another genetic disorder attributed to an autosomal recessive disorder closely associated with CBAVD [27] which affects 1% of infertile men [28]. Therefore in infertile patients with CBAVD, testing for CF in both parents and referral to a genetic counselor should be offered [13]. Additional consideration for genetic evaluation in Klinefelter's syndrome is warranted, as this is the most common chromosomal abnormality (affecting one in 600 phenotypic males) accounting for approximately 15% of nonobstructive azoospermia [29]. The non-mosaic "classical" form (47,XXY) accounts for 80–90% of Klinefelter's syndrome cases [30]. Clinically, these men have small, firm testicles (volume <5 cm³) [31] and may demonstrate normal virilization, with scant or a typical female hair distribution.

Radiographic studies have a limited role in the evaluation of azoospermic men. In men with suspected ejaculatory duct obstruction, transrectal ultrasound (TRUS) may identify dilation of seminal vesicles. Likewise, testicular biopsy also has limited indication for azoospermia evaluation. If testicular biopsy is planned, a simultaneously cryopreservation of sperm should be included to enable future ICSI.

9.4.2   Oligoasthenoteratospermia (OATS)

OATS implies defect in sperm density, motility, and morphology, and often associated with varicocele. Additional causes of OATS are endocrinologic abnormality, environmental gonadotoxins, medications, and cryptorchidism.

9.4.3   Asthenospermia

Asthenospermia implies defect in sperm movement. This may be manifested by a low sperm motility or poor forward progression. Prolonged abstinence periods, genital tract infections associated with pyospermia, antisperm antibodies (ASA), spermatozoal ultrastructural defects, partial ejaculatory duct obstruction, varicoceles, defective transport through the genital ductal system, and idiopathic causes may result in asthenospermia. If antisperm antibodies (ASA) are present, patients may be treated with immunosuppressive steroids; however, the effectiveness of this medical treatment is low and there is risk of serious side effects such as aseptic hip necrosis; more commonly, patients are directed towards IUI or ICSI. In addition, spermatozoal ultrastructural defects should also be considered when evaluating asthenospermia particularly if a high proportion of viable sperm with extremely low motility are noted. The most common of such sperm abnormality includes primary ciliary dyskinesia (immotile cilia syndrome); when this disorder presents with situs inversus, it is known as Kartagener syndrome.

9.4.4 Teratoazoospermia

Teratoazoospermia signifies defects in sperm morphology. Although the methods for routine measurement of sperm concentration and motility have changed little during the past two decades, sperm morphology assessment has evolved considerably. The 1999 WHO criteria for scoring sperm morphology and the Kruger (Tygerberg) strict criteria are both widely used [14, 15]. When any strict criteria are applied to the evaluation of sperm morphology, relatively few sperm are classified as having normal morphology, even in semen from fertile men. Sperm morphology might be an indicator of function and has been used to identify couples who have a poor chance of fertilization with IVF, and a better chance of fertilization with ICSI [15, 32]. The majority of teratoazoospermia cases are liked genetically determined, and repair of varicoceles and correction of scrotal temperature insults rarely improve sperm morphology. Rare ultrastructural defects, such as the presence of round-headed sperms (globozoospermia) are characterized by an absence of acrosome [19, 33]. While IVF ICSI is a treatment option, fertility outcome has been poor.

9.5 Additional Laboratory Tests

9.5.1 Post-ejaculatory Urinalysis (PEU)

Ejaculation involves a coordinated series of events including the deposition of semen in the posterior urethra, opening of its external sphincter, and closure of the bladder neck. Ejaculatory dysfunction can be found in diabetic men or spinal cord injury patients. The presence of sperm in the post-ejaculate urinalysis (PEU) is usually considered diagnostic of retrograde ejaculation. However, there is no consensus on the minimum number required for a PEU to be considered positive [34]. Moreover, the presence of sperm in the PEU may be due to either true retrograde ejaculation or residual sperm in the urethra that are washed out with voiding. Additionally, low-volume or absent antegrade ejaculate suggests incomplete semen collection, lack of emission, or ejaculatory duct obstruction. It is important also to determine whether an improper or incomplete collection or a very short abstinence interval (<1 day) might be the cause. After ruling out collection error, PEU should be performed in men with low ejaculate volume <1.0 mL. PEU is performed by centrifuging the urine specimen for 10 min at 300g, followed by microscopic examination of the pellet at ×400 magnification.

9.6   Imaging

Options include ultrasound (US), magnetic resonance imaging (MRI), or more invasive methods including vasography.

9.6.1   Scrotal Ultrasound (US)

Careful clinical examination can identify most scrotal pathology including varicoceles, spermatoceles, absent vasa, epididymal induration, and testicular masses. Scrotal US can also verify testis size, and observe for absence of structures as well as for evidence of obstruction including spermatocele or dilatation of vas/epididymis/rete testis or occult varicocele [10]. Scrotal US can be helpful if the physical examination is difficult because of body habitus, testicular pain or if the examination findings are equivocal or ambiguous. Scrotal US should be considered for men presenting with risk factors for malignancy, such as abnormal testicular exam, cryptorchidism, or a previous testicular cancer.

9.6.2   Transrectal Ultrasound (TRUS)

TRUS is most useful to identify ejaculatory duct obstruction, dilated seminal vesicles or ejaculatory ducts and/or midline cystic prostatic structures. An anterior-posterior diameter of the seminal vesicle greater than 15 mm is suggestive of ejaculatory duct obstruction [35]. US-guided aspiration of the vesicles with a 22G needle can be simultaneously performed, and more than one to two sperm per high power field suggests obstruction [36]. TRUS-guided aspiration can also be a useful sperm retrieval technique in select cases to enable ICSI.

9.6.3   Renal Ultrasound

Patients with CBAVD usually have hypoplastic seminal vesicles with abnormal mullerian duct structures and often present with renal agenesis requiring renal US for evaluation [20, 21]. Similarly, renal US should also be performed when unilateral absence of the vas is noted—20% will have ipsilateral renal agenesis [37].

9.6.4   Magnetic Resonance Imaging (MRI)

MRI can help identify ejaculatory duct/prostatic cysts. It enables evaluation of the vas deferens and seminal vesicles in high resolution and may indicate a point of obstruction [38]. The role for routine utilization of MRI is not yet established.

9.6.5   Vasography

Vasography is an invasive investigation used to identify the site of vasal obstruction. It is rarely used in purely diagnostic situations and requires microsurgical skills. It is an open procedure, usually undertaken as part of a therapeutic intervention during vasal reconstruction. It can also localize the site of obstruction due to iatrogenic injury such as post inguinal hernia repair. Several methods have been described including vasopuncture, hemisection as well as endoscopic retrograde vasography. Vasopuncture involves placement of a fine needle into the lumen of the vas to inject contrast. Alternatively, hemisection of the vas can be performed under an operating microscope with a micro-knife. The vasal fluid should be examined—if no sperm are present, the etiology is either epididymal obstruction or nonobstructive azoospermia. Normal saline (via a 24G cannula) can then be injected into the distal segment—if it passes easily, there is likely to be no obstruction. Indigo carmine can be injected and a cystoscopy or indwelling catheter can confirm the presence of dye, indicative of a patent system. Contrast vasography is rarely indicated as most etiologies can be diagnosed by the preoperative investigations as well as the above maneuvers. If hernia mesh is thought to be the culprit, a prolene suture can be passed down the vas to measure the distance to the obstruction. Once vasography is complete, the defect (if hemisection performed) can be closed with 8-0 to 10-0 nylon suture. Complications include hematoma, granuloma, and stricture—the procedure can itself cause vasal obstruction [39]. If the injected saline/indigo carmine reaches the urine, then epididymal obstruction is diagnosed and vasoepididymostomy (VE) should be performed [37].

9.6.6   Adjunct Semen and Sperm Tests

In selected settings, specialized tests for semen can be performed to improve the diagnostic evaluation of the infertile male when the previously noted evaluations fail to identify an infertility etiology. Generally, such specialized tests should be reserved for circumstances where results would clearly influence treatment.

9.7   Pyospermia

Pyospermia implies the presence of white blood cells (WBC) in semen, often associated with deficiencies in sperm function and motility. Under wet-mount microscopy, WBC and immature germ cells appear quite similar and are both properly described as "round cells." Hence, it is the responsibility of the treating physician to differentiate between the two types when evaluating infertile men, utilizing special cytologic staining and immunohistochemical techniques [40]. Men with true pyospermia (>1 M leukocytes/mL) should be specifically evaluated to exclude genital tract infection or inflammation. Although controversial, suggested treatments have included empiric antibiotic therapy, anti-inflammatory medications, frequent ejaculation, and prostatic massage. Despite a lack of proven efficacy, consideration may be given to semen processing to remove WBC and the processed sperms may be then utilized for IUI or IVF [41].

9.8   Antisperm Antibodies (ASA)

Despite the availability of ASA assays for many years, the indications for testing, interpretation of results, and management of the immunogenic infertility remain a topic of controversy. Traditionally, ASA test has been performed when the SA reveals an isolated asthenospermia (with normal sperm concentration), sperm agglutination, or unexplained infertility. ASA can be found in the serum, in the seminal plasma, or bound directly to sperm. ASA can form when there is a breach in the blood-testis barrier and the immune system is exposed to large quantities of sperm antigens, or after vasectomy. Additional risk factors for ASA formation include prior testicular trauma, torsion, biopsy, orchitis, testicular cancer, and vasectomy. Whereas indirect antibody agglutination assays are used to detect ASA in serum or seminal plasma, a direct immunobead test is used to detect ASA (IgG and IgA) bound to the sperm head or tail. Sperm-bound antibodies are thought to be clinically important because they can decrease motility, block penetration of the cervical mucus, and prevent fertilization, thereby decreasing the likelihood for conception [42]. Management strategies have ranged from attempts to decrease the production of ASA to semen processing technique to remove ASA, or the use of ICSI to bypass potential problems induced by the ASA [43].

9.9   Sperm Viability

Sperm viability can be assessed by mixing fresh semen with a supravital dye such as eosin or trypan blue, or by the use of the hypoosmotic swelling (HOS) test [12]. These assays determine whether non-motile sperm are viable by identifying which sperm have intact cell membranes. In dye tests, viable sperm actively exclude the dye and remain colorless, whereas nonviable sperm readily take up the stain. Immotile but viable sperm, as determined by the HOS test, may be used successfully for ICSI. The role of sperm viability testing is limited in the modern era of ART.

9.10   Sperm Deoxyribonucleic Acid (DNA) Integrity Test

DNA integrity testing refers to a variety of assays utilized to evaluate the degree of sperm DNA fragmentation. In addition to poor reproductive outcomes, sperm DNA damage is also associated with increased rate of spontaneous recurrent miscarriage.

Although contemporary data relating to the relationship between abnormal DNA integrity and reproductive outcomes are limited, the effect of abnormal sperm DNA fragmentation on the value of IUI or IVF and ICSI results may be clinically informative [44, 45]. A study by Bungum et al. has suggested that abnormal DNA integrity in the sample used for IUI was highly predictive of pregnancy [46]. Without further studies, there is inadequate evidence to suggest the assay has prognostic value when performed prior to initiation of IUI. A meta-analysis of published studies has found a small statistically significant predictive effect of DNA integrity results upon pregnancy rates for IVF with or without ICSI [47, 48]. Of note, sperm retrieved from the testis were shown to have reduced DNA fragmentation in men with abnormal ejaculated sperm DNA integrity [49]. There is growing evidence suggesting improved IVF outcomes using testicular sperm in men with abnormal sperm DNA fragmentation in cases of miscarriage or failed previous ART [45]. However, the effect of an abnormal DNA integrity test on pregnancy rates is too small to warrant routine testing prior to ART at the present time.

9.11 Miscellaneous Tests

A number of biochemical tests of sperm function have been studied, including measurement of sperm creatine kinase and reactive oxygen species (ROS). ROS appear to be generated by both seminal leukocytes and sperm cells and can interfere with sperm function by peroxidation of sperm lipid membranes and creation of toxic fatty acid peroxides [50, 51]. Additionally, ROS have not been shown to be predictive of pregnancy independent of routine semen parameters nor are there any proven therapies to correct an abnormal test result. There is insufficient data to support the routine use of reactive oxygen species testing in the management of the male partner of an infertile couple. Other tests and procedures have been used to select sperm for ICSI and may identify sperms with better quality, including hyaluronic acid binding, membrane maturity testing, apoptotic evaluation, and magnified sperm examination [52]. However, these tests have a very limited role in the evaluation of male infertility because they have limited clinical utility and typically do not affect treatment.

9.12 Functional Assays

The standard SA measures objective parameters of semen such as sperm count, motility, and seminal volume. Although these variables may correlate with fertilization, they do not directly measure any processes required for fertilization. For fertilization to occur in vivo, a sperm must be able to reach the site of the ovum by traversing the cervical mucus, undergo capacitation and the acrosome reaction, fuse with the oolemma, and be incorporated into the ooplasm. There are currently a variety of functional assays that measure the ability of the sperms to progress through these various stages.

9.12.1 Sperm–Cervical Mucus Interaction Test

The post-coital test (PCT) is the microscopic examination of the cervical mucus, performed shortly before expected ovulation and within hours after intercourse, to identify the presence of motile sperm in the mucus. Although PCT is the traditional method for identifying cervical factors which may contribute to infertility, an abnormal cervical mucus or abnormal sperm/cervical mucus interaction is rarely the primary cause of infertility. Despite its controversies, some clinicians advocate that PCT may help in identifying ineffective coital practices or perhaps some cervical factor not otherwise suspected on the basis of history and physical examination [53]. Nonetheless, contemporary infertility treatments such as ovarian hyperstimulation with IUI or IVF with ICSI can effectively negate any unrecognized cervical factor.

9.12.2 Zona-Free Hamster Oocyte Test

The sperm penetration assay (SPA) entails the removal of the zona pellucida from hamster oocytes, which allows human sperm to fuse with hamster ova. For penetration to occur, sperm must undergo capacitation, the acrosome reaction, fusion with the oolemma, and incorporation into the ooplasm [54]. This test now has a very limited role in modern ART and should only be reserved for patients in whom results will influence treatment strategy.

9.13 Miscellaneous

The acrosome reaction of human sperm can be detected using specialized staining techniques. Rates of spontaneous acrosome reactions and acrosome reactions induced by agents such as calcium ionophore and progesterone are well documented, and samples from infertile men tend to demonstrate lower induced acrosome reaction levels than fertile men [55]. These tests are important investigative tools, but are not clinically useful to be incorporated into routine evaluation of the infertile men.

9.14 Genetic Testing

A number of genetic disorders may result in infertility by affecting sperm production or sperm transport. Classically, there are at least three genetic factors known to be related to male infertility: (1) cystic fibrosis gene mutations associated with congenital absence of the vas deferens; (2) chromosomal abnormalities resulting in impaired testicular function; and (3) Y-chromosome microdeletions associated with isolated spermatogenic impairment. Genetic testing is an important part of the workup for azoospermia, especially when considering nonobstructive azoospermia, as there is an increased frequency of chromosomal translocations, duplications, deletions, and inversions [13].

9.14.1 Autosomal Disorders: Cystic Fibrosis (CF)

Cystic fibrosis (CF) is an autosomal recessive disorder that affects 1/2500 Caucasian newborns and has a carrier frequency of 4%. CF is characterized by the presence of thick and viscid secretions in the lungs, pancreas, intestines, and liver. Such abnormal secretions result in the formation of plugs that obstruct the ductal lumens in these organs, causing dilatations, frequent infections, and fibrosis. The viscid secretions result from a failure of epithelial cells to transport chloride, sodium ions, and water to the lumen of epithelial tubes. This dysfunction itself is in turn due to a mutation in the CFTR gene, which encodes a chloride channel protein. It should be noted that CF gene mutations are the most common genetic error resulting in azoospermia. Moreover, CF is due to a mutation often associated with congenital bilateral agenesis of the vas deferens (CBAVD) in at least 95% of men [27]. The condition affects at least 6% of cases of obstructive azoospermia and 1% of infertile men [28]. Patients with CBAVD due to CFTR mutations are at risk of having both male and female offspring with CF and male offspring with CBAVD, given the relatively high carrier rate of CFTR mutations (e.g., 4% in the Caucasian population). For this reason, both partners should be screened prior to ART to estimate risk for transmitting CFTR mutations to offspring [13].

9.14.2 Gonosomal Abnormalities: Klinefelter's Syndrome

Klinefelter's syndrome is the most common chromosomal abnormality (affecting one in 600 phenotypic males) and accounts for approximately 15% of nonobstructive azoospermia [29]. The non-mosaic "classical" form (47,XXY) accounts for 80–90% of KS cases [30]. Clinically, these men have small firm testicles (less than 5 cm³) [31] and may demonstrate normal virilization, scant or typical female hair distribution. The mechanisms of infertility associated with Klinefelter's syndrome include a lack of testicular growth, premature degeneration of the primordial germ cells before puberty, and the early or late maturation arrest of spermatogenesis at the primary spermatocyte stage. Later stages of sperm development can also be affected [56]. In addition to small firm testes, gynecomastia (40%) and features of male hypogonadism are also present, such as sparse facial and pubic hair growth, loss of libido, and erectile dysfunction. Low testosterone is observed in as many as 80% of men, an effect attributed to small testicular growth despite the presence of Leydig cell hyperplasia. Several studies have demonstrated that Klinefelter's syndrome patients exhibit a high incidence of aneuploid gametes, rendering them at risk for producing offspring with chromosomal abnormalities [57]. Interestingly, the successful fathering of 60 children has been achieved by TESE and ICSI in men with Klinefelter's syndrome. Karyotype studies that were performed on approximately 50 children revealed no chromosomal abnormalities [58, 59]. Further clarification was provided by Sciurano et al., who detected spermatogenesis foci in testicular biopsies of 6/11 men with non-mosaic Klinefelter's [60]. Whereas the majority of seminiferous tubules are devoid of germ cells, 8–24% do contain germ cells. In addition, Sciurano et al. examined the chromosomal complements of 92 meiotic spermatocytes using fluorescent in situ hybridization (FISH). These spermatocytes exhibited euploidy and the ability to form haploid gametes [60]. These novel findings may explain the high rate of normal children who are born following TESE and ICSI. Notwithstanding this high rate of children born with no detectable genetic imbalance, there is still a risk of genetic defects in the offspring. Thus it is advised that a preimplantation genetic screening (PGS) be offered prior to ART to ensure that the offspring are not aneuploid [56].

9.14.3   Y-chromosome Abnormalities

Three microdeletions (AZFa, AZFb, and AZFc) on the long arm of the Y-chromosome (Yq) account for ~7% of severely oligospermic/azoospermic males [22]. AZFa (associated with Sertoli cell only syndrome) and AZFb (associated with maturation arrest) patients are azoospermic [23]. AZFc has a variable phenotype ranging from azoospermia to oligospermia [24]. Men with nonobstructive azoospermia should be tested for microdeletions—if ICSI is utilized, these aberrations will be passed onto male children [25]. In certain countries, preimplantation embryo sex selection may be utilized in such cases. If AZFa or AZFb microdeletions are detected, it is highly unlikely that any sperm will be found and thus microTESE is not indicated [26]. However, there is up to 70% chance of finding sperm with AZFc and thus micro-TESE may be considered [23].

9.15   Conclusion

The goal of the male fertility evaluation is to identify any correctable factors, identify any potential life-threatening conditions, and minimize the complexity of any ART required. Initial clinical evaluation is based on complete medical history, clinical examination, and semen analysis. Limitations still exist in the understanding of male infertility. Advancements in laboratory medicine have provided additional sperm function testing with an evolving role. Despite the popular belief that ICSI is a cure for all cases of infertility, optimal fertility outcomes can only be achieved when male and female fertility specialists work collaboratively.

References

1. Zegers-Hochschild F, Adamson GD, de Mouzon J, Ishihara O, Mansour R, Nygren K, et al. International Committee for Monitoring Assisted Reproductive Technology (ICMART) and the World Health Organization (WHO) revised glossary of ART terminology, 2009. Fertil Steril. 2009;92:1520–4.
2. Practice Committee of the American Society for Reproductive Medicine. Definitions of infertility and recurrent pregnancy loss. Fertil Steril. 2008;90(5 Suppl):S60.
3. Stephen EH, Chandra A. Declining estimates of infertility in the United States: 1982–2002. Fertil Steril. 2006;86:516–23.
4. Thonneau P, Marchand S, Tallec A, Ferial ML, Ducot B, Lansac J, et al. Incidence and main causes of infertility in a resident population (1,850,000) of three French regions (1988–1989). Hum Reprod. 1991;6(6):811.
5. Carlsen E, Giwercman A, Keiding N, Skakkebaek NE. Evidence for decreasing quality of semen during past 50 years. BMJ. 1992;305:609–13.
6. Auger J, Kunstmann JM, Czyglik F, Jouannet P. Decline in semen quality among fertile men in Paris during the past 20 years. N Engl J Med. 1995;332:281–5.
7. Lackner J, Schatzl G, Waldhör T, Resch K, Kratzik C, Marberger M. Constant decline in sperm concentration in infertile males in an urban population: experience over 18 years. Fertil Steril. 2005;84(6):1657.
8. Swan SH. Semen quality in fertile US men in relation to geographical area and pesticide exposure. Int J Androl. 2006;29:62–8.
9. Jarow J, Sigman M, Koletttis PN, Lipshultz LI, McClure RD, Nangia AK, Naughton CK, Prins GS, Sandlow JI, Schlegel PN. Optimal evaluation of the infertile male: AUA best practice statement. AUA Publication; 2010. p. 1–38.
10. Practice Committee of the American Society for Reproductive Medicine. Diagnostic evaluation of the infertile male: a committee opinion. Fertil Steril. 2015;103(3):e18–25.
11. Lipshultz LI, Howards SS, Niederberger CS. Infertility in the male. 4th ed. New York: Cambridge University Press; 2009.
12. Kumanov P, Nandipati K, Tomova A, Agarwal A. Inhibin B is a better marker of spermatogenesis than other hormones in the evaluation of male factor infertility. Fertil Steril. 2006;86:332–8.
13. American Urological Association. The management of obstructive azoospermia: AUA Best Practice Statement 2010. https://www.auanet.org/education/guidelines/male-infertility. Accessed Feb 2016.
14. World Health Organization. WHO laboratory manual for the examination of human semen and sperm-cervical mucus interaction. 4th ed. New York: Cambridge University Press; 1999.
15. Kruger TF, Acosta AA, Simmons KF, et al. Predictive value of abnormal sperm morphology in in vitro fertilization. Fertil Steril. 1988;49:112.
16. Suarez SS, Ho HC. Hyperactivation of mammalian sperm. Cell Mol Biol. 2003;49(3):351–6.
17. Amann RP, Katz DF. Reflections on CASA after 25 years. J Androl. 2004;25(3):317–25.
18. Corea M, Campagnone J, Sigman M. The diagnosis of azoospermia depends on the force of centrifugation. Fertil Steril. 2005;83(4):920–2.
19. Jarow JP, Espeland MA, Lipshultz LI. Evaluation of the azoospermic patient. J Urol. 1989;142(1):62–5.
20. Oates RD, Amos JA. The genetic basis of congenital bilateral absence of the vas deferens and cystic fibrosis. J Androl. 1994;15(1):1–8.
21. Schlegel PN, Shin D, Goldstein M. Urogenital anomalies in men with congenital absence of the vas deferens. J Urol. 1996;155(5):1644–8.

22. Stahl PJ, Masson P, Mielnik A, Marean MB, Schlegel PN, Paduch DA. A decade of experience emphasizes that testing for Y microdeletions is essential in American men with azoospermia and severe oligozoospermia. Fertil Steril. 2010;94(5):1753–6.
23. Hotaling JM. Genetics of male infertility. Urol Clin North Am. 2014;41(1):1–17.
24. Krausz C. Y chromosome and male infertility. Andrologia. 2005;37(6):219–23.
25. Lynch M, Cram DS, Reilly A, et al. The Y chromosome gr/gr subdeletion is associated with male infertility. Mol Hum Reprod. 2005;11(7):507–12.
26. Jungwirth A, Giwercman A, Tournaye H, et al. European Association of Urology guidelines on male infertility: the 2012 update. Eur Urol. 2012;62(2):324–32.
27. Chillón M, Casals T, Mercier B, et al. Mutations in the cystic fibrosis gene in patients with congenital absence of the vas deferens. N Engl J Med. 1995;332(22):1475–80.
28. Yu J, Chen Z, Ni Y, Li Z. CFTR mutations in men with congenital bilateral absence of the vas deferens (CBAVD): a systemic review and meta-analysis. Hum Reprod. 2012;27(1):25–35.
29. Ghorbel M, Gargouri Baklouti S, Ben Abdallah F, et al. Chromosomal defects in infertile men with poor semen quality. J Assist Reprod Genet. 2012;29(5):451–6.
30. Bojesen A, Gravholt CH. Klinefelter syndrome in clinical practice. Nat Clin Pract Urol. 2007;4(4):192–204.
31. Yoshida A, Miura K, Shirai M. Cytogenetic survey of 1,007 infertile males. Urol Int. 1997;58(3):166–76.
32. Pisarska MD, Casson PR, Cisneros PL, et al. Fertilization after standard in vitro fertilization versus intracytoplasmic sperm injection in subfertile males using sibling oocytes. Fertil Steril. 1999;71:627.
33. Singh G. Ultrastructural features of round-headed human spermatozoa. Int J Fertil. 1992;37(2):99–102.
34. Mehta A, Jarow JP, Maples P, Sigman M. Defining the "normal" postejaculate urinalysis. J Androl. 2012;33:917–20.
35. Jarow JP. Transrectal ultrasonography of infertile men. Fertil Steril. 1993;60:1035–9.
36. Engin G, Celtik M, Sanli O, Aytac O, Muradov Z, Kadioglu A. Comparison of transrectal ultrasonography and transrectal ultrasonography-guided seminal vesicle aspiration in the diagnosis of the ejaculatory duct obstruction. Fertil Steril. 2009;92(3):964–70.
37. Sigman M, Jarow JP. Male infertility. In: Campbell MF, Wein AJ, Kavoussi LR, editors. Campbell-Walsh urology. 9th ed. Philadelphia: Saunders; 2007. p. 638.
38. Ammar T, Sidhu PS, Wilkins CJ. Male infertility: the role of imaging in diagnosis and management. Br J Radiol. 2012;85(Spec No 1):S59–68.
39. Poore RE, Schneider A, DeFranzo AJ, Humphries ST, Woodruff RD, Jarow JP. Comparison of puncture versus vasotomy techniques for vasography in an animal model. J Urol. 1997;158(2):464–6.
40. Wolff H, Anderson DJ. Immunohistologic characterization and quantitation of leukocyte subpopulations in human semen. Fertil Steril. 1988;49:497–504.
41. Yanushpolsky EH, Politch JA, Hill JA, Anderson DJ. Antibiotic therapy and leukocytospermia: a prospective, randomized, controlled study. Fertil Steril. 1995;63(1):142–7.
42. Ayvaliotis B, Bronson R, Rosenfeld D, Cooper G. Conception rates in couples where autoimmunity to sperm is detected. Fertil Steril. 1985;43:739–42.
43. Check ML, Check JH, Katsoff D, Summers-Chase D. ICSI as an effective therapy for male factor with antisperm antibodies. Arch Androl. 2000;45:125–30.
44. Spano M, Bonde JP, Hjollund HI, et al. Sperm chromatin damage impairs human fertility. The Danish First Pregnancy Planner Study Team. Fertil Steril. 2000;73:43.
45. Collins JA, Barnhart KT, Schlegel PN. Do sperm DNA integrity tests predict pregnancy with in vitro fertilization? Fertil Steril. 2008;89:823–31.
46. Bungum M, Humaidan P, Axmon A, et al. Sperm DNA integrity assessment in prediction of assisted reproduction technology outcome. Hum Reprod. 2007;22:174.
47. Evenson DP, Wixon R. Data analysis of two in vivo fertility studies using sperm chromatin structure assay-derived DNA fragmentation index vs. pregnancy outcome. Fertil Steril. 2008;90:1229.

48. Zini A, Sigman M. Are tests of sperm DNA damage clinically useful? Pros and cons. J Androl. 2009;30:219.
49. Greco E, Scarselli F, Iacobelli M, Rienzi L, Ubaldi F, Ferrero S, et al. Efficient treatment of infertility due to sperm DNA damage by ICSI with testicular spermatozoa. Hum Reprod. 2005;20:226–30.
50. Huszar G, Vigue L, Morshedi M. Sperm creatine phosphokinase M-isoform ratios and fertilizing potential of men: a blinded study of 84 couples treated with in vitro fertilization. Fertil Steril. 1992;57:882–8.
51. Kim JG, Parthasarathy S. Oxidation and the spermatozoa. Semin Reprod Endocrinol. 1998;16:235–9.
52. Said TM, Land JA. Effects of advanced selection methods on sperm quality and ART outcome: a systematic review. Hum Reprod Update. 2011;17:719–33.
53. Glatstein IZ, Harlow BL, Hornstein MD. Practice patterns among reproductive endocrinologists: further aspects of the infertility evaluation. Fertil Steril. 1998;70:263.
54. Smith RG, Johnson A, Lamb D, et al. Functional tests of spermatozoa. Sperm penetration assay. Urol Clin North Am. 1987;14:451.
55. Liu de Y, Liu ML, Garrett C, et al. Comparison of the frequency of defective sperm-zonapellucida (ZP) binding and the ZP-induced acrosome reaction between subfertile men with normal and abnormal semen. Hum Reprod. 2007;22:1878.
56. Georgiou I, Syrrou M, Pardalidis N, Karakitsios K, Mantzavinos T, Giotitsas N, et al. Genetic and epigenetic risks of intracytoplasmic sperm injection method. Asian J Androl. 2006;8(6):643–73.
57. Ron-El R, Strassburger D, Gelman-Kohan S, Friedler S, Raziel A, Appelman Z. A 47,XXY fetus conceived after ICSI of spermatozoa from a patient with non-mosaic Klinefelter's syndrome: case report. Hum Reprod. 2000;15(8):1804–6.
58. Schiff JD, Palermo GD, Veeck LL, Goldstein M, Rosenwaks Z, Schlegel PN. Success of testicular sperm extraction [corrected] and intracytoplasmic sperm injection in men with Klinefelter syndrome. J Clin Endocrinol Metab. 2005;90(11):6263–7.
59. Staessen C, Tournaye H, Van Assche E, Michiels A, Van Landuyt L, Devroey P, et al. PGD in 47,XXY Klinefelter's syndrome patients. Hum Reprod Update. 2003;9(4):319–30.
60. Sciurano RB, Luna Hisano CV, Rahn MI, Brugo Olmedo S, Rey Valzacchi G, Coco R, et al. Focal spermatogenesis originates in euploid germ cells in classical Klinefelter patients. Hum Reprod. 2009;24(9):2353–60.

Chapter 10
Intracytoplasmic Morphologically Selected Sperm Injection (IMSI): An Overview

Daniel Luna Origgi and Javier García-Ferreyra

10.1 Introduction

In assisted reproductive technologies (ART), intracytoplasmic sperm injection (ICSI) is an alternative for couples with male factor infertility and low or absent fertilization rate in previous conventional in vitro fertilization (IVF) cycles [1]. ICSI outcome depends on several factors that include oocyte quality, patient age, and the quality of the spermatozoa selected to be injected into the oocyte. The selection of sperm for injection is performed under an inverted microscope with magnification of ×200–×400 that allows assessment of both motility and normal morphology [2, 3]. Several studies have shown that subtle morphological malformations of sperm nuclei are related to low fertilization rates [4], reduced blastocyst formation [5], and poor clinical outcomes [6, 7]. The optics used for visualization of spermatozoa do not provide sufficient resolution to allow identification of small defects and morphological abnormalities, which play a major role in fertilization, implantation, and pregnancy [8]. Bartoov et al. [9] introduced the motile sperm organelle morphology examination (MSOME) using high-power differential interference contrast optics, allowing the implementation of a new method for sperm handling: intracytoplasmic morphologically selected sperm injection (IMSI). This high-magnification approach permitted identification of spermatozoa with morphologically normal nuclei, which have a symmetrical and oval shape with homogeneous chromatin mass and have no more than one vacuole occupying less than 4% of the nuclear area.

Presence of nuclear vacuoles in the injected spermatozoa was reported to be the most relevant parameter that might significantly impact the clinical results of ICSI [10] since vacuoles are a possible indicator of sperm DNA damage (fragmentation or denaturation) [11] and can negatively affect embryo development. The origin of these vacuoles is unclear; several researchers support a nuclear origin, some link the

D.L. Origgi (✉) • J. García-Ferreyra
FERTILAB Laboratory of Assisted Reproduction, Lima, Peru
e-mail: dluna@fertilab.pe

© Springer International Publishing AG 2018   143
G.D. Palermo, E.S. Sills (eds.), *Intracytoplasmic Sperm Injection*,
https://doi.org/10.1007/978-3-319-70497-5_10

presence of large nuclear vacuoles (LNV) with increased DNA fragmentation, while other studies implicate chromatin condensation defects.

Several studies have demonstrated that IMSI significantly improves embryo quality, implantation and pregnancy rates when compared to ICSI; however, the results are controversial. Numerous publications have reported that IMSI is positively associated with implantation and/or pregnancy rates in couples with previous and repeated implantation failures and in patients with male factor infertility. Furthermore, the effect of IMSI on the chromosomal status or aneuploidy of the embryos is still controversial since many studies comparing ICSI and IMSI show conflicting results.

10.2 Sperm Nuclear Vacuoles and Nuclear Morphology: Significance, Origins, and Fertility Implications

Classical parameters of sperm quality are not always related to good prognosis and fertility since sperm DNA fragmentation and head vacuoles may be present. This problem can be addressed through sperm selection under high magnification or IMSI. Patients undergoing ICSI would benefit from sperm selection under high magnification [12]. The benefits of IMSI to improve outcomes in cases of male infertility patients have already been published [6, 13, 14]. The IMSI procedure improves embryo development prior to and immediately following activation of the embryonic genome, as the presence (and size) of vacuoles appears to influence ART outcome [12]. The MSOME observation technique allows embryologists to assess a spermatozoon's morphology and a better visualization of sperm head vacuoles, which are structures that are not visible under a conventional ICSI magnification microscope. Sperm head vacuoles can be classified by size, position, depth, and number. Vacuoles can be found in samples with normal semen parameters as well as in specimens with abnormal ones, and vacuole size has been negatively correlated with poor sperm morphology [15].

Two different studies showed that the injection of morphometrically normal spermatozoa with no vacuoles or only one small vacuole was associated with significantly higher blastocyst [5] and/or pregnancy rates [5, 16] (relative to the injection of morphometrically abnormal spermatozoa or morphometrically normal spermatozoa with two or more small vacuoles or one large vacuole). Cassuto et al. [17] established a score that took into account sperm head morphology, base morphology, and vacuole number. Figure 10.1 shows vacuole grading as described by Vanderzwalmen [5]. The researchers reported that pregnancy rate varied as a function of the score, with lower rates obtained for abnormal spermatozoa with vacuoles. Although one group has reported that the injection of vacuole-free spermatozoa was associated with lower blastocyst rates, the cohort was very small and azoospermia was present in one-third of the patients [18]. Thus, it seems that the presence of

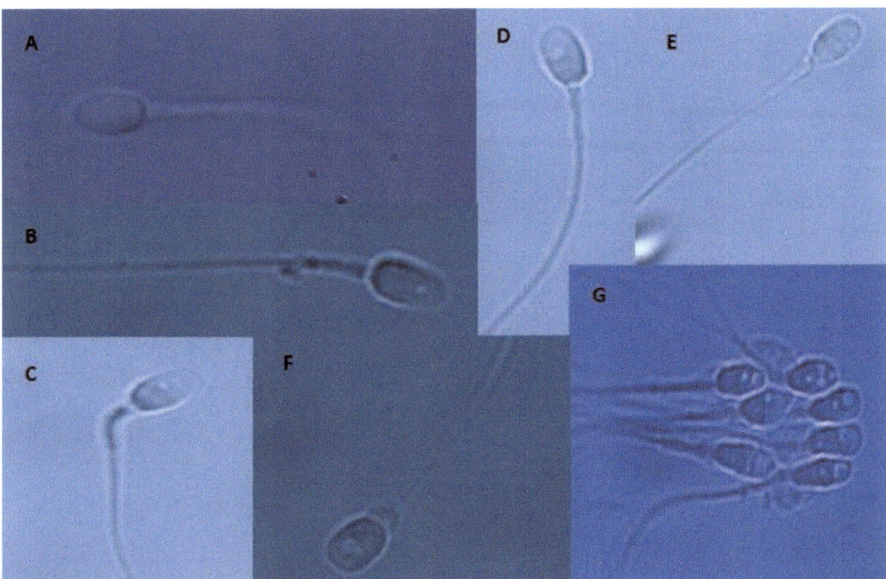

Fig. 10.1 Grading of spermatozoa into four groups according to the presence or size of vacu-oles. Grade I: normal form and no vacuoles (**a**). Grade II: normal form with less than or equal to two small vacuoles (**b**, **c**). Grade III: normal form with more than two small vacuoles or at least one large vacuole (**d**, **e**). Grade IV: large vacuole and abnormal head shapes or other abnor-malities (**f**, **g**)

one or more sperm nuclear vacuoles can influence blastocyst development and preg-nancy rates.

Several studies indicate that the injection of DNA-damaged or vacuolated sper-matozoa is related to a blockage of embryo development before and after implanta-tion, reflecting a late paternal effect [19, 20]. These findings provide more evidence to support the fact that the standard ICSI technique might generate a lower quality embryo and poorer clinical outcomes compared to IMSI because of the chance of injecting highly vacuolated and DNA-damaged sperm into the ooplasm [21]. This is due to the fact that sperm DNA integrity, chromosomal constitution, and nuclear morphology cannot be assessed in a sperm used for ICSI. An adverse late paternal effect can be characterized by poor embryo development to the blastocyst stage, implantation failure, and pregnancy loss as observed in the ICSI group. Furthermore, a high percentage of abnormal spermatozoa with LNV, according to MSOME crite-ria, were observed in male patients older than 40 years [22], and up to 65% of sper-matozoa that were deemed suitable for ICSI by conventional methods were subsequently deselected after MSOME [23]. In addition, LNV are closely associ-ated with chromatin condensation failure and a potential increase in susceptibility to DNA damage during the IMSI/ICSI procedure [24], thereby explaining the reduced potential of success of the ICSI procedures.

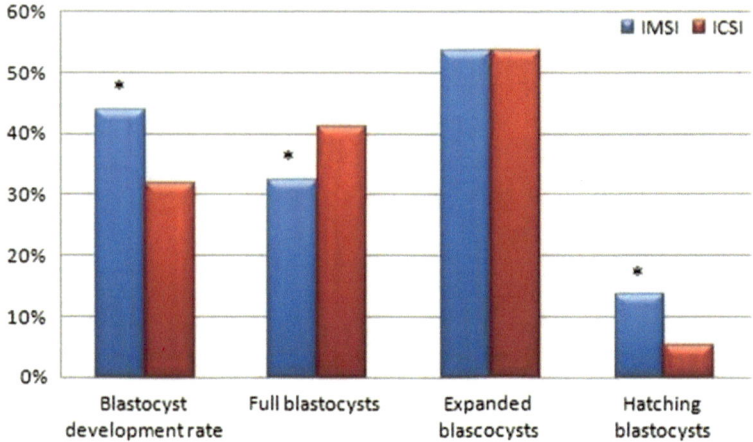

Fig. 10.2 Blastocyst quality in the IMSI and ICSI cycles

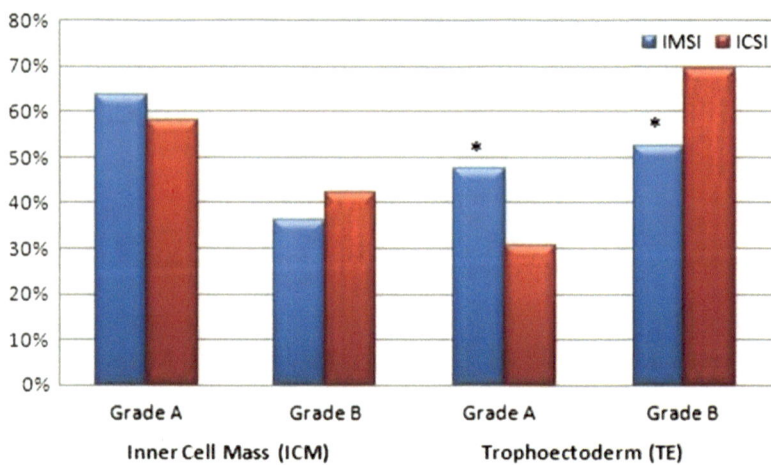

Fig. 10.3 Comparison of ICM and TE from blastocysts between IMSI and ICSI groups

Furthermore, the blastocysts from the IMSI group showed a tendency for better ICM quality and a better TE quality by an increment on grade A when compared with those from the conventional ICSI (Figs. 10.2 and 10.3) [12]. This in an indication that might explain the better outcomes of IMSI in cases of male factor infertility since the initial contact between the blastocyst and maternal tissues is by adhesion of the trophoblast to the uterine epithelium and cell-to-cell interaction [25, 26]. This interaction is believed to be critical for implantation, so the trophoblast quality highly influences the chances of embryo implantation and reduces the chances of miscarriage (Fig. 10.4).

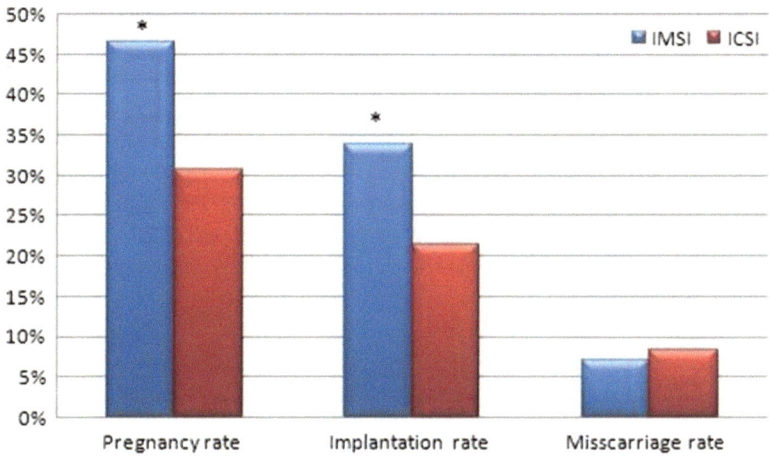

Fig. 10.4 Clinical outcomes in the IMSI and ICSI cycles

10.2.1   Sperm Nuclear Vacuoles: Age, Sperm Morphology, and DNA Fragmentation

Male aging has been associated with a decrease in serum steroid levels, testicular volume, progressive motility, daily sperm production, inhibin B/FSH ratio, alteration in testicular histomorphology, risk of chromosomal disorders [27, 28], and a significant increase in spermatic DNA fragmentation particularly in men >50 years [29, 30]. According to the presence of nuclear vacuoles in human sperm head, Silva et al. [22] showed that the percentages of LNV spermatozoa increases significantly with subject age (33.8% in men ≥41 years old vs. 28.6 and 31.1% in men ≤35 years and 36–40 years, respectively; $p < 0.05$). Similar results were observed by de Almeida Ferreira Braga et al. [21] and Wogatzky et al. [31]. In contrast, Fekonja et al. [32] did not identify a correlation between sperm head vacuoles and patient age.

The relationship between nuclear vacuoles and sperm morphology has previously been studied with controversial results. Bartoov et al. [4] did not observe any relationship, while other investigators reported a significant positive correlation between large vacuoles and the frequency of abnormal morphology in sperm [32–34]. De Vos et al. [35] analyzed 330 semen samples under high magnification, in which 54.4% of amorphous sperm had large vacuoles compared to 27.5% in normally shaped spermatozoa. Perdrix et al. [15] analyzed 10,975 spermatozoa from 440 males and found that the relative vacuolar area, defined as vacuole area (μm^2)/head area (μm^2) × 100, was the most discriminative MSOME criterion between normal vs. abnormal sperm and was negatively correlated with poor sperm morphology ($r = 0.53$; $p < 0.001$) [15]. Regarding acrosome morphology, spermatozoa with small acrosomes exhibit large vacuoles that cause deformities of the nucleus and the head shape [36], which are more frequent in infertile males with an excess of sperm precursors [37]. In addition, Montjean et al. [38] incubated 35 semen samples with follicular fluid and hyaluronic acid and showed that the presence of vacuoles negatively influences sperm capacity to undergo the acrosome reaction. This observation suggests that most nuclear vacuoles are of acrosomal origin, and a reflection of sperm physiology, rather than an expression of nuclear abnormalities [38]. Similarly, Kacem et al. [39] reported that of all acrosome-reacted sperm analyzed, 70.9% had no vacuoles, whereas in those sperms showing incomplete acrosome reaction or an intact acrosome the corresponding percentage was 39.3%.

Conversely, previous studies based on electron microscopy data [4, 6, 14] have suggested an association between nuclear vacuoles and chromatin damage, and the presence of large vacuoles reflects some underlying chromosomal or DNA defect [6] affecting mitochondrial function, chromatin status, and aneuploidy rate [11]. Moreover, LNV have been associated to abnormal chromatin packaging [40], increased level of chromatin immaturity [34, 41], increased DNA fragmentation and denaturation [11, 40, 42] and DNA damage [23, 43]. Further studies [11, 41, 44, 45] have reported an increase in aneuploid spermatozoa associated with the presence of vacuoles, but results were not statistically significant. The absence of vacuoles after MSOME analysis was not a guarantee of chromosomally normal sperm in the setting of macrocephalic sperm head syndrome [46, 47]. Finally, Hammoud et al. [42] evaluated spermatozoa from eight patients with elevated sperm DNA fragmentation and found vacuole-free spermatozoa to have a significantly lower incidence of DNA fragmentation (4.4 ± 1.1%) than other types of spermatozoa.

10.2.2   IMSI and Embryo Aneuploidy

It has been reported that total aneuploidy rate was not statistically different between IMSI and ICSI procedures, but there was a significantly high incidence of sex chromosome aneuploidy among ICSI embryos [48]. It is important to point out that aneuploidy is independent of embryo appearance since a good morphology blastocyst can still be aneuploid and the pregnancy most likely will result in a miscarriage [49]. This phenomenon was observed in PGD reports (see Table 10.1) where a significant number of embryos achieving the blastocyst stage were aneuploid and unsuitable for transfer after either IMSI or ICSI (16% and 22%, respectively; $p > 0.05$). Moreover, PGD diagnosis by FISH provides information on only a limited number of chromosomes, whereas a more robust method such as CGH and its 24-chromosome resolution is associated with better clinical outcome and more

Table 10.1 Aneuploidy rate in those patients from IMSI and ICSI cycles with PGD

	IMSI	ICSI
No. of genetically analyzed embryos	39	86
Aneuploidy rate (%)	76.9	70.9
Aneuploid blastocyst (%)	16.0	22.0

accurate PGD results [50]. It may be that in a non-PGS setting, there is a higher probability of normal embryo selection for transfer based on morphological criteria in cases of embryos derived from sperm selected by high magnification.

A study on embryo aneuploidy reported that the proportion of abnormal embryos increases with the severity of male factor condition, but the type of defect depends on the sperm characteristics [51]. There is little information available regarding the comparison of aneuploidy rates between ICSI and IMSI, with one study reporting that autosomal aneuploidy was not affected by the sperm selection method, but there was a higher sex chromosomal aneuploidy in IMSI. Aneuploidy rates have also been compared in cleavage stage embryos and blastocysts utilizing FISH [52], and comparative genomic hybridization (CGH) showed no differences between ICSI and IMSI. Aneuploidy rate remain the same between the IMSI and ICSI groups, implying that the additional time required to select the suitable MSOME-graded spermatozoon on a PVP microdroplet is not detrimental to DNA integrity, and does not lead to lower embryo quality or lower blastocyst development rates [12]. Furthermore, since no damage to DNA is done, the IMSI procedure is adequate for patients with elevated DNA fragmentation in order to select sperm with better morphology, but without increasing the underlying DNA fragmentation since it is related to poor semen parameters [53] and clinical outcomes [54].

10.3 IMSI Procedure Indication: ICSI or IMSI?

10.3.1 Paternal Effect: Semen Quality (Poor Semen Quality)

Sperm of poor quality can negatively affect embryo developmental events like fertilization, cleavage, and blastocyst development. ICSI is the best procedure for couples with severely compromised seminal parameters. Oligo-, astheno-, and teratozoospermia are semen parameters considered to indicate ICSI. However, the presence of nuclear vacuoles in sperm head [18] as a new parameter for sperm quality leads to a preference for the IMSI procedure in males with poor semen quality. Knez et al. [55] evaluated the effect of IMSI in 57 couples with poor semen quality and previous ICSI cycles where all their embryos had arrested development (IMSI = 20; ICSI = 37). This research revealed a higher number of blastocysts (0.80 vs. 0.65) and implantation (17.1% vs. 6.8%) and pregnancy rates (25.0% vs. 8.1%) in IMSI cycles compared to ICSI, respectively. On the other hand, Leandri et al. [56] compared IMSI and ICSI in oligozoospermic patients (motile sperm count $<1 \times 10^6$ after selection, but at least 3×10^6 spermatozoa per ejaculate) but did not find important differences in implantation (24% vs. 23%) or clinical pregnancy (31% vs. 33%) rates. However, a prospective study including 500 couples undergoing first IVF and male factor infertility showed that IMSI increased the likelihood of fertilization, implantation, and pregnancy in patients with oligoasthenozoospermia compared to ICSI cycles [57]. With regard to teratozoospermia, La Sala et al. [58]

prospectively evaluated 121 patients with <4% normal morphology and showed similar clinical pregnancy per embryo transferred in IMSI vs. ICSI cycles (32.3% vs. 23.4%; respectively).

10.3.2 Recurrent Implantation Failure (RIF)

Implantation failure is the principal cause of unsuccessful ART procedures. The outcome of ICSI is positively associated with overall sperm morphology [8], while early miscarriage rates are associated with nuclear morphology [59]. Oliveira et al. [60] compared the effect of IMSI in 200 couples with repeated implantation failure and did not observe significant improvement in clinical outcomes compared to patients that underwent standard ICSI. There were clear trends for lower miscarriage rates, higher rates of ongoing pregnancies and live births within the IMSI group but these were not significant. In a prospective study in which 75 couples acted as their own controls, IMSI was carried out after at least two previous IVF or ICSI failures. The women in the study group had better quality embryos at day 2, more cycles with extended embryo culture, and higher mean number of blastocysts compared to previous IVF/ICSI cycles [61]. Conversely, a meta-analysis in 13 studies comparing ICSI vs. IMSI in couples with previous ICSI failures showed that IMSI increases the odds of implantation by 50% and pregnancy by 60% [62]. However, as no randomized evidence exists, such studies are needed to validate IMSI benefits in couples with implantation failures.

10.3.3 Poor Responders

The poor ovarian response is defined as the retrieval of low number of oocytes despite adequate ovarian stimulation in an assisted conception cycle [63]. Normally, a depletion of the ovarian pool of non-growing follicles occurs, leading to a decline in oocyte quantity and quality. A potential strategy to increase the success of the procedure involves ICSI and/or IMSI, through which zygotes and embryos can be obtained. Setti et al. [64] compared the outcomes of ICSI and IMSI in 414 women with poor ovarian response divided in two groups: poor-responder patients ($\leq$4 oocytes retrieved) and normoresponder patients (>4 oocytes retrieved). Patients who underwent IMSI were matched with patients who underwent ICSI in the same period, and outcomes were compared. In the poor-responder group, fertilization rate (53.9% vs. 79.8%) and number of transferred embryos (1.5 ± 0.8 vs. 1.9 ± 0.7) were significantly lower in IMSI compared with ICSI. Implantation, pregnancy, and miscarriage rates were similar when IMSI or ICSI was performed. In the normoresponder group, there was no difference in cycle outcomes. These data suggest that poor ovarian responder patients do not benefit from IMSI.

10.4 The IMSI Procedure Advantages

At the beginning of the IMSI era, its possible advantages in clinical outcomes were overestimated. Several studies have shown that IMSI significantly improves embryo quality [5, 6], but in term of implantation, pregnancy, and miscarriage rates, there are conflicting reports. A review by Nadalina et al. [65] reported higher fertilization, implantation, and pregnancy rates in IMSI compared to ICSI procedures. In a prospective randomized trial on male infertility patients, higher clinical pregnancy rates with IMSI compared to ICSI were reported, whereas miscarriage rates were no different between both procedures [7]. Using exclusively teratozoospermic samples, a prospective non-randomized observational study showed higher implantation and clinical pregnancy rates with IMSI [66]. A systematic review with meta-analysis that compared IMSI with ICSI in couples with ICSI failures [62] demonstrated improved clinical outcomes in patients who underwent IMSI. Implantation rate was threefold higher [OR 2.88; 95% CI 2.13–3.89], pregnancy rate twofold improved (OR 2.07; 95% CI 1.22–3.50), and miscarriage rate was reduced by 70% (OR 0.31; 95% CI 0.14–0.67) in IMSI compared to ICSI cycles [62].

Yet, in a randomized controlled trial, La Sala et al. [58] found significantly different clinical pregnancy and live birth delivery rates in 48 IMSI cycles compared to 73 ICSI procedures. From this, it was concluded that there is no rationale for routine use of IMSI in clinical practice. Similar results were observed by Balaban et al. [67] and Leandri et al. [56]. A Cochrane Review based on nine prospective randomized controlled trials evaluated 1002 IMSI and 1012 ICSI cycles and found no differences in live birth [Risk Ratio (RR) 1.14] or abortion rates (RR 0.82) in the IMSI technique [68]. De Vos et al. [8] prospectively studied more than 3000 sibling-oocytes in 350 ICSI cycles with a high-magnification sperm selection method to evaluate the role of IMSI in clinical outcomes. Fertilization rate, blastocyst development, and implantation rates per embryo transferred were similar for IMSI and ICSI cycles.

References

1. Practice Committees of the American Society for Reproductive Medicine and Society for Assisted Reproductive Technology. Intracytoplasmic sperm injection (ICSI) for non-male factor infertility: a committee opinion. Fertil Steril. 2012;98:1395–9.
2. Kruger TF, Haque D, Acosta AA, et al. Correlation between sperm morphology, acrosin, and fertilization in an IVF program. Arch Androl. 1988;20:237–41.
3. Bartoov B, Eltes F, Pansky M, et al. Improved diagnosis of male fertility potential via a combination of quantitative ultramorphology and routine semen analyses. Hum Reprod. 1994;9:2069–75.
4. Bartoov B, Berkovitz A, Eltes F, Kogosowski A, Menezo Y, Barak Y. Real-time fine morphology of motile human sperm cells is associated with IVF-ICSI outcome. J Androl. 2002;23:1–8.

5. Vanderzwalmen P, Hiemer A, Rubner P, et al. Blastocyst development after sperm selection at high magnification is associated with size and number of nuclear vacuoles. Reprod Biomed Online. 2008;17:617–27.
6. Berkovitz A, Eltes F, Lederman H, et al. How to improve IVF-ICSI outcome by sperm selection. Reprod Biomed Online. 2006;12:634–8.
7. Antinori M, Licata E, Dani G, et al. Intracytoplasmic morphologically selected sperm injection: a prospective randomized trial. Reprod Biomed Online. 2008;16:835–41.
8. De Vos A, Van De Velde H, Joris H, Verheyen G, Devroey P, Van Steirteghem A. Influence of individual sperm morphology on fertilization, embryo morphology, and pregnancy outcome of intracytoplasmic sperm injection. Fertil Steril. 2003;79:42–8.
9. Bartoov B, Berkovitz A, Eltes F. Selection of spermatozoa with normal nuclei to improve the pregnancy rate with intracytoplasmic sperm injection. N Engl J Med. 2001;345:1067–8.
10. Berkovitz A, Eltes F, Ellenbogen A, Peer S, Feldberg D, Bartoov B. Does the presence of nuclear vacuoles in human sperm selected for ICSI affect pregnancy outcome? Hum Reprod. 2006;21:1787–90.
11. Garolla A, Fortini D, Menegazzo M, et al. High-power microscopy for selecting spermatozoa for ICSI by physiological status. Reprod Biomed Online. 2008;17:610–6.
12. Luna D, Hilario R, Dueñas-Chacón J, et al. The IMSI procedure improves laboratory and clinical outcomes without compromising the aneuploidy rate when compared to the classical ICSI procedure. Clin Med Insights Reprod Health. 2015;9:29–37.
13. Knez K, Zorn B, Tomazevic T, Vrtacnik-Bokal E, Virant-Klun I. The IMSI procedure improves poor embryo development in the same infertile couples with poor semen quality: a comparative prospective randomized study. Reprod Biol Endocrinol. 2011;9:123.
14. Berkovitz A, Eltes F, Yaari S, et al. The morphological normalcy of the sperm nucleus and pregnancy rate of intracytoplasmic injection with morphologically selected sperm. Hum Reprod. 2005;20:185–90.
15. Perdrix A, Saidi R, Menard JF, Gruel E, Milazzo JP, Mace B, Rives N. Relationship between conventional sperm parameters and motile sperm organelle morphology examination (MSOME). Int J Androl. 2012;35:491–8.
16. Knez K, Tomazevic T, Zorn B, Vrtacnik-Bokal E, Virant-Klun I. Intracytoplasmic morphologically selected sperm injection improves development and quality of preimplantation embryos in teratozoospermia patients. Reprod Biomed Online. 2012;25:168–79.
17. Cassuto NG, Bouret D, Plouchart JM, Jellad S, Vanderzwalmen P, Balet R, Larue L, Barak Y. A new real-time morphology classification for human spermatozoa: a link for fertilization and improved embryo quality. Fertil Steril. 2009;92:1616–25.
18. Tanaka A, Nagayoshi M, Tanaka I, Kusunoki H. Human sperm head vacuoles are physiological structures formed during the sperm development and maturation process. Fertil Steril. 2012;98:315–20.
19. Tesarik J, Greco E, Mendoza C. Late, but not early, paternal effect on human embryo development is related to sperm DNA fragmentation. Hum Reprod. 2004;19:611–5.
20. Borini A, Tarozzi N, Bizzaro D, et al. Sperm DNA fragmentation: paternal effect on early post-implantation embryo development in ART. Hum Reprod. 2006;21:2876–81.
21. Ferreira d A, Braga DP, Setti AS, Figueira RC, et al. Sperm organelle morphologic abnormalities: contributing factors and effects on intracytoplasmic sperm injection cycles outcomes. Urology. 2011;78:786–91.
22. Silva LF, Oliveira JB, Petersen CG, et al. The effects of male age on sperm analysis by motile sperm organelle morphology examination (MSOME). Reprod Biol Endocrinol. 2012;10:19.
23. Wilding M, Coppola G, di Matteo L, Palagiano A, Fusco E, Dale B. Intracytoplasmic injection of morphologically selected spermatozoa (IMSI) improves outcome after assisted reproduction by deselecting physiologically poor quality spermatozoa. J Assist Reprod Genet. 2011;28:253–62.
24. Boitrelle F, Guthauser B, Alter L, et al. The nature of human sperm head vacuoles: a systematic literature review. Basic Clin Androl. 2013;23:3.

25. Thie M, Denker HW. In vitro studies on endometrial adhesiveness for trophoblast: cellular dynamics in uterine epithelial cells. Cells Tissues Organs. 2002;172:237–52.
26. Aplin JD, Kimber SJ. Trophoblast-uterine interactions at implantation. Reprod Biol Endocrinol. 2004;2:48.
27. Handelsman DJ, Staraj S. Testicular size: the effect of aging, malnutrition, and illness. J Androl. 1985;6:144–51.
28. Mahmoud AM, Goemaere S, El-Garem Y, Van Potterlberrgh I, Comhaire FH, Kaufman JM. Testicular volume in relation to hormonal indices of gonadal function in community-dwelling elderly men. J Clin Endocrinol Metab. 2003;88:179–84.
29. García-Ferreyra J, Romero R, Hilario R, Dueñas-Chacón J. High levels of DNA fragmentation observed in an infertile population attending a fertility center are related to advanced paternal age. J Fert In Vitro. 2012;2:1–5.
30. García-Ferreyra J, Villegas L, Romero R, Zavala P, Hilario R, Casafranca G, Dueñas-Chacón J. Sperm DNA fragmentation is significantly increased in those men with morphologically abnormal spermatozoa. J Fert In Vitro. 2014;2:1–5.
31. Wogatzky J, Wirleitner B, Stecher A, Vanderzwalmen P, Neyer A, Spitzer D, Schuff M, Schechinger B, Zech NH. The combination matters—distinct impact of life factors on sperm quality: a study on semen analysis of 1683 patients according to MSOME criteria. Reprod Biol Endocrinol. 2012;10:115.
32. Fekonja N, Štrus J, Tušek Žnidarič M, Knez K, Vrtacnik Bokal E, Verdenik I, Virant-Klun I. Clinical and structural features of sperm head vacuoles in men included in the in vitro fertilization programme. Biomed Res Int. 2014;2014:927841.
33. Oliveira JB, Massaro FC, Mauri AL, Petersen CG, Nicoletti AP, Baruffi RL, Franco JG Jr. Motile sperm organelle morphology examination is stricter tan Tygerberg criteria. Reprod Biomed Online. 2009;18:320–6.
34. Perdrix A, Travers A, Chelli MH, Escalier D, Do Rego JL, Milazzo JP, Mousset-Siméon N, Macé B, Rives N. Assessment of acrosome and nuclear abnormalities in human spermatozoa with large vacuoles. Hum Reprod. 2011;26:47–58.
35. De Vos A, Van de Velde H, Bocken G, Eylenbosch G, Franceus N, Meersdom G, Tistaert S, Vankelecom A, Tournaye H, Verheyen G. Does intracytoplasmic morphologically selected sperm injection improve embryo development? A randomized sibling-oocyte study. Hum Reprod. 2013;28:617–26.
36. Zamboni L. The ultrastructural pathology of the spermatozoon as a cause of infertility: the role of electron microscopy in the evaluation of semen quality. Fertil Steril. 1987;47:711–34.
37. Mundy AJ, Ryder TA, Edmonds DK. A quantitative study of sperm head ultrastructure in subfertile males with excess sperm precursors. Fertil Steril. 1994;61:751–4.
38. Montjean D, Belloc S, Benkhalifa M, Dalleac A, Menezo Y. Sperm vacuoles are linked to capacitation and acrosomal status. Hum Reprod. 2012;27:2927–32.
39. Kacem O, Sifer C, Barraud-Lange V, Ducot B, De Ziegler D, Poirot C, Wolf J. Sperm nuclear vacuoles, as assessed by motile sperm organellar morphological examination, are mostly of acrosomal origin. Reprod Biomed Online. 2010;20:132–7.
40. Franco JG, Baruffi RL, Mauri AL, Petersen CG, Oliveira JB, Vagnini L. Significance of large nuclear vacuoles in human spermatozoa: implications for ICSI. Reprod Biomed Online. 2008;17:42–5.
41. Boitrelle F, Ferfouri F, Petit JM, Segretain D, Tourain C, Bergere M, Bailly M, Vialard F, Albert M, Selva J. Large human sperm vacuoles observed in motile spermatozoa under high magnification: nuclear thumbprints linked to failure of chromatin condensation. Hum Reprod. 2011;26:1650–8.
42. Hammoud I, Boitrelle F, Ferfouri F, Vialard F, Bergere M, Wainer B, Bailly M, Albert M, Selva J. Selection of normal spermatozoa with a vacuole-free head (x6300) improves selection of spermatozoa with intact DNA in patients with high sperm DNA fragmentation rates. Andrologia. 2013;45:163–70.

43. Oliveira JB, Massaro FC, Baruffi RL, Mauri AL, Petersen CG, Silva LF, Vagnini LD, Franco JG Jr. Correlation between semen analysis by motile sperm organelle morphology and sperm DNA damage. Fertil Steril. 2010;94:1937–40.
44. Watanabe S, Tanaka A, Fujii S, Mizunuma H, Fukui A, Fuluhara R, Nakamura R, Yamada K, Tanaka I, Awata S, Nagayoshi M. An investigation of the potential effect of vacuoles in human sperm on DNA damage using a chromosome assay and the TUNEL assay. Hum Reprod. 2011;26:978–86.
45. Perdrix A, Rives N. Motile sperm organelle morphology examination (MSOME) and sperm head vacuoles: state of art in 2013. Hum Reprod Update. 2013;19:527–41.
46. Chelli MH, Albert M, Ray PF, Guthauser B, Izard V, Hammoud I, Selva J, Vialard F. Can intracytoplasmic morphologically selected sperm injection be used to select normal-sized sperm heads in infertile patients with macrocephalic sperm head syndrome? Fertil Steril. 2010;93:1347.e1–5.
47. Cassuto NG, le Foll N, Chantot-Bastaraud S, Balet R, Bouret D, Rouen A, Bhouri R, Hyon C, Siffroi JP. Sperm fluorescence in situ hybridization study in nine men carrying a Robertsonian or a reciprocal translocation: relationship between segregation modes and high-magnification sperm morphology examination. Fertil Steril. 2011;96:826–32.
48. Figueira Rde C, Braga DP, Setti AS, Iaconelli A Jr, Borges E Jr. Morphological nuclear integrity of sperm cells is associated with preimplantation genetic aneuploidy screening cycle outcomes. Fertil Steril. 2011;95:990–3.
49. Sandalinas M, Sadowy S, Alikani M, Calderon G, Cohen J, Munné S. Developmental ability of chromosomically abnormal human embryos to develop to the blastocyst stage. Hum Reprod. 2001;16:1954–8.
50. Keltz MD, Vega M, Sirota I, et al. Preimplantation genetic screening (PGS) with comparative genomic hybridization (CGH) following day 3 single cell blastomere biopsy markedly improves IVF outcomes while lowering multiple pregnancies and miscarriages. J Assist Reprod Genet. 2013;30(10):1333–9.
51. Magli MC, Gianaroli L, Ferraretti AP, Gordts S, Fredericks V, Crippa A. Paternal contribution to aneuploidy in preimplantation embryos. Reprod Biomed Online. 2009;18:536–42.
52. Fragouli E, Alfarawati S, Spath K, Wells D. Morphological and cytogenetic assessment of cleavage and blastocyst stage embryos. Mol Hum Reprod. 2014;20(2):117–26.
53. Boushaba S, Belaaloui G. Sperm DNA fragmentation and standard semen parameters in Algerian infertile male partners. World J Mens Health. 2015;33(1):1–7.
54. Jin J, Pan C, Fei Q, et al. Effect of sperm DNA fragmentation on the clinical outcomes for in vitro fertilization and intracytoplasmic sperm injection in women with different ovarian reserves. Fertil Steril. 2015;103(4):910–6.
55. Knez K, Zorn B, Tomazevic T, Vrtacnik-Bokal E, Virant-Klun I. The IMSI procedure improves poor embryo development in the same infertile couples with poor semen quality: a comparative prospective randomized study. Reprod Biol Endocrinol. 2011;9:123.
56. Leandri RD, Gachet A, Pfeffer J, Celebi C, Rives N, Carre-Pigeon F, Kulski O, Mitchell C, Parinaud J. Is intracytoplasmic morphologically selected sperm injection (IMSI) beneficial in the first ART cycle? A multicéntrico randomized controlled trial. Andrology. 2013;1:692–7.
57. Setti AS, Figueira Rde C, Braga DP, Iaconelli A Jr, Borges E Jr. intracytoplasmic morphologically selected sperm injection benefits for patients with oligoasthenozoospermia according to the 2010 World Health Organization references values. Fertil Steril. 2011;95:2711–4.
58. La Sala GB, Nicoli A, Fornaciari E, Falbo A, Rondini I, Morini D, Valli B, Villani MT, Palomba S. Intracytoplasmic morphologically selected sperm injection versus conventional intracytoplasmic sperm injection: a randomized controlled trial. Reprod Biol Endocrinol. 2015;13:97.
59. Bartoov B, Berkovitz A, Eltes F, Kogosovsky A, Yagoda A, Lederman H, Artzi S, Gross M, Barak Y. Pregnancy rates are higher with intracytoplasmic morphologically selected sperm injection than with conventional intracytoplasmic injection. Fertil Steril. 2003;80:1431–19.

60. Oliveira JB, Cavagna M, Petersen CG, Mauri AL, Massaro FC, Silva LFL, Baruffi ELR, Franco JG Jr. Pregnancy outcomes in women with repeated implantation failures after intracytoplasmic morphologically selected sperm injection (IMSI). Reprod Biol Endrocrinol. 2011;9:1–7.
61. Delaroche L, Yazbeck C, Gout C, Kahn V, Oger P, Rougier N. Intracytoplasmic morphologically selected sperm injection (IMSI) after repeated IVF or ICSI failures: a prospective comparative study. Eur J Obstet Gynecol Reprod Biol. 2013;167:76–80.
62. Setti AS, Braga DP, Figueira RC, Iaconelli A, Borgues E. Intracytoplasmic morpgologically selected sperm injection results in improved clinical outcomes in couples with previous ICSI failures or male factor infertility: a meta-analysis. Eur J Obstet Gynecol Reprod Biol. 2014;183:96–103.
63. Jeve YB, Harich MB. Effective treatment protocol for poor ovarian response: a systematic review and meta-analysis. J Hum Reprod Sci. 2016;9:70–81.
64. Setti AS, Braga DPAF, Figueira RCS, Iaconelli A, Borges E. Poor-responder patients do not benefit from intracytoplasmic morphologically selected sperm injection. J Assist Reprod Genet. 2015;32(3):445–50.
65. Nadalina M, Tarozzi N, Distratis V, Scaravelli G, Borini A. Impact of intracytoplasmic morphologically selected sperm injection on assisted reproduction outcome: a review. Reprod Biomed Online. 2009;19:45–55.
66. El Khattabi L, Dupont C, Sermondade N, Hughes JN, Poncelet C, Porcher R, Cedrin-Dumerin I, Lévy R, Sifer C. Is intracytoplasmic morphologically selected sperm injection effective in patients with infertility related to teratozoospermia or repeated implantation failure? Fertil Steril. 2013;100:62–8.
67. Balaban B, Yakin K, Alatas C, Oktem O, Isklar A, Urman B. Clinical outcome of intracytoplasmic injection of spermatozoa morphologically selected under high magnification: a prospective randomized study. Reprod Biomed Online. 2011;22:472–6.
68. Texeira DM, Barbosa MA, Ferriani RA, Navarro PA, Raine-Fenning N, Nastri CO, Martins WP. Regular (ICSI) versus ultra-high magnification (IMSI) sperm selection for assisted reproduction. Cochrane Database Syst Rev. 2013;(7):CD010167.

Chapter 11
Implications of Sperm Source on ICSI Outcome: Assessment of TESE and Other Surgical Sperm Retrieval Methods

Nikita Abhyankar, Samuel Ohlander, and Martin Kathrins

Abbreviations

ART	Assisted reproductive technology
CBAVD	Congenital bilateral absence of the vas deferens
CI	Confidence interval
DFI	DNA fragmentation index
DNA	Deoxyribonucleic acid
ICSI	Intracytoplasmic sperm injection
IVF	In vitro fertilization
MESA	Micro-epididymal sperm aspiration
microTESE	Microdissection testicular sperm extraction
PESA	Percutaneous epididymal sperm aspiration
RR	Relative risk
SSR	Sperm retrieval rate
TESA	Testicular sperm aspiration
TESE	Testicular sperm extraction
TUNEL	dUTP nick end labelling

N. Abhyankar (✉) • S. Ohlander
Department of Urology, University of Illinois at Chicago, Chicago, IL, USA
e-mail: nikitaa@uic.edu; sohlande@uic.edu

M. Kathrins
Harvard Medical School, Brigham and Women's Hospital, Boston, MA, USA
e-mail: mkathrins@bwh.harvard.edu

© Springer International Publishing AG 2018   157
G.D. Palermo, E.S. Sills (eds.), *Intracytoplasmic Sperm Injection*,
https://doi.org/10.1007/978-3-319-70497-5_11

11.1   Introduction

The advent of intracytoplasmic sperm injection (ICSI) offers couples with severe semen abnormalities the opportunity to conceive their own biologic child, without reliance on anonymous donor sperm. The question of the optimal source of sperm to use for ICSI is a controversial one and a definitive answer remains elusive. This chapter will seek to explore what options exist for sperm source, its acquisition, and outcomes data.

11.2   Sperm Source and ICSI Outcomes Theories

Ejaculated, epididymal, and testicular sperm have differing characteristics with regard to motility, morphology, and maturity [1–3]. It is postulated that ICSI bypasses the need for some of these developmental properties; however, some key differences remain. One of these differences is the DNA fragmentation index (DFI). DFI reflects the fraction of sperm in a sample with fragmented chromatin and is a surrogate for sperm DNA damage. DNA damage has been postulated to occur during sperm transit through the male genital tract, resulting from oxidative insults to spermatic DNA by reactive oxidative species, leading to lower ejaculated sperm quality [4–10]. This theory was supported by topographic DFI mapping performed at discrete locations along the male reproductive tract [11]. Ejaculated sperm demonstrated the highest DFI, followed by vasal sperm, then epididymal sperm, and finally testicular sperm having the lowest DFI [11]. A more recent study compared epididymal sperm to testicular sperm in men with obstructive azoospermia using dUTP nick end labelling (TUNEL) assay to measure DFI [12]. The authors also found the lowest DFI to be testicular sperm, then caput epididymis, and highest DFI to be the corpus epididymal sperm, supporting previously published work which demonstrated increasing DFIs as sperm progressed through the reproductive tract [12]. No difference was found between causes of obstructive azoospermia and sperm DFI at any location. To date, all investigations of DFI through the reproductive tract has demonstrated the smallest degree of DNA damage to be at the testicular source and increases during transit to the ejaculate [13–15].

A sample analysis obtained from 2586 men showed higher DFI to be associated with lower sperm concentration, motility, and morphology [16]. Other studies have similarly shown a positive correlation between sperm DNA damage and abnormal semen parameters [17, 18]. Several studies have shown a correlation between DFI and assisted reproductive technology (ART) outcomes. Benchaib et al. performed a prospective study analyzing fertilization rates using ejaculated sperm for ICSI/IVF and found a statistically significantly impaired fertilization rate in those with DFI > 10% [19]. Similarly, Cozzubbo et al. [11] found higher fertilization rates in ICSI cycles using testicular sperm with a lower DFI compared to ejaculated sperm; however, this study included only men with high ejaculated sperm DFI [8]. Additional studies support these findings and have shown lower fertilization rates, pregnancy rates, embryo quality, and implantation rates in men with high DFI [20, 21]. A systematic review and meta-analysis by Robinson et al. found a positive correlation when evaluating miscarriage rates and DNA fragmentation [22]. In contrast, Lin et al. performed a review of 223 couples undergoing IVF using ejaculated sperm and found no correlation between DFI and fertilization or pregnancy rates [23]. Another smaller prospective study comparing fertilization rates with DFI in 34 couples also showed no correlation, so our understanding of the clinical significance of elevated DFI remains somewhat unclear [24].

11.3 Surgical Techniques for Sperm Extraction

Sperm can be obtained from the ejaculate, vas deferens, epididymis, or testicle. Surgical extraction from the epididymis or testes can be done percutaneously, or by open surgery with or without the use of a surgical microscope. A 2008 Cochrane review concluded that there is insufficient evidence to recommend any one particular method of sperm retrieval [25].

Various methods of surgical retrieval for testicular sperm exist. The conventional testicular sperm extraction (TESE) is a commonly used technique first described in 1993 and remains a mainstay in therapy [26]. In this approach, the testicle is incised to expose the seminiferous tubules for retrieval. In the andrology lab, sperm are then isolated from the extracted tissue. In 1999, Schlegel demonstrated the use of a surgical microscope to identify the tubules most likely to contain sperm [27]. This technique known as microdissection testicular sperm extraction (microTESE or mTESE) improved sperm retrieval rates (SSR) from 32 to 45% with the traditional TESE to 57–63% [27, 28]. Testicular sperm aspiration (TESA) has also been described [29]. TESA is performed using a large bore needle to create negative pressure allowing percutaneous retrieval of a small volume of seminiferous tubules. A recent systematic review compared these three techniques of testicular sperm extraction (TESA, TESE, microTESE) [30]. Fifteen studies were included for analysis. In the comparison of microTESE and conventional TESE, the SSR for conventional TESE was 35% (95% CI 30–40%) and microTESE was 52% (95% CI 47–58%). Therefore, microTESE was 1.5 times more likely to yield sperm (95% CI 1.4–1.6). In the comparison of conventional TESE and TESA, the SSR for TESA was 28% (95% CI 10–39%) and for conventional TESE was 56% (95% CI 50–61%). Therefore, conventional TESE was twice more likely to yield sperm than TESA (95% CI 1.8–2.2).

Epididymal sperm can similarly be extracted by percutaneous aspiration or microsurgical extraction. Percutaneous epididymal sperm aspiration (PESA) was first described in 1994 [31]. PESA involves needle aspiration of sperm from the epididymis. Micro-epididymal sperm extraction (MESA) is performed via scrotal incision to expose the epididymis and using an operative microscope to identify dilated epididymal tubules for incision and aspiration of tubular fluid [32]. Higher pregnancy rates have been published using MESA rather than PESA [33, 34]. The cost-effectiveness of MESA has also been shown to be superior to PESA [35].

11.4   Epididymal Versus Testicular Sperm for ICSI

Epididymal or testicular sperm are options for ICSI in men with obstructive azoospermia. The benefit of using epididymal sperm over testicular is that; often more sperm can be retrieved and the sperm are more likely to be motile, acting as a surrogate for viability [36]. On the other hand, chances of reconstruction in the future are limited by scarring of the epididymis after surgical extraction of sperm. Therefore, the use of epididymal sperm in men with obstructive azoospermia typically is reserved for cases where reconstruction is impossible or undesired. In addition, epididymal sperm may not always be available due to the absence or fibrosis of the epididymis. The issue of higher DFI in epididymal sperm compared to testicular is also a contributing factor in deciding between these sperm sources, as previously discussed [15].

There are several studies comparing ICSI outcomes using testicular vs. epididymal sperm. van Wely et al. compared microsurgical epididymal sperm aspiration to testicular sperm for ICSI in 374 patients with obstructive azoospermia due to congenital bilateral absence of the vas deferens (CBAVD) and vasectomy [36]. The authors showed a higher live birth rate and pregnancy rate with MESA compared to TESE [36]. This remained true when each pathologic subset, CBAVD and vasectomy, was analyzed separately. Similarly, Ketabchi investigated men with cryptozoospermia who were randomly assigned to testicular, epididymal, or ejaculated sperm extraction and showed the highest pregnancy rate and embryo quality when using epididymal sperm [37]. Conversely, another prospective study compared ejaculated sperm from men with severe oligoasthenoteratozoospermia, epididymal sperm from men with obstructive azoospermia and testicular sperm from men with azoospermia due to spermatogenic dysfunction and found no differences in fertilization or pregnancy rates between these sperm sources [38]. However, an argument can be made for these differing pathologies confounding the results. Additional studies support these findings, demonstrating no statistical difference in pregnancy and fertilization rates between testicular and epididymal sperm sources for ICSI [39, 40]. Furthermore, there does not appear to be a demonstrable difference in birth defects in children born after ICSI using PESA (percutaneous epididymal sperm extraction) and TESE [41]. Unfortunately, the optimal source remains unclear due to conflicting data.

Obstructive azoospermia may be acquired or congenital, and outcomes and sperm source may vary based on type of obstructive azoospermia [42]. Common acquired causes include vasectomy, post-infectious and post-surgical. CBAVD is, by definition, a congenital cause. It is rare, occurring in 0.1% of the male population [43]. Using epididymal sperm aspiration, Chen et al. demonstrated higher pregnancy rates in men with congenital compared to acquired obstructive azoospermia, yet fertilization rates were similar [42]. Epididymal sperm extraction for ART in men with CBAVD was first described in 1987 and has been found to be reasonably successful with sperm retrieval rates of 43.5% [44, 45]. Llabador et al. [45] investigated sperm source outcomes in this cohort and found statistically similar fertilization and pregnancy rates using epididymal and testicular sperm; however, Beauvillard et al. showed better outcomes in men with epididymal sperm over testicular [46]. Given its rare occurrence, comparative outcome studies on sperm source for men with CBAVD are very limited and therefore definitive superiority of either source cannot be established.

11.5   Testicular vs. Ejaculated Sperm for ICSI

There is much debate over whether testicular or ejaculated sperm should be used for ICSI in men with cryptozoospermia [38, 47]. Cryptozoospermia is defined by the World Health Organization as spermatozoa absent from fresh preparations, but observed in a centrifuged pellet [48]. There are inherent problems with the use of ejaculated sperm in men with cryptozoospermia. Preparation of such ejaculated samples requires thorough examination and prolonged preparation time [49]. Repeated centrifugation to locate sperm can increase the production of reactive oxidative species, particularly when motile sperm are present. This may lead to reduced sperm quality by increasing DFI and possibly worsened assisted reproductive outcomes, as previously discussed [50]. The inconsistent presence of sperm in the ejaculate of cryptozoospermic men—often referred to as virtual azoospermia—and technical difficulties of cryopreservation in this population may lead to mis-timing of oocyte retrieval [51–53]. Moreover, microTESE while well tolerated, does carry inherent risks of surgical complications as well as possible long-term hypoandrogenism necessitating hormone replacement therapy [54, 55]. Such risks may not be justifiable if outcomes are no different. It has been suggested that testicular sperm should be used for ICSI after failure to achieve a pregnancy using ejaculated sperm; however, limited data exist to support this [56, 57].

Ben-Ami et al. preformed a retrospective cohort study of 17 patients with cryptozoospermia undergoing 116 ICSI cycles [58]. The patients in this study all underwent ICSI using ejaculated sperm first and then testicular sperm. The authors found testicular sperm to have higher implantation rates, pregnancy rates, and take home baby rates. However, the results of this study may be skewed since the patients had all failed ICSI using ejaculated sperm first. In 2008, Bendikson et al. also compared ejaculated vs. sperm in men with cryptozoospermia. They retrospectively reviewed 16 couples undergoing 48 ICSI cycles and compared outcomes in men who had undergone cycles with both ejaculated and testicular sperm. Unpaired analysis showed no difference in pregnancy or fertilization rates within the two groups. However, paired analysis of chronologically close cycles did demonstrate a higher rate of normal (*2pn*) fertilization in the TESE group (60.9% vs. 48.5%, $p < 0.05$) and a trend towards higher delivery rates (50% using testicular sperm vs. 14.3% with ejaculated sperm). Hauser et al. and Weissman similarly found better fertilization rates using testicular sperm than with ejaculated sperm [57, 59].

A 2016 meta-analysis of available evidence showed no demonstrable statistical difference in the fertilization or pregnancy rates for testicular versus ejaculated sperm from men with cryptozoospermia when undergoing ICSI [60]. This research included five cohort studies examining either pregnancy or fertilization rates using both testicular and ejaculated sperm in men with cryptozoospermia, encompassing 272 ICSI cycles and 2547 injected oocytes [57–59, 61, 62]. A set of four studies included data on fertilization rates [57–59, 62] and another distinct set of four studies [58, 59, 61, 62] included data on pregnancy rates. There were no differences in the ICSI pregnancy rates (RR = 0.53, 95% CI: 0.19–1.42, p = 0.21, I^2 = 67%) or fertilization rates (RR = 0.91, 95% CI: 0.78–1.06, p = 0.21, I^2 = 73%). The between-study variance was relatively higher in the pregnancy rates analysis (Tau^2 = 0.64). There was low variance between studies used in the fertilization rates analysis (Tau^2 = 0.02). Post hoc power analysis revealed pβ < 20% for pregnancy rate analysis and pβ <10% for fertilization rate analysis. Thus, the risk of Type II error is acceptably low. Limitations of this work include the retrospective nature of the included studies, the studies included in the pregnancy rates analysis had a small sample sizes, and there are only a small number of available studies. In addition, there were higher maternal and paternal ages in the testicular sperm groups although this would seem to favor the ejaculated sperm cohort.

There may be other rationales to proceed with testicular sperm extraction in the setting of cryptozoospermia, including the unreliable presence of sperm in the ejaculate in preparation for an in vitro fertilization cycle, an inadequate absolute number of sperm available in the ejaculate, or abnormal ejaculated sperm DFI. In addition, freezing low volumes of ejaculated sperm can lead to loss of sperm on thawing at the time of ICSI [63]. MicroTESE is an effective method to retrieve sperm in men with cryptozoospermia. One study reported a 96% successful surgical sperm retrieval rate, with a subsequent pregnancy rate of 33% [64]. This is significantly better than reported surgical sperm retrieval rates for men with azoospermia due to spermatogenic dysfunction [65]. Although microTESE is a safe and effective procedure, adverse events may occur including hematoma, infection, or pain [66]. Short-term changes in testosterone levels have also been shown after microTESE. One study demonstrated testosterone levels returned to 80% of their preoperative levels by 3–6 months, and rose to 95% of baseline levels after 18 months [28]. However, if testicular sperm offers no demonstrable fertility advantage over ejaculated sperm, patients may rightly opt to forgo surgery.

11.6 Cryopreservation and Sperm Source

Cryopreservation of sperm is an important consideration when evaluating sperm sources. There are several important reasons why cryopreserved sperm are used. In the case of ejaculated sperm, there is significant variability in sperm parameters over time and an optimal fresh specimen cannot be guaranteed at the time of ICSI. Similarly, for surgically extracted sperm, retrieval rates are not 100%. Cryopreserved sperm can be kept as a "back up" if fresh sperm are unavailable at the time of ICSI; it also avoids mis-timing with the female cycle. Freezing surgically extracted sperm allows for multiple ICSI cycles to be undertaken using sperm from a single operation. In addition, geographic location of services and logistics may make timed fresh cycles a challenge.

Men with severe oligozoospermia or cryptozoospermia may be encouraged to cryopreserve ejaculated sperm in anticipation of IVF due to the risk of transient azoospermia, which may exceed 50% [51, 67]. It is currently thought that conventional techniques of cryopreservation may represent a barrier to men with severe male factor infertility due to perceived diminished post-thaw sperm recovery [68]. A systematic review of 30 studies quantifying sperm loss after cryopreservation of very low numbers of ejaculated sperm had post-thaw retrieval rates ranging from 59 to 100% [68]. This may represent a disadvantage of the use of ejaculated sperm in these men.

Epididymal sperm has been frozen given the abundance with each aspiration. Janzen et al. reported their outcomes of 141 couples undergoing ICSI using frozen and fresh epididymal sperm retrieved by MESA [69]. No difference in pregnancy or fertilization rates were identified between the fresh or frozen sperm groups despite some post-thaw sperm loss [69]. Other studies have similarly shown no differences in fertilization and pregnancy rates when using fresh or frozen sperm [70–72]. The method of epididymal sperm retrieval may be of relevance when cryopreserving sperm. Rosenlund et al. reported a 33% rate of sufficient sperm from cryopreservation using PESA to retrieve sperm, whereas Janzen et al. reported a 100% rate of sufficient sperm from MESA [69, 73].

Testicular sperm is also frequently cryopreserved to allow for multiple cycles to be performed from a single surgery. A 2014 meta-analysis compared ICSI outcomes using fresh and frozen testicular sperm in men with azoospermia due to spermatogenic dysfunction [74]. Eleven studies were included in the pregnancy rate analysis and ten for the fertilization rate analysis. 28.7% of ICSI cycles using fresh testicular sperm resulted in clinical pregnancy compared to 28.1% of ICSI cycles when frozen testicular sperm was used (RR = 1.0, 95% CI 0.92–1.02). Similarly, for fertilization rates no difference was found when fresh or frozen testicular sperm was used (53.9% vs. 54%, RR 0.97, 95% CI 0.92–1.02) [73]. In men with obstructive azoospermia, cryopreservation of testicular sperm also does not appear to reduce pregnancy or fertilization rates [75].

11.7   Conclusion

The question of optimal sperm source for ICSI is complex and inconclusively answered. ICSI allows even samples with very small amounts of sperm to fertilize an egg. Possible sperm sources for ICSI include the ejaculate, epididymis, and testicle. In the setting of azoospermia, options include epididymal or testicular sperm. Procurement of epididymal sperm can cause scarring and therefore is reserved for men for whom reconstruction is not possible or not desired. Literature comparing outcomes using epididymal and testicular sperm for ICSI having varying results, and therefore it is not clear which source is optimal. For men with low volumes of ejaculated sperm such as cryptozoospermia or severe oligozoospermia, ejaculated, epididymal, or testicular sperm can be used. Current evidence does not demonstrate any difference in pregnancy or fertilization rates using ejaculated or testicular sperm. Testicular, epididymal, and ejaculated sperm can all be cryopreserved with outcomes comparable to using fresh sperm. However, low volumes can be associated with sperm loss post thaw, and therefore should be a consideration.

References

1. Lu Y, Gao H, Li B, Zheng Y, Ye Y, Qian Y, et al. Different sperm sources and parameters can influence intracytoplasmic sperm injection outcomes before embryo implantation. J Zhejiang Univ Sci B [Internet]. 2012;13:1–10. http://www.ncbi.nlm.nih.gov/pmc/articles/PMC3251746/
2. Bedford JM, Calvin H, Cooper GW. The maturation of spermatozoa in the human epididymis. J Reprod Fertil Suppl. 1973;18:199–213.
3. Hinrichsen MJ, Blaquier JA. Evidence supporting the existence of sperm maturation in the human epididymis. J Reprod Fertil. 1980;60:291–4.
4. Suganuma R, Yanagimachi R, Meistrich ML. Decline in fertility of mouse sperm with abnormal chromatin during epididymal passage as revealed by ICSI. Hum Reprod. 2005;20:3101–8.
5. Aitken RJ, Krausz C. Oxidative stress, DNA damage and the Y chromosome. Reproduction. 2001;122:497–506.
6. Greco E, Romano S, Iacobelli M, Ferrero S, Baroni E, Minasi MG, et al. ICSI in cases of sperm DNA damage: beneficial effect of oral antioxidant treatment. Hum Reprod. 2005;20:2590–4.
7. Greco E, Scarselli F, Iacobelli M, Rienzi L, Ubaldi F, Ferrero S, et al. Efficient treatment of infertility due to sperm DNA damage by ICSI with testicular spermatozoa. Hum Reprod. 2005;20:226–30.
8. Muratori M, Tamburrino L, Marchiani S, Cambi M, Olivito B, Azzari C, et al. Investigation on the origin of sperm DNA fragmentation: role of apoptosis, immaturity and oxidative stress. Mol Med. 2015;21:109–22.
9. Aitken RJ, Bronson R, Smith TB, De Iuliis GN. The source and significance of DNA damage in human spermatozoa; a commentary on diagnostic strategies and straw man fallacies. Mol Hum Reprod. 2013;19:475–85.
10. Aitken RJ, Baker MA. Oxidative stress, sperm survival and fertility control. Mol Cell Endocrinol. 2006;250:66–9.
11. Cozzubbo T, Neri QV, Goldstein M, Rosenwaks Z, Palermo GD. Topographic mapping of sperm DNA fragmentation within the male genital tract. Fertil Steril [Internet]. 2014;102:e188. http://linkinghub.elsevier.com/retrieve/pii/S0015028214012618
12. Hammoud I, Bailly M, Bergere M, Wainer R, Izard V, Vialard F, et al. Testicular spermatozoa are of better quality than epididymal spermatozoa in patients with obstructive azoospermia. Urology. 2017; 103:106–111.
13. Esteves SC, Sánchez-Martín F, Sánchez-Martín P, Schneider DT, Gosálvez J. Comparison of reproductive outcome in oligozoospermic men with high sperm DNA fragmentation undergoing intracytoplasmic sperm injection with ejaculated and testicular sperm. Fertil Steril [Internet]. 2015;104(6):1398–405. http://www.sciencedirect.com/science/article/pii/S0015028215018749
14. Mehta A, Bolyakov A, Schlegel PN, Paduch DA. Higher pregnancy rates using testicular sperm in men with severe oligospermia. Fertil Steril [Internet]. 2015;104(6):1382–7. http://www.sciencedirect.com/science/article/pii/S0015028215017628

15. O'Connell M, McClure N, Lewis SEM. Mitochondrial DNA deletions and nuclear DNA fragmentation in testicular and epididymal human sperm. Hum Reprod. 2002;17:1565–70.
16. Moskovtsev SI, Willis J, White J, Mullen JB. Sperm DNA damage: correlation to severity of semen abnormalities. Urology [Internet]. 2009;74:789–93. http://www.sciencedirect.com/science/article/pii/S0090429509007043
17. Moskovtsev SI, Willis J, White J, Mullen JBM. Sperm DNA damage: correlation to severity of semen abnormalities. Urology. 2009;74:789–93.
18. Giwercman A, Lindstedt L, Larsson M, Bungum M, Spano M, Levine RJ, et al. Sperm chromatin structure assay as an independent predictor of fertility in vivo: a case-control study. Int J Androl. 2010;33(1):e221–7.
19. Benchaib M. Sperm DNA fragmentation decreases the pregnancy rate in an assisted reproductive technique. Hum Reprod [Internet]. 2003;18:1023–8. http://humrep.oxfordjournals.org/cgi/content/long/18/5/1023
20. Simon L, Liu L, Murphy K, Ge S, Hotaling J, Aston KI, et al. Comparative analysis of three sperm DNA damage assays and sperm nuclear protein content in couples undergoing assisted reproduction treatment. Hum Reprod. 2014;29:904–17.
21. Larson-Cook KL, Brannian JD, Hansen KA, Kasperson KM, Aamold ET, Evenson DP. Relationship between the outcomes of assisted reproductive techniques and sperm DNA fragmentation as measured by the sperm chromatin structure assay. Fertil Steril. 2003;80:895–902.
22. Robinson L, Gallos ID, Conner SJ, Rajkhowa M, Miller D, Lewis S, et al. The effect of sperm DNA fragmentation on miscarriage rates: a systematic review and meta-analysis. Hum Reprod. 2012;27:2908–17.
23. Lin M-H, Kuo-Kuang Lee R, Li S-H, C-H L, Sun F-J, Hwu Y-M. Sperm chromatin structure assay parameters are not related to fertilization rates, embryo quality, and pregnancy rates in in vitro fertilization and intracytoplasmic sperm injection, but might be related to spontaneous abortion rates. Fertil Steril. 2008;90:352–9.
24. Gandini L, Lombardo F, Paoli D, Caruso F, Eleuteri P, Leter G, et al. Full-term pregnancies achieved with ICSI despite high levels of sperm chromatin damage. Hum Reprod. 2004;19:1409–17.
25. Van Peperstraten A, Proctor ML, Johnson NP, Philipson G. Techniques for surgical retrieval of sperm prior to intra-cytoplasmic sperm injection (ICSI) for azoospermia. Cochrane Database Syst Rev 2008;(2):CD002807.
26. Schoysman R, Vanderzwalmen P, Nijs M, Segal L, Segal-Bertin G, Geerts L, et al. Pregnancy after fertilisation with human testicular spermatozoa. Lancet. 1993;342(8881):1237.
27. Schlegel PN. Testicular sperm extraction: microdissection improves sperm yield with minimal tissue excision. Hum Reprod. 1999;14:131–5.
28. Ramasamy R, Yagan N, Schlegel PN. Structural and functional changes to the testis after conventional versus microdissection testicular sperm extraction. Urology. 2005;65:1190–4.
29. Lewin A, Weiss DB, Friedler S, Ben-Shachar I, Porat-Katz A, Meirow D, et al. Delivery following intracytoplasmic injection of mature sperm cells recovered by testicular fine needle aspiration in a case of hypergonadotropic azoospermia due to maturation arrest. Hum Reprod. 1996;11:769–71.
30. Bernie AM, Mata DA, Ramasamy R, Schlegel PN. Comparison of microdissection testicular sperm extraction, conventional testicular sperm extraction, and testicular sperm aspiration for nonobstructive azoospermia: a systematic review and meta-analysis. Fertil Steril. 2015;104:1093–9.
31. Shrivastav P, Nadkarni P, Wensvoort S, Craft I. Percutaneous epididymal sperm aspiration for obstructive azoospermia. Hum Reprod. 1994;9:2058–61.
32. Silber SJ, Balmaceda J, Borrero C, Ord T, Asch R. Pregnancy with sperm aspiration from the proximal head of the epididymis: a new treatment for congenital absence of the vas deferens. Fertil Steril. 1988;50:525–8.

33. Meniru GI, Gorgy A, Podsiadly BT, Craft IL. Results of percutaneous epididymal sperm aspiration and intracytoplasmic sperm injection in two major groups of patients with obstructive azoospermia. Hum Reprod. 1997;12:2443–6.
34. Friedler S, Raziel A, Soffer Y, Strassburger D, Komarovsky D, Ron-El R. The outcome of intracytoplasmic injection of fresh and cryopreserved epididymal spermatozoa from patients with obstructive azoospermia—a comparative study. Hum Reprod. 1998;13(7):1872.
35. Pavlovich CP, Schlegel PN. Fertility options after vasectomy: a cost-effectiveness analysis. Fertil Steril. 1997;67:133–41.
36. van Wely M, Barbey N, Meissner A, Repping S, Silber SJ. Live birth rates after MESA or TESE in men with obstructive azoospermia: is there a difference? Hum Reprod. 2015;30:761–6.
37. Ketabchi AA. Intracytoplasmic sperm injection outcomes with freshly ejaculated sperms and testicular or epididymal sperm extraction in patients with idiopathic cryptozoospermia. Nephrourol Mon. 2016;8:e41375.
38. Ghazzawi IM, Sarraf MG, Taher MR, Khalifa FA. Comparison of the fertilizing capability of spermatozoa from ejaculates, epididymal aspirates and testicular biopsies using intracytoplasmic sperm injection. Hum Reprod [Internet]. 1998;13:348–52. http://www.ncbi.nlm.nih.gov/pubmed/9557836
39. Silber SJ, Nagy Z, Liu J, Tournaye H, Lissens W, Ferec C, et al. The use of epididymal and testicular spermatozoa for intracytoplasmic sperm injection: the genetic implications for male infertility. Hum Reprod. 1995;10:2031–43.
40. Nagy Z, Liu J, Cecile J, Silber S, Devroey P, Van Steirteghem A. Using ejaculated, fresh, and frozen-thawed epididymal and testicular spermatozoa gives rise to comparable results after intracytoplasmic sperm injection. Fertil Steril. 1995;63:808–15.
41. Meijerink AM, Oomen RE, Fleischer K, IntHout J, Woldringh GH, Braat DDM. Effect of maternal and treatment-related factors on the prevalence of birth defects after PESA-ICSI and TESE-ICSI: a retrospective cohort study. Acta Obstet Gynecol Scand. 2015;94:1245–53.
42. Chen CS, Chu SH, Soong YK, Lai YM. Epididymal sperm aspiration with assisted reproductive techniques: difference between congenital and acquired obstructive azoospermia? Hum Reprod. 1995;10:1104–8.
43. Wagenknecht LV, Lotzin CF, Sommer HJ, Schirren C. Vas deferens aplasia: clinical and anatomical features of 90 cases. Andrologia. 1983;15 Spec No:605–13.
44. Silber S, Ord T, Borrero C, Balmaceda J, Asch R. New treatment for infertility due to congenital absence of vas deferens. Lancet. 1987;2(8563):850–1.
45. Llabador MA, Pagin A, Lefebvre-Maunoury C, Marcelli F, Leroy-Martin B, Rigot JM, et al. Congenital bilateral absence of the vas deferens: the impact of spermatogenesis quality on intracytoplasmic sperm injection outcomes in 108 men. Andrology. 2015;3:473–80.
46. Beauvillard D, Perrin A, Drapier H, Ravel C, Freour T, Ferec C, et al. [Congenital bilateral absence of vas deferens: from diagnosis to assisted reproductive techniques—the experience of three centers]. Gynecol Obstet Fertil. 2015;43:367–74.
47. Göker EN, Sendag F, Levi R, Sendag H, Tavmergen E. Comparison of the ICSI outcome of ejaculated sperm with normal, abnormal parameters and testicular sperm. Eur J Obstet Gynecol Reprod Biol. 2002;104:129–36.
48. Edition F. Examination and processing of human semen. World Health [Internet]. 2010; Edition, F:286. http://whqlibdoc.who.int/publications/2010/9789241547789_eng.pdf
49. Swanton A, Itani A, McVeigh E, Child T. Azoospermia: is sample centrifugation indicated? A national survey of practice and the Oxford experience. Fertil Steril [Internet]. 2007;88:374–8. http://www.sciencedirect.com/science/article/pii/S0015028206046619
50. Agarwal A, Ikemoto I, Loughlin KR. Effect of sperm washing on levels of reactive oxygen species in semen. Arch Androl. 1994;33:157–62.
51. Koscinski I, Wittemer C, Lefebvre-Khalil V, Marcelli F, Defossez A, Rigot JM. Optimal management of extreme oligozoospermia by an appropriate cryopreservation programme. Hum Reprod [Internet]. 2007;22:2679–84. http://humrep.oxfordjournals.org/cgi/content/long/22/10/2679

52. Ron-El R, Strassburger D, Friedler S, Komarovski D, Bern O, Soffer Y, et al. Extended sperm preparation: an alternative to testicular sperm extraction in non-obstructive azoospermia. Hum Reprod. 1997;12(6):1222.
53. Palermo GD, Neri QV, Schlegel PN, Rosenwaks Z. Intracytoplasmic SPERM Injection (ICSI) in extreme cases of male infertility. PLoS One [Internet]. 2014;9:e113671. http://dx.plos.org/10.1371/journal.pone.0113671
54. Schlegel PN, Su LM. Physiological consequences of testicular sperm extraction. Hum Reprod. 1997;12:1688–92.
55. Everaert K, De Croo I, Kerckhaert W, Dekuyper P, Dhont M, Van der Elst J, et al. Long term effects of micro-surgical testicular sperm extraction on androgen status in patients with non obstructive azoospermia. BMC Urol. 2006;6:9.
56. Hayden RP, Wright DL, Toth TL, Tanrikut C. Selective use of percutaneous testis biopsy to optimize IVF-ICSI outcomes: a case series. Fertil Res Pract [Internet]. 2016;2:7. http://fertilityresearchandpractice.biomedcentral.com/articles/10.1186/s40738–016–0020-y
57. Weissman A, Horowitz E, Ravhon A, Nahum H, Golan A, Levran D. Pregnancies and live births following ICSI with testicular spermatozoa after repeated implantation failure using ejaculated spermatozoa. Reprod Biomed Online [Internet]. 2008;17:605–9. https://doi.org/10.1016/S1472-6483(10)60306-9.
58. Ben-Ami I, Raziel A, Strassburger D, Komarovsky D, Ron-El R, Friedler S. Intracytoplasmic sperm injection outcome of ejaculated versus extracted testicular spermatozoa in cryptozoospermic men. Fertil Steril [Internet]. 2013;99:1867–71. http://www.sciencedirect.com/science/article/pii/S0015028213002975
59. Hauser R, Bibi G, Yogev L, Carmon A, Azem F, Botchan A, et al. Virtual azoospermia and cryptozoospermia—fresh/frozen testicular or ejaculate sperm for better IVF outcome? J Androl. 2011;32:484–90.
60. Abhyankar N, Kathrins M, Niederberger C. Use of testicular versus ejaculated sperm for intracytoplasmic sperm injection among men with cryptozoospermia: a meta-analysis. Fertil Steril. 2016;105:1469–1475.e1.
61. Amirjannati N, Heidari-Vala H, Akhondi MA, Hosseini Jadda SH, Kamali K, Sadeghi MR, et al. Comparison of intracytoplasmic sperm injection outcomes between spermatozoa retrieved from testicular biopsy and from ejaculation in cryptozoospermic men. Andrologia [Internet]. 2012;44(Suppl 1):704–9. http://www.ncbi.nlm.nih.gov/pubmed/12206925
62. Bendikson KA, Neri QV, Takeuchi T, Toschi M, Schlegel PN, Rosenwaks Z, et al. The outcome of intracytoplasmic sperm injection using occasional spermatozoa in the ejaculate of men with spermatogenic failure. J Urol [Internet]. 2008;180:1060–4. http://www.sciencedirect.com/science/article/pii/S0022534708012457
63. O'Connell M, McClure N, Lewis SEM. The effects of cryopreservation on sperm morphology, motility and mitochondrial function. Hum Reprod. 2002;17:704–9.
64. Alrabeeah K, Wachter A, Phillips S, Cohen B, Al-Hathal N, Zini A. Sperm retrieval outcomes with microdissection testicular sperm extraction (micro-TESE) in men with cryptozoospermia. Andrology [Internet]. 2015;3(3):462–6. http://doi.wiley.com/10.1111/andr.12000
65. Bernie AM, Ramasamy R, Schlegel PN. Predictive factors of successful microdissection testicular sperm extraction. Basic Clin Androl [Internet]. 2013;23:25. https://doi.org/10.1186/2051-4190-23-5. http://www.ncbi.nlm.nih.gov/pmc/articles/PMC4346292/
66. Amer M, Ateyah A, Hany R, Zohdy W. Prospective comparative study between microsurgical and conventional testicular sperm extraction in non-obstructive azoospermia: follow-up by serial ultrasound examinations. Hum Reprod. 2000;15:653–6.
67. Montagut M, Gatimel N, Bourdet-Loubere S, Daudin M, Bujan L, Mieusset R, et al. Sperm freezing to address the risk of azoospermia on the day of ICSI. Hum Reprod. 2015;30:2486–92.
68. AbdelHafez F, Bedaiwy M, El-Nashar SA, Sabanegh E, Desai N. Techniques for cryopreservation of individual or small numbers of human spermatozoa: a systematic review. Hum Reprod Update. 2009;15:153–64.

69. Janzen N, Goldstein M, Schlegel PN, Palermo GD, Rosenwaks Z, Hariprashad J. Use of elec-
    tively cryopreserved microsurgically aspirated epididymal sperm with IVF and intracytoplas-
    mic sperm injection for obstructive azoospermia. Fertil Steril. 2000;74:696–701.
70. Cayan S, Lee D, Conaghan J, Givens CA, Ryan IP, Schriock ED, et al. A comparison of ICSI
    outcomes with fresh and cryopreserved epididymal spermatozoa from the same couples. Hum
    Reprod. 2001;16:495–9.
71. Hutchon S, Thornton S, Hall J, Bishop M. Frozen-thawed epididymal sperm is effective for
    intracytoplasmic sperm injection: implications for the urologist. Br J Urol. 1998;81:607–11.
72. Madgar I, Hourvitz A, Levron J, Seidman DS, Shulman A, Raviv GG, et al. Outcome of in vitro
    fertilization and intracytoplasmic injection of epididymal and testicular sperm extracted from
    patients with obstructive and nonobstructive azoospermia. Fertil Steril. 1998;69:1080–4.
73. Rosenlund B, Westlander G, Wood M, Lundin K, Reismer E, Hillensjo T. Sperm retrieval
    and fertilization in repeated percutaneous epididymal sperm aspiration. Hum Reprod.
    1998;13:2805–7.
74. Ohlander S, Hotaling J, Kirshenbaum E, Niederberger C, Eisenberg ML. Impact of fresh ver-
    sus cryopreserved testicular sperm upon intracytoplasmic sperm injection pregnancy outcomes
    in men with azoospermia due to spermatogenic dysfunction: a meta-analysis. Fertil Steril.
    2014;101:344–9.
75. Karacan M, Alwaeely F, Erkan S, Cebi Z, Berberoglugil M, Batukan M, et al. Outcome of
    intracytoplasmic sperm injection cycles with fresh testicular spermatozoa obtained on the day
    of or the day before oocyte collection and with cryopreserved testicular sperm in patients with
    azoospermia. Fertil Steril. 2013;100:975–80.

Chapter 12
Intracytoplasmic Sperm Injection (ICSI): Applications and Insights

Toru Suzuki and Anthony C.F. Perry

12.1 Introduction

Intracytoplasmic sperm injection (ICSI) was originally developed in sea urchins [1] and has classically described the injection of a sperm into an unfertilized, metaphase II (mII) oocyte [2]. ICSI has now been extended to at least 17 mammalian species and has become a key technique for the production of embryos and offspring [3, 4]. It is currently the most prevalent method of human assisted reproduction, accounting for approximately two-thirds of cycles [5]. Since its first application in the mouse [3], ICSI has been harnessed to dissect gamete function [6, 7], adapted for the production of genome modified animals with transgenes [8–10] or following genome editing [11] and to inject materials other than sperm into oocytes, including somatic cell nuclei [12, 13], secondary spermatocyte nuclei [14], round spermatid nuclei [15], and microbeads [16]. This chapter describes ICSI in the mouse and how it has recently been extended to sperm injection into embryos including parthenogenotes [16].

12.2 Outline of the Method

In the first reported mammalian ICSI, golden hamster or human sperm were injected into golden hamster oocytes [17]. A similar method has been used for other mammalian species, but although the mouse is perhaps the most important mammalian model, the development of mouse ICSI has been slow because mouse mII oocytes are extremely fragile and typically do not survive conventional injection. This

T. Suzuki • A.C.F. Perry (✉)
Laboratory of Mammalian Molecular Embryology, Department of Biology and Biochemistry, University of Bath, Bath, UK
e-mail: T.Suzuki@bath.ac.uk; acfp20@bath.ac.uk

© Springer International Publishing AG 2018
G.D. Palermo, E.S. Sills (eds.), *Intracytoplasmic Sperm Injection*,
https://doi.org/10.1007/978-3-319-70497-5_12

situation changed in 1995 with the application of piezo-actuated microinjection (simply referred to below as piezo) to mouse ICSI [3]. Piezo is thought to drive the tip of a pipette housed in a piezo-actuating unit to make a relatively neat wound in the mouse mII oocyte plasma membrane from which it can recover, in contrast to manually produced breaks generated by conventional methods. The result is improved survival following sperm injection, from 16% in conventional ICSI, to 80% with piezo-ICSI [3]. This is accompanied by increases in development to the blastocyst stage in vitro from 33 to 68% (of starting one-cell embryos), with 30% of two-cell embryos produced by piezo developing to term [3]. While our basic piezo methodology is based on the first report of mouse ICSI [3], its modifications [4] can give success rates of over 80% (offspring per transferred two-cell embryo) in the case of hybrid B6D2F1 crosses [16].

With the advent of mouse ICSI, it was rapidly established that injecting sperm heads into MII oocytes efficiently supported full-term development [18]. In our protocol, demembranated sperm heads [6] are freshly prepared from cauda epididymidal sperm just prior to use (see Fig. 12.1a) [4, 19]. Typically, one sexually mature male contains sufficient sperm for a single microinjection session lasting up to 2–3 h. Epididymides are isolated and minced with fine scissors in nuclear isolation medium (NIM; [6]) to liberate the sperm inside. Sperm preparation is performed in the presence of a detergent such as CHAPS, which demembranates the sperm heads. This removes acrosomal and other contents that do not normally enter the oocyte during fertilization and which may be harmful, and either causes head-tail detachment (facilitating subsequent ICSI) or makes detachment easier during micromanipulation. Treated sperm are washed in NIM to remove the CHAPS, although CHAPS appears to be relatively nontoxic [6]. Freshly prepared sperm head suspensions in NIM are mixed with long-chain polyvinylpyrrolidone (PVP) to give a typical PVP concentration of 4–5% (w/v) and sperm density of $1.0e^5$–$4.0e^7$/mL. The PVP stabilizes the pipette during injection and acts as a lubricant, but although higher PVP concentrations facilitate micromanipulation, they can have a toxic effect on embryo development, so there is a technical and biological trade-off. From collection of the cauda epididymidis to the preparation of the working sperm suspension in PVP takes less than 15 min.

Unlike the glass pipettes used in conventional microinjection which are beveled, piezo uses sharp, flush-ended tips (with an internal diameter of ~6 μm) made of relatively hard borosilicate glass (see Fig. 12.1a). Oil in the injection line can be messy and water is preferred, but in either case, piezo is applied to drill through the zona pellucida and then (with a different piezo setting) to puncture the MII oocyte plasma membrane (see Fig. 12.1b) [4]. Piezo allows coinjection of other materials with the sperm, for example linearized DNA fragments for transgenesis [8] or Cas9 cRNA plus gRNA for targeted mutagenesis [11]. Recently, we adapted ICSI to incorporate sperm chromatin into mouse parthenogenetic embryos [16], which is described next.

Fig. 12.1 Sperm injection
into mouse MII oocytes
and haploid
parthenogenotes at the first
mitosis. (**a**) Sperm heads
and glass needle used for
microinjection (left; scale
bar, 25 μm) and enlarged
sperm heads (scale bar,
5 μm). (**b**) Mouse MII
oocyte and sperm head
within needle (left) and just
before the needle
penetrates the oocyte
plasma membrane in
ICSI. Genomic DNA in
oocytes and sperm heads is
stained with Hoechst
33342 (blue). (**c**) Mouse
haploid parthenogenote
and sperm head in glass
needle (left) and just prior
to penetrating the
parthenogenote membrane
by the needle in phICSI-13.
Genomic DNA in
parthenogenotes and sperm
heads are stained with
Hoechst 33342 and colored
blue. Scale bar, 50 μm

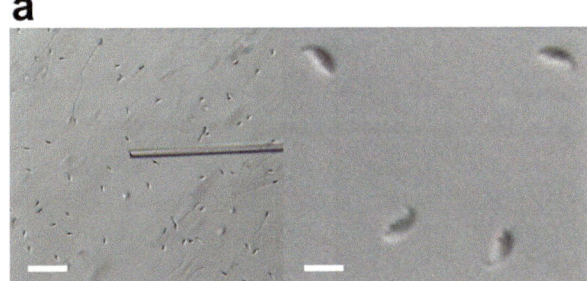

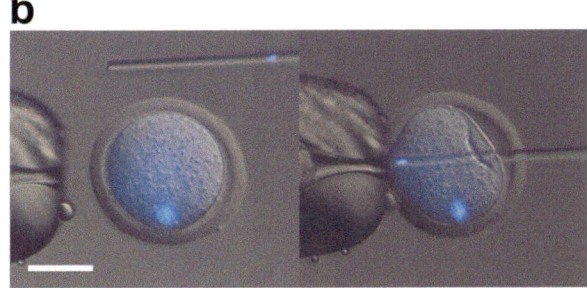

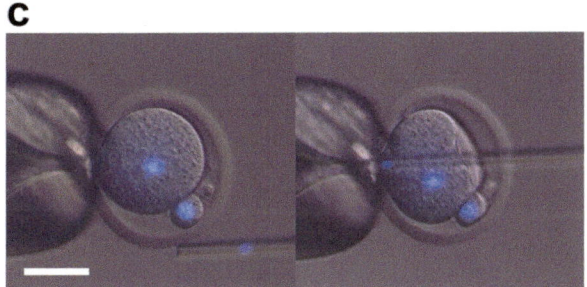

12.3 Sperm Reprogramming to Totipotency

Totipotency refers to the developmental ability of a cell to engender an entire individual [20]. In the mouse, only two cell types are totipotent: the zygote and blastomeres of a two-cell embryo. Blastomeres of four-cell or later-stage mouse embryos
(or derivatives such as embryonic stem cells) are not totipotent in that single cells
from these stages cannot support full-term development. The union of MII oocyte
and sperm results in the formation of a totipotent zygote, but the underlying mechanisms instating totipotency are poorly understood. Do oocytes contribute anything
special to establish embryonic totipotency?

Ovulated mouse oocytes awaiting fertilization are arrested at MII [21] until
sperm entry triggers meiotic resumption and paternal chromatin reprogramming to
developmental competence. From previous work on the mouse, it has been inferred

that sperm chromatin must be incorporated into MII oocytes with the correct timing for full-term embryo development to occur; this window of opportunity soon closes (within 3 h), suggesting that critical cytoplasmic changes occur rapidly after fertilization to transform the oocyte into a nascent embryo [22–24]. This finding seemed at odds with reports of reprogramming of ES cell chromatin and of partial reprogramming of differentiated somatic cell chromatin by later-stage one- and two-cell mouse embryos [25, 26]. Although term development was not supported by the differentiated somatic cell nuclei, these findings did at least raise the possibility of sperm chromatin reprogramming by developing embryos, which we decided to investigate.

12.4   The Acid Test of Totipotency

Perhaps the strictest test of complete sperm chromatin reprogramming to totipotency [20] is to demonstrate that it results in living animals. The gametes of eutherian mammals undergo parent-of-origin imprinting during their genesis, and this results in a strict requirement for balanced maternal and paternal autosomal contributions (one chromosome set from each parent) for development to occur beyond implantation. Mouse ICSI is a powerful tool with which to dissect this because it enables accurate manipulation in the context of well-understood embryology and developmental biology. With ICSI, it is possible to manipulate mouse oocytes and embryos with low trauma and to adjust the timing of sperm chromatin incorporation into recipient cells. In addition, full-term development takes only 18–19 days, making it easy to produce living animals in a relatively short time. We harnessed these features of mouse ICSI to design an experimental protocol in which sperm genome incorporation into embryonic cells can generate diploid cells with the potential to develop. Features of ICSI are likely to have been important for efficient sperm chromatin reprogramming and the high subsequent developmental potential of reconstructed embryos.

12.5   Sperm Reprogramming in Mitotic Haploid Parthenogenotes

We wished to know whether sperm chromatin could be remodeled in developing haploid parthenogenotes to form paternal (pro)nuclei and contribute to embryonic development in vitro [16]. Parthenogenetic activation of MII oocytes induced second polar body extrusion, degradation of Geminin-Venus (which also occurs in G1 of somatic cells), and maternal pronucleus (pn) formation. Maternal pn membrane breakdown occurred during entry into the first mitotic cleavage, about 13 h after the start of parthenogenetic activation. Using piezo, we introduced sperm heads into these haploid parthenogenotes at 7, 10, and 13 h (with pn membrane break down,

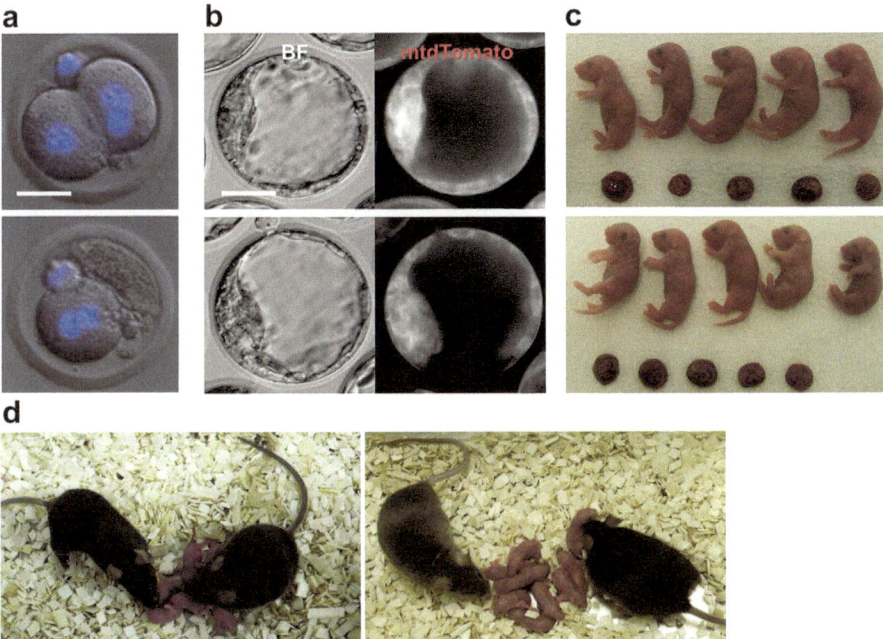

Fig. 12.2 Embryos and newborn phICSI-13 offspring. (**a**) Mouse embryos at the two-cell stage produced by phICSI-13. The embryo comprised one blastomere with a haploid maternal nucleus and another with haploid maternal nucleus and a paternal nucleus. A second polar body is present above the embryo. The lower panel shows a phICSI-13 two-cell embryo after destruction of the haploid (monoparental) blastomere (phICSI-13-1bla). Genomic DNA is stained with Hoechst 33342 (blue). (**b**) Blastocysts on day four produced by ICSI (upper) or phICSI-13 using sperm carrying an *mtdTomato* transgene. This allows visualization of cells carrying a contribution from the sperm-derived genome. Cells in phICSI-13 embryos are partially positive for mtdTomato. (**c**) Newborn pups and their associated placentae 19 days after embryo transfer of ICSI (upper) or phICSI-13-1bla two-cell stage embryo to pseudopregnant mothers. (**d**) Adults generated from phICSI-13 (left image) and phICSI-13-1bla embryos with their 3-day-old pups, produced as a result of natural mating

pnMBD) after parthenogenetic activation; we refer to this method as phICSI (see Fig. 12.1c for phICSI-13). Little, if any, sperm chromatin remodeling was detected in phICSI-7 or -10 (prior to pnMBD), but it began within 1 h after pnMBD for phICSI-7, -10, and -13.

After the first mitotic (one- to two-cell) division, phICSI two-cell embryos were placed into four categories based on nuclear configuration. One class comprised two-cell embryos containing one blastomere which was biparental and binuclear, and the other that was uniparental (maternal) and mononuclear; we refer to this class as 2 + 1 (Fig. 12.2a). Overall, 34.1–37.2% of phICSI (-7, -10, and -13) embryos developed to the blastocyst stage, compared with 73.1% for mock-injected haploid parthenogenotes and 94.0% for ICSI controls (see Table 12.1). A genetic contribution from sperm to phICSI blastocysts was demonstrated by the expression of paternal (sperm-borne) transgenes encoding pCAG-mtdTomato (see Fig. 12.2b),

Table 12.1 Embryo development

		In vitro			In vivo	
	Cultured (n)	Blastocyst (%)	Transferred (n)	Pups (n)	Pups (%)
1NPA (mock)	85	73.1 ± 5.6	–	–	–
ICSI	84	94.0 ± 1.8	106	85	82.5 ± 9.5
ICSI-1bla	198	90.7 ± 3.3	237	107	43.3 ± 15.1
phICSI-7	104	34.1 ± 7.9	465	5	1.0 ± 1.7
phICSI-10	105	35.5 ± 4.4	384	7	1.8 ± 1.4
phICSI-13	113	37.2 ± 4.0	259	21	8.1 ± 1.8
phICSI-13-1bla	149	21.5 ± 6.5	232	24	10.4 ± 3.1
phICSI-*PiV*	nd	nd	154	2	1.2 ± 1.2
ROSI	nd	nd	50	16	31.7 ± 1.6
phROSI-pnMBD-2h	nd	nd	213	6	2.6 ± 1.0

Abbreviations are explained in the text. *nd* no data

pNanog-GFP, and pOct4-mCherry, confirming that mitotically reprogrammed sperm chromatin contributed to blastocyst stage preimplantation development.

To evaluate phICSI embryo development in vivo, we non-selectively transferred wild-type (wt) phICSI two-cell embryos to the oviducts of pseudopregnant females. Viable offspring were obtained at 1.0% (offspring per embryo transferred) for phICSI-7, 1.8% for phICSI-10, and 8.1% for phICSI-13 (see Fig. 12.2c for phICSI-13 pups); the comparable rate for ICSI two-cell embryos was 82.5%, and 43.3% for ICSI two-cell embryos in which one of the two blastomeres had been destroyed by puncturing (see Table 12.1). Compared to controls, phICSI-derived offspring were indistinguishable in terms of birth-weight, placental size, fertility (see Fig. 12.2d), and longevity. We also produced healthy phICSI offspring by injecting B6D2F1 sperm into haploid parthenogenotes spontaneously arising from *Plcz-ires-Venus* transgenic females [27]. Collectively then, this work employed piezo to show that sperm chromatin reprogramming can occur in mitotic embryos with an efficiency that increased the closer sperm injection was to mitotic M-phase.

12.6 Lineage Fates in Postimplantation phICSI Embryos

A biparental genome is essential for full-term natural development in mice and probably all mammals [28, 29]. Since phICSI introduced sperm heads into haploid parthenogenotes, we reasoned that developmentally competent two-cell phICSI embryos comprised one biparental blastomere (from which offspring developed) and one uniparental one. To test this supposition and track blastomere contributions in development, we performed phICSI using parthenogenotes that expressed a *flox*ed, membrane-targeted Tomato (mtdT) that blocked ubiquitous expression of a downstream membrane-targeted GFP (mGFP) from the same transgene. The parthenogenotes were injected with sperm from males homozygous for a ubiquitously expressed Cre recombinase transgene. Since biparental blastomeres (or at least, cells containing maternal and paternal chromosomes) after sperm injection contained Cre, they underwent Cre-mediated deletion of *mtdT* and a switch from red-to-green fluorescence, whereas the uniparental maternal blastomeres remained red fluorescent. By 11.5 or 12.5 days after fertilization, phICSI embryos in these experiments were largely green fluorescent (control embryos lacking Cre remained red) suggesting that the contribution of uniparental cells in phICSI embryos is negligible.

This result suggested that the uniparental blastomere made little, if any, contribution to lineages surviving after 11.5 days, but it did not address whether the uniparental blastomere was required for full-term development or conversely, whether it had a negative impact. To evaluate this, we destroyed uniparental blastomeres of two-cell phICSI embryos (which we referred to as phICSI-13-1bla; see Fig. 12.2a) and monitored development in vivo of the remaining biparental blastomere; our control comparator was ICSI two-cell embryos in which one of the blastomeres had been randomly abolished (ICSI-1bla). The raw phICSI-13-1bla developmental rate to term was 10.4%, which was 24% of the rate of the ICSI-1bla controls (see Fig. 12.2c and Table 12.1). This suggests that biparental blastomeres in phICSI two-cell embryos are embryo-autonomously capable of supporting term development; that is, they are totipotent.

12.7 Parthenogenetic Reprogramming of Nucleosomal Chromatin; phROSI

The protein component of mouse sperm chromatin almost entirely (at least 98%) comprises the noncanonical nucleoprotein, protamine, which is restricted to sperm (and sperm precursors) and which packages the paternal genome in torroids, rather than histone-containing nucleosomes typical of other chromatin [30, 31]. The ability of mitotic parthenogenotes to remodel protaminic sperm chromatin was unexpected and led us to ask whether they could also remodel nucleosomal chromatin present in round spermatids, which are postmeiotic haploid sperm precursors. We therefore applied the phICSI protocol to round spermatid injection (ROSI); phROSI. Injection of control sperm from *mtdT* transgenic males into wt parthenogenotes at increasing times after pnMBD resulted in decreasing rates of development in vitro, but in phROSI, the developmental rate increased, with the highest blastocyst developmental rate (26.8% Tomato-positive blastocysts) when injection was 2.0–2.5 h after pnMBD (phROSI-pnMBD-2h). This suggests that the optimal time window for efficient mitotic reprogramming partly depends on architecture of the incoming nucleus that is being remodeled. Following two-cell transfer to pseudopregnant females, phROSI-pnMBD-2h embryos produced healthy offspring at a rate of 2.6% per transferred embryo (see Table 12.1). This shows that nucleosomal chromatin in male haploid germ cells can also be reprogrammed for full-term development in mitotic haploid parthenogenotes.

12.8   Chromatin Remodeling in phICSI

Given the clear differences between oocytes/ICSI and parthenogenotes/phICSI (for example, in the molecular components that drive their respective cell cycles), we analyzed molecular and morphological remodeling of sperm chromatin in phICSI and ICSI embryos at similar times after sperm injection in each case. To follow protamine removal, we injected sperm from transgenic males in which protamine 2 was expressed as an mCherry fusion (Prm2-mCherry). Prm2-mCherry disappeared from sperm chromatin within 2 h of injection in phICSI-13 and ICSI. In phICSI-7, injected sperm head morphology altered little, if at all, for 5 h prior to pnMBD, suggesting that sperm decondensation failed in phICSI-7.

The size ratio of paternal-to-maternal nuclei in phICSI-13 two-cell embryos was 66.7% that of ICSI controls, because phICSI paternal nuclei were smaller than maternal ones in marked contrast to the situation in normal fertilization (Fig. 12.3a). This gross difference hints at major chromatin remodeling differences between phICSI and controls, which we investigated further on a molecular level.

The incorporation of histone H3.3-mCherry into sperm chromatin occurred more slowly in phICSI-13 than that in ICSI controls. The modification of core nucleosomal histones at the same times after sperm injection in phICSI-13 and ICSI revealed similarities (for example, H4K12ac), differences at first that subsequently recovered (for example, H3K4me3 and H3K27me3), and sustained differences (for example, H3K9me2).

Fertilization results in unusual DNA methylation dynamics in both parental genomes that are a hallmark of epigenetic regulation in one-cell embryos (see Fig. 12.3a, b) [32–35]. We therefore pursued this for phICSI. In ICSI one-cell controls, 5′-hydroxymethylcytosine (5hmC) accumulated more in paternal than maternal pronuclei, but after a comparable period following sperm injection in phICSI-13, the paternal:maternal ratio was *lower* (55%; see Fig. 12.3b) and remained after cell division. It is thus likely that atypical sperm chromatin remodeling in phICSI affected paternal genomic 5hmC. To investigate the possibility that this was due to 5hmC-inhibitory sperm components, we bound magnetic microbeads to DNA produced in vitro with or without cytosine methylation (5mC) and injected them into mII oocytes or embryos (see Fig. 12.4a). As a control, the methylDNA beads (meDNA-beads) were detected by 5mC immunofluorescence microscopy (IFM) after they had been injected into mII oocytes. However, the beads were not labeled by 5hmC after 7 h. When oocytes were artificially activated following DNA-beads injection, both 5mC and 5hmC were detected in a methyl DNA-dependent manner (see Fig. 12.4b). In addition, 5hmC was present on the meDNA-beads in two-cell embryos. Injection of (me)DNA-beads into parthenogenotes with timing analogous to sperm injection in phICSI-13, there was almost no 5hmC accumulation on them (see Fig. 12.4b). These results strongly suggest that the control of genomic 5hmC synthesis is time- and 5mC-dependent and involves meiotic progression.

Epigenetic regulation closely prescribes gene expression to ensure that it occurs at the right loci with the correct timing and to the proper degree. It was therefore

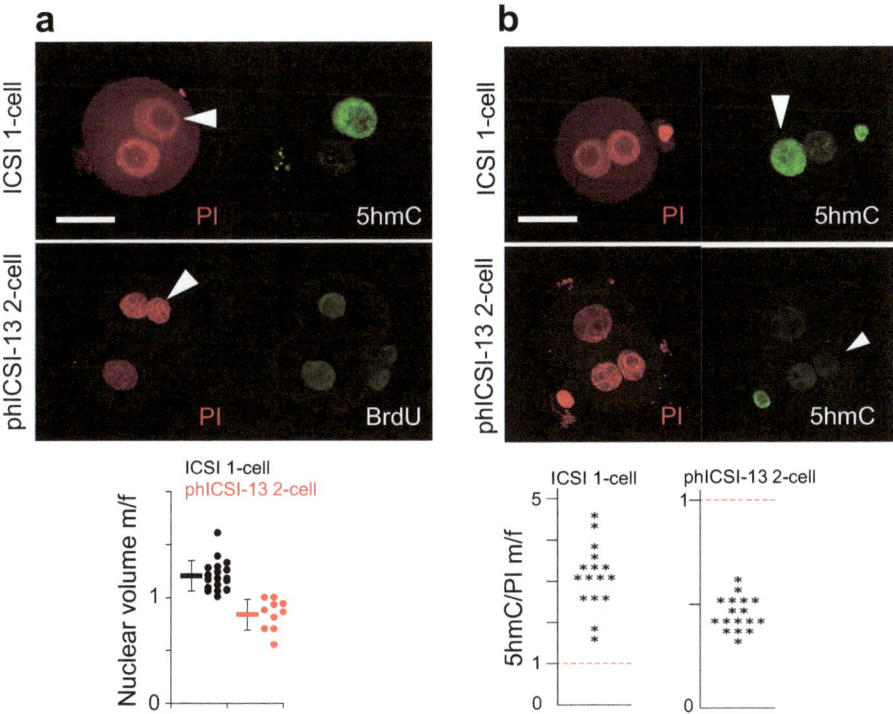

Fig. 12.3 Nuclear architecture and DNA 5′-hydroxymethylcytosine (5hmC) modification in ICSI-and phICSI-13-derived embryos. (**a**) Nuclear sizes of paternal nuclei in ICSI (one-cell stage) and phICSI-13 (two-cell stage) embryos in relation to their corresponding maternal nuclei. Nuclear DNA is stained with propidium iodide (PI, red) and 5hmC with anti-5hmC antibodies in ICSI one-cell embryos (green) or BrdU with anti-BrdU antibodies in (phICSI-13 two-cell embryos green) to discriminate paternal and maternal nuclei. The relative nuclear volumes (male/female) in ICSI one-cell and phICSI-13 two-cell embryos are plotted below. (**b**) Nuclear DNA stained with PI (red) and 5hmC (green) in ICSI one-cell or phICSI-13 two-cell embryos. The male/female (paternal:maternal) ratio of 5hmC intensities (relative to PI) is plotted below. All values in ICSI one-cell embryos were >1, but in phICSI-13 two-cell embryos they were <1. Arrowheads in (**a**) and (**b**) indicate paternal (sperm-derived) nuclei. Scale bars, 50 μm

possible that the distinctive epigenetic trajectories of phICSI embryos produced gene expression dysregulation. Indeed, upregulation of a paternally inherited, Oct4 promoter-driven mCherry transgene was delayed in phICSI-13 embryos. To analyze gene expression more completely, we performed microarray transcriptome analyses of phICSI-13 biparental blastomeres and ICSI control blastomeres at the two-cell stage, corresponding to the major wave of zygotic gene activation [36]. Pairs of blastomeres from any given ICSI-derived two-cell embryo exhibited similar global gene expression patterns, consistent with our previous work [37]. However, clear differences in global gene expression existed between ICSI blastomeres and those from phICSI-13 embryos: 73 genes were expressed at significantly higher or lower

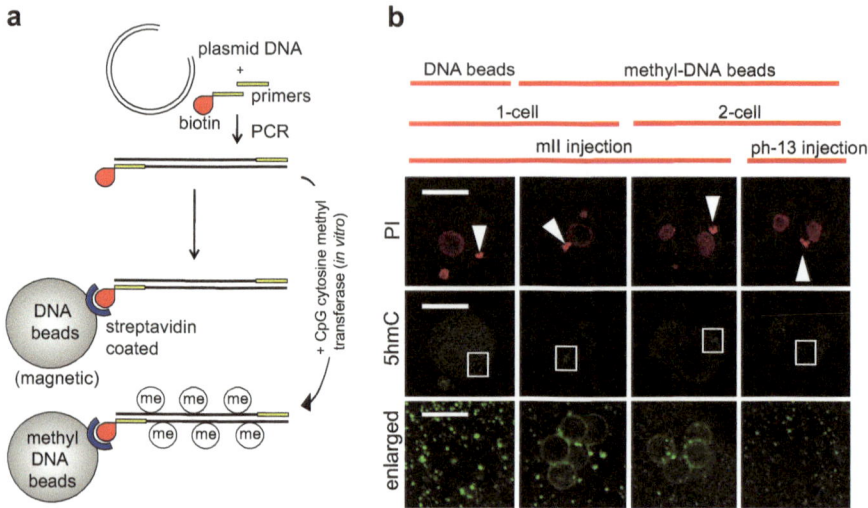

Fig. 12.4 Intracellular DNA bead assay for 5′-hydroxymethylcytosine (5hmC) production. (**a**) Schematic representation of in vitro production of DNA-bound magnetic microbeads. Double-strand DNA is amplified from plasmid DNA with sequence-specific primers one of which is labeled at its 5′ end with biotin so that the resulting amplimer can bind streptavidin-coated micro-beads via a biotin-streptavidin interaction. Some of the amplified DNA may be methylated in vitro at CpG dinucleotides with M.SssI methyl transferase prior to beads mixing. (**b**) (Methyl) DNA beads are injected into MII oocytes or haploid parthenogenotes at the first mitosis at the same timing to phICSI-13 (they are ph-13 haploid parthenogenotes produced by artificial activation of MII oocytes with SrCl$_2$). Samples were labeled with propidium iodide (PI) for DNA (red) or anti-5hmC antibodies for 5hmC (green) at one- or two-cell stages. Enlarged images (bottom, corresponding to the white squares in panels respectively above) are shown for injected beads labeled as described above to show 5hmC (green). Arrowheads show injected (methyl) DNA beads. Scale bars, 50 μm, except lowest panels (5 μm)

levels between the two groups. We also analyzed the expression of endogenous pluripotency regulatory genes in phICSI and control ICSI embryos at the morula stage. Expression of transgenes and of endogenous *Oct4* and *Cdx2* genes were delayed or lower in phICSI-13 embryos. These findings suggested that phICSI induced dysregulation of endogenous gene expression in phICSI-13 embryos.

12.9   Summary and Future Directions

Piezo-ICSI is a robust and reliable method by which to incorporate sperm chromatin into oocytes. Its low trauma and high success rates mean that it is applicable not only in the mouse, in which it is practicably essential, but it is advantageous in many other species, even where it is not. We have extended piezo in a new direction, and uncovered what is for us the interesting result that viable and fertile offspring can be produced by injecting sperm chromatin into haploid mitotic parthenogenotes. This finding has several clear implications:

- That it is possible to circumvent the intracellular events of the first 13 h of normal fertilization for sperm chromatin reprogramming sufficient for full-term development. Although we have shown that the events bypassed in phICSI are not essential for full development, it is possible that they are critical for optimal reprogramming efficiency.
- That reprogramming of sperm chromatin to participate in totipotency is not a function that is exclusive to meiotic cells (i.e., MII oocytes), as the parthenogenotes in phICSI are mitotic. It would be beneficial to unveil the mechanisms underlying "meiotic" and "mitotic" reprogramming to establish whether they overlap and if so, how, and the better to understand how they lead to totipotency.
- That it is possible for full development to follow distinctive epigenetic pathways and gene expression at the one-to-two-cell stage and the question is open as to whether or not early embryos are uniquely flexible in this regard or if this flexibility is exhibited widely.

One reason for our success may be the strict control of sperm injection timing in phICSI. Today, the molecular mechanisms and technological potential of mitotic sperm reprogramming are largely unknown, but using the control enabled by piezo, we hope to reveal them in the near future.

Acknowledgements The authors thank Animal Facility support staff for ensuring the welfare of animals used in this work, Dr. Maki Asami for immunofluorescence images, and we acknowledge Project Grant support from the Medical Research Council, UK (G1000839 and MR/N000080/1) to A.C.F.P.

References

1. Hiramoto Y. Microinjection of the live spermatozoa into sea urchin eggs. Exp Cell Res. 1962;27:416–26.
2. Palermo G, Joris H, Devroey P, Van Steirteghem AC. Pregnancies after intracytoplasmic injection of single spermatozoon into an oocyte. Lancet. 1992;340:17–8.
3. Kimura Y, Yanagimachi R. Intracytoplasmic sperm injection in the mouse. Biol Reprod. 1995;52:709–20.
4. Yoshida N, Perry ACF. Piezo-actuated mouse intracytoplasmic sperm injection (ICSI). Nat Protoc. 2007;2:296–304.
5. Dyer S, Chambers GM, de Mouzon J, Nygren KG, Zegers-Hochschild F, Mansour R, Ishihara O, Banker M, Adamson GD. International Committee for Monitoring Assisted Reproductive Technologies world report: Assisted Reproductive Technology 2008, 2009 and 2010. Hum Reprod. 2016;31:1588–609.
6. Perry ACF, Wakayama T, Yanagimachi R. A novel *trans*-complementation assay suggests full mammalian oocyte activation is coordinately initiated by multiple, submembrane sperm compartments. Biol Reprod. 1999;60:747–55.
7. Shoji S, Yoshida N, Amanai M, Ohgishi M, Fukui T, Fujimoto S, Nakano Y, Kajikawa E, Perry ACF. Mammalian Emi2 mediates cytostatic arrest and transduces the signal for meiotic exit *via* Cdc20. EMBO J. 2006;25:834–45.
8. Perry ACF, Wakayama T, Kishikawa H, Kasai T, Okabe M, Toyoda Y, Yanagimachi R. Mammalian transgenesis by intracytoplasmic sperm injection. Science. 1999;284:1180–3.

9. Perry ACF, Rothman A, de las Heras JI, Feinstein P, Mombaerts P, et al. Efficient metaphase II transgenesis with different transgene archetypes. Nat Biotechnol. 2001;19:1071–3.
10. Perry ACF. Metaphase II transgenesis. Reprod Biomed Online. 2002;4(3):279–84.
11. Suzuki T, Asami M, Perry ACF. Asymmetric parental genome engineering by Cas9 during mouse meiotic exit. Sci Rep. 2014;4:7621.
12. Wakayama T, Perry ACF, Zuccotti M, Johnson KR, Yanagimachi R. Full-term development of mice from enucleated oocytes injected with cumulus cell nuclei. Nature. 1998;394:369–74.
13. Onishi A, Iwamoto M, Akita T, Mikawa S, Takeda K, et al. Pig cloning by microinjection of fetal fibroblast nuclei. Science. 2000;289:1188–90.
14. Kimura Y, Yanagimachi R. Development of normal mice from oocytes injected with secondary spermatocyte nuclei. Biol Reprod. 1995;53:855–62.
15. Kimura Y, Yanagimachi R. Mouse oocytes injected with testicular spermatozoa or round spermatids can develop into normal offspring. Development. 1995;121:2397–405.
16. Suzuki T, Asami M, Hoffmann M, Lu X, Gužvić M, et al. Mice produced by mitotic reprogramming of sperm injected into haploid parthenogenotes. Nat Commun. 2016;7:12676.
17. Uehara T, Yanagimachi R. Microsurgical injection of spermatozoa into hamster eggs with subsequent transformation of sperm nuclei into male pronuclei. Biol Reprod. 1976;15:467–70.
18. Kuretake S, Kimura Y, Hoshi K, Yanagimachi R. Fertilization and development of mouse oocytes injected with isolated sperm heads. Biol Reprod. 1996;55:789–95.
19. Suzuki T, Yoshida N, Suzuki E, Okuda E, Perry ACF. Full-term mouse development by abolishing Zn^{2+}-dependent metaphase II arrest without Ca^{2+} release. Development. 2010;137:2659–69.
20. Condic ML. Totipotency: what it is and what it is not. Stem Cells Dev. 2014;23:796–812.
21. Perry ACF, Verlhac M-H. Second meiotic arrest and exit in frogs and mice. EMBO Rep. 2008;9:246–51.
22. Maleszewski M, Borsuk E, Koziak K, Maluchnik D, Tarkowski AK. Delayed sperm incorporation into parthenogenetic mouse eggs: sperm nucleus transformation and development of resulting embryos. Mol Reprod Dev. 1999;54:303–10.
23. Kishigami S, Wakayama S, Nguyen VT, Wakayama T. Similar time restriction for intracytoplasmic sperm injection and round spermatid injection into activated oocytes for efficient offspring production. Biol Reprod. 2004;70:1863–9.
24. Yang H, Shi L, Chen CD, Li J. Mice generated after round spermatid injection into haploid two-cell blastomeres. Cell Res. 2011;21:854–8.
25. Egli D, Rosains J, Birkhoff G, Eggan K. Developmental reprogramming after chromosome transfer into mitotic mouse zygotes. Nature. 2007;447:679–85.
26. Kang E, et al. Nuclear reprogramming by interphase cytoplasm of two-cell mouse embryos. Nature. 2014;509:101–4.
27. Yoshida N, Amanai M, Fukui T, Kajikawa E, Brahmajosyula M, Iwahori A, Nakano Y, Shoji S, Diebold J, Hessel H, Huss R, Perry ACF. Broad, ectopic expression of the sperm protein, PLCZ1 induces parthenogenesis and ovarian tumours in mice. Development. 2007;134:3941–52.
28. McGrath J, Solter D. Completion of mouse embryogenesis requires both the maternal and paternal genomes. Cell. 1984;37:179–83.
29. Barton SC, Surani MA, Norris ML. Role of paternal and maternal genomes in mouse development. Nature. 1984;311:374–6.
30. Balhorn R, Gledhill BL, Wyrobek AJ. Mouse sperm chromatin proteins: quantitative isolation and partial characterization. Biochemistry. 1977;16:4074–80.
31. Hud NV, Allen MJ, Downing KH, Lee J, Balhorn R. Identification of the elemental packing unit of DNA in mammalian sperm cells by atomic force microscopy. Biochem Biophys Res Commun. 1993;193:1347–54.
32. Mayer W, Niveleau A, Walter J, Fundele R, Haaf T. Demethylation of the zygotic paternal genome. Nature. 2000;403:501–2.
33. Gu TP, et al. The role of Tet3 DNA dioxygenase in epigenetic reprogramming by oocytes. Nature. 2012;477:606–10.

34. Iqbal K, Jin S-G, Pfeifer GP, Szabó PE. Reprogramming of the paternal genome upon fertilization involves genome-wide oxidation of 5-methylcytosine. Proc Natl Acad Sci U S A. 2011;108:3642–7.
35. Wossidlo M, et al. 5-Hydroxymethylcytosine in the mammalian zygote is linked with epigenetic reprogramming. Nat Commun. 2011;2:241.
36. Hamatani T, Carter MG, Sharov AA, Ko MS. Dynamics of global gene expression changes during mouse preimplantation development. Dev Cell. 2004;6:117–31.
37. VerMilyea MD, Maneck M, Yoshida N, Blochberger I, Suzuki E, et al. Transcriptome asymmetry within mouse zygotes but not between early embryonic sister blastomeres. EMBO J. 2011;30:1841–51.

Chapter 13
The Human Y-chromosome: Evolutionary Directions and Implications for the Future of "Maleness"

Darren K. Griffin and Peter J.I. Ellis

13.1 Introduction

The human Y chromosome is an iconic image. As a symbol of maleness, it has been depicted in many different forms and the consequences of deletion, mutation, or rearrangement extensively documented in the literature and seen in infertility clinics, notably among men undergoing ICSI. The human Y chromosome is however simply the best known example of a range of sex chromosome systems. Both XY sex determination, where the male has two distinct (heterogametic) sex chromosomes and the female has two identical sex chromosomes, and ZW sex determination—where the reverse holds—are commonplace in different taxa. Both XY and ZW systems have evolved independently several times. The best-studied XY system is that seen in mammals—for which humans represent just one example of a myriad of mammalian Y chromosomes that come in all shapes and sizes. For ZW systems, birds are the best-cited example, but Lepidoptera (butterflies and moths), some snakes, fish, and reptiles also have ZW sex chromosomes. In certain animal groups, both ZW and XY systems are apparent [1, 2], even within the same genera [3–6] or species [7]. A key observation in both XY and ZW systems is that one of the sex chromosomes is only seen in the heterogametic sex: for example, in mammals the Y is passed clonally from father to son, while in birds the W is passed clonally from mother to daughter. These chromosomes are thus only ever present as a single copy and cannot undergo recombination, and it is this failure to recombine that leads to the genetic degradation that distinguishes Y from X chromosomes, or W from Z.

Numerous species have only partially differentiated sex chromosomes including pythons [8], ratite birds [9, 10], tilapia [3, 5], and European tree frogs. There are several reports of insects [11, 12], plants [13, 14], and vertebrates (mostly fish) with novel sex chromosome systems close to the beginning of the degenerative process

D.K. Griffin (✉) • P.J.I. Ellis
School of Biosciences, University of Kent, Canterbury, Kent, UK
e-mail: d.k.griffin@kent.ac.uk; p.j.i.ellis@kent.ac.uk

© Springer International Publishing AG 2018
G.D. Palermo, E.S. Sills (eds.), *Intracytoplasmic Sperm Injection*,
https://doi.org/10.1007/978-3-319-70497-5_13

[15, 16], but newly formed sex chromosomes are rarely reported in mammals or indeed insects [17–19].

Sex chromosome differentiation is a commonplace, perhaps inevitable, consequence of the evolution of genetically determined sex. The prevailing wisdom is that the mammalian (including human) Y chromosome was once identical to its partner, and that the appearance of a dominant sex-determining gene *SRY* was the starting point distinguishing the proto-Y from the proto-X chromosomes. Following this, a series of events played out that led to degradation of the newly formed Y chromosome. These events include a reduction in genetic recombination around the sex-determining region that could have initially been a consequence of a de novo expansion of heterochromatin (non-coding DNA) [4]. Loss of euchromatin (coding DNA) and an expansion of heterochromatin resulted in further reduction of recombination, creating a vicious cycle that led to a much degraded Y [20]. The contemporary human sex chromosomes retain shadows of their evolutionary past with the euchromatic portion of the male-specific region of the Y chromosome (MSY) roughly 17% the size of the X with only 8% of the gene count [21, 22]. In short: the Y chromosome is a degraded X chromosome—an understanding that goes back almost to the birth of modern genetics, in the work of Hermann Muller in 1918, subsequently refined by Susumo Ohno in 1967.

The question that seems to extend beyond the learned genetic journals and into the popular press however, is whether this degradation will continue until the Y reaches oblivion, or has the Y chromosome reached a point of equilibrium where it can go no further? Sometimes that discussion gets a little extrapolated and exaggerated.

13.2   Why the Y Will Not Degrade

The main proponents of the notion of why the Y will *not* degrade (let's call them "the remainers" to use a Brexit analogy) base their view mostly on Y chromosome analyses of three primates (human, chimpanzee, and rhesus macaque) [21, 23, 24]. Due to the quantity of repeated DNA, sequencing the Y is a laborious process when the so-called BAC-by-BAC approach is used—a state-of-the-art technique before the arrival of next-generation sequencing, which is often the best. Another reason why Y chromosome sequencing groups had to go back to the drawing board is that many sequencing projects started with a female reference individual.

The notion that the Y is actually a degraded X is not in dispute: There are ~1000 genes on the 180Mb X chromosome [22], but only 78 genes on the 23Mb Y chromosome [21]. Indeed, the degeneration of the Y chromosome probably occurred because of the absence of meiotic recombination partner over most of its length. Recombination suppression between the proto sex chromosomes appears to have been selectively advantageous initially as the evolving Y was a good place for male-benefit genes to reside, and subsequent recombination suppression kept these genes linked to the male-determining *SRY* locus [25].

The human Y chromosome was the first of its kind to be fully sequenced and assembled [21]. It well established that it has a large heterochromatic region; however, the focus of research has been on the euchromatic portion of the "male-specific Y" (MSY; i.e., not the pseudoautosomal regions (those that recombine during meiosis) at the tips). This portion consists of three sequence classes. The "X-transposed" region a ~3-Mb block of gene-poor sequence that was transferred from the X to the Y about 3–4 million years ago [26]. The "X-degenerate" regions, which can be thought of degenerate X chromosome component of the MSY and constitute a little greater than half of its euchromatic content. These regions have 16 single-copy genes, most of which have ubiquitous expression patterns. Finally, the "ampliconic" or repeat-rich regions make up the largest portion of these regions are rich in multi-copy genes that are expressed exclusively in testes, implying a role in spermatogenesis. All the X-degenerate genes and some of the ampliconic genes have a shared X–Y homology and it is these that often, when deleted or mutated, lead to male infertility phenotypes. Moreover, several of the ampliconic genes have been translocated from autosomes [27, 28].

In this context, what is the fate of the genes on the Y that, in the absence of meiotic recombination, are at risk of deletion or mutation? From a detailed analysis of the euchromatic Y chromosome the argument is that this chromosome has evolved several mechanisms to ensure its survival. Much of the ampliconic region is made up of palindromic structures, i.e., closely spaced inverted repeats sharing close to 100% identity [21]. It is argued that a process of non-reciprocal recombination (essentially bits of the Y undergoing recombination with itself) first of all maintains this high level (nearly 100%) of identity within the repeat units themselves. It is also argued that this probably protects the integrity of male-only genes that reside within them in the absence of "normal" crossing over [29]. What happens to the single-copy genes on the Y chromosome that are not protected by this process still is the subject of further research.

Concentrating on the chimpanzee Y-specific sequence provides insight into the recent evolutionary history of the human Y. At both a gross cytogenetic and molecular level, the human and chimp Ys are very different indeed, despite evolving only 6 million years ago. Compare this to the similarly sized human chromosome 21 and chimp chromosome 22, which are near identical from the perspective of gene order [30]. Clearly, the Y chromosomes of ourselves and our nearest neighbors have rearranged considerably and the nature of these changes are deletions, insertions, inversions, and duplications [23]. Moreover, the degree of rearrangement is considerably higher in the amplified regions when compared to the X-degenerate regions and this applies also to the amount of sequence present in one species but not the other (~50% vs. ~9%) [23]. Despite the fact that, when looking down the microscope, the total size of the chimpanzee Y is significantly smaller than the human (this is because it lacks a large heterochromatic region) the ampliconic sequence is larger and more complex in chimps. The proportion of the MSY sequence that is ampliconic, 45% in human, is 57% in chimpanzee, and the chimp has over twice as many palindromes.

Concerning gene loss, Hughes and colleagues have compared gene content, assembly and annotation in both species, suggesting that there has been no gene loss from the human lineage since the two diverged [23, 31]. In other words, the chimpanzee MSY contains no genes that are missing in the human sequence and has lost at least six of these, while the human has not [23, 31]. Why did this happen in chimp but not human? Perhaps unfavorable mutations have become fixed by being linked to a favorable one? The chimpanzee has a highly promiscuous mating system [32], which vastly increases sperm competition compared to humans. The suggestion is that, in chimps, there is positive selection on a mutation in a gene or genes that greatly increase the output of spermatogenesis and this outweighs the comparatively weaker purifying selection on other genes with less strong effects [23, 31]. Work has continued on the rhesus macaque [24], an Old World monkey that diverged from us around 25 million years ago, and more distant mammals, including marmoset, mouse, rat, bull, and opossum. Taken together, evidence suggests that the human Y has held up well in terms of gene content.

The "remainers" argue that the processes they describe will ultimately save the Y and natural selection will remove those regions of the chromosome that contain mutated copies of genes deleterious to sex determination and male fertility. They argue that comparison of orthologous palindrome sequences in chimpanzee and human that palindromes suggests that they are evolving much more slowly than other sequences [29] suggesting a drive to maintain the status quo. Furthermore, simulation-based models and population genetics suggest that even low levels of gene conversion can maintain the integrity of Y-linked genes [33, 34] and genes that don't undergo this process (single-copy, X-degenerate genes) are under considerable purifying selection. These genes have not decayed in 6 million (or, if Macaque comparisons are to be believed, 25 million) years, close to 20% of the mammalian MSY history. Finally, Y chromosome resequencing of men from different ethnic backgrounds suggests conservation of coding sequence within the X-degenerate genes [35], which also supports the notion that MSY genes are indispensable, not only for sex determination, but for spermatogenesis and other crucial biological functions.

In conclusion, the remainers' argument is as follows:

- The human Y has not disappeared yet and has been around, in terms of gene content, for hundreds of millions of years.
- Without "normal" crossing over the human Y has evolved mechanisms to cling on to life through palindromic sequences that recombine with one another
- The majority of human Y genes display purifying selection during primate evolution.
- The human Y has added more than eight different genes. Some of these have then expanded in copy number.
- The human Y has not lost any genes since the human and chimpanzee lineages diverged ~6 million years ago.

13.3 Why the Y Will Leave Us

The proponents of the notion that the Y is going to disappear (the "leavers") make the fundamental "common sense" point that it has been degenerating for millions of years and claim it is inevitable that it will disappear completely. Rather than focusing on a small number of species closely related to humans, the "leavers" take a wider perspective and argue that while the homology between the mammalian X and Y chromosomes is well established in that most Y genes have X orthologues, the gene content of the Y differs between mammalian species. That is, some genes have been deleted in certain lineages whereas others have disappeared [36]. Therefore, the remainers' argument that genes with important functions cannot be lost from the Y is shown to be false, and even genes with an important function can disappear from a lineage and subsequently be replaced. If all the important Y genes become inactivated, the Y can be lost completely. There are several possible fates of Y chromosomal genes [20] including:

- They could of course remain intact and functional (this would apply to genes in the pseudoautosomal region).
- They could be mutated.
- They could inactivated and become pseudogenes.
- They could duplicate.
- They could be deleted.
- New genes could be introduced from other chromosomes.

Three models to describe the Y chromosome have been proposed [37]—the "dominant Y" exerting a massive influence over the phenotype despite its small size, the "selfish Y" acquiring genes from other chromosomes, and the "wimpy Y," a shadow of its former self. We know however that the dominant Y model describes only the influence on male phenotype of a single gene *SRY*, which alone can induce testis differentiation and activate hormones that masculinize the embryo. The "selfish" model well describes the Drosophila Y chromosome, which originated as a heterochromatic element and imported copies of many fertility genes [19]—see below. It is suggested however that this describes only a handful of genes on the mammalian Y, as most have a homologue on the X. The "wimpy Y" is the model favored by Jenny Graves and her colleagues.

The basic premise of why Y chromosomes will eventually disappear is that high variation on Y chromosome leads to many mutations, deletions, and insertions. The Y chromosome is handed down the male generations (and hence always in a testis but never in an ovary). This is a harsh environment for cell division, with many opportunities for DNA damage, and a setting where DNA repair is limited [38, 39] in the absence of genetic recombination [40]. Selection is difficult on single loci, which could therefore lead to selection against the whole chromosome. In other words, an evolutionarily advantageous variant on an otherwise bad Y chromosome is unlikely to survive; however, a disadvantageous variant could be passed on easily [41].

The Graves lab has studied the sex chromosomes of numerous of vertebrates, but particularly mammals. Comparative genomics of human and marsupial X chromosome genes has identified an X-conserved region and an X-added region, which is autosomal in marsupials. Not including the X–Y pairing regions, the human Y contains genes (around 7) from the X-conserved region but most (12) from the X-added region. In contrast, the kangaroo Y contains around 12 genes all with "brains and balls" X homologues on the X-conserved region. The mammalian XY system is relatively young in evolutionary terms and other systems exist, e.g., birds and reptiles. Indeed, distantly related reptiles (geckos and turtles) have bird-like ZW chromosomes suggesting an ancient lineage ancestral to reptiles. Indeed in monotremes (platypus and echidna), the complex sex chromosome system bears similarities to the ancestral ZW chromosomes, not the XY of the other mammals—marsupials and eutherians [36, 42]. The mammalian XY system probably evolved recently (i.e., 160 million years ago), the time at which other mammals diverged from monotremes.

If the Y is indeed disappearing, then the question arises of how long it will actually take. Taking X chromosome gene number, it is reasonable to deduce that the ancestral Y used to have around 1700 genes whereas now it has 78. Given a linear rate of loss, it may be surmised that the Y chromosome would vanish in around 4.6 million years. So perhaps we don't need to worry. There are other possibilities besides a linear degradation [36], including an initial linear loss but with subsequent slow down due to an evolutionary advantage to retention of certain genes. It is argued however that this is unlikely to affect total protection against loss due to the fact that certain gene combinations are retained in specific lineages. Various models based on a reduction of Y chromosome size exist and some are more in-depth than others [43]. A two-stage degradation of first the X-conserved, and then the X-added regions has been proposed as the most realistic model [36]. A second model [44] is that the disappearance will happen relatively soon in evolutionary time, as evidenced by two lineages of rodents which have already survived the complete loss of the Y chromosome (Japanese spiny rats and mole voles). Japanese spiny rats (Genus *Tokudaia*) [45] comprise three species that live on islands off the coast of Japan. One has retained the Y chromosome (the Okinawa spiny rat *T. muenninki*), but the other two (the Amami spiny rat *T. osimensis* and the Tokunoshima spiny rat *T. tokunoshimensis*) have lost their Y chromosomes completely and do not appear to have *sry*. *T. muenninki*, although retaining a Y chromosome containing *sry*, this doesn't bind DNA particularly efficiently. To compensate for this, it has undergone multiple gene duplications in a last ditch attempt to hang on to life [46]. Among some species, *E. fuscocapillus* has XY males and XX females; *E. lutescens* has XO males and XO females; while *E. tancrei* features XX males and XX females—interestingly, none have *sry*.

The "leavers" argue that some *Drosophila* species are on their third Y chromosome and *D. melanogaster* has already completely lost its Y, replaced by a mass of heterochromatin that, in other *Drosophila* species, has been moved to an autosome, also under degradation [19, 47]. They argue that this process of loss and reformation of one of the sex chromosomes is an inevitable fact of life for species with differentiated sex chromosomes. They argue that gene conversion can result in conversion of a mutant to an undamaged copy, *and* from a good copy to a mutant copy and, in the latter case, once it's gone, it's gone. They argue that some palindromic arms show evidence of degradation, e.g., the human Y has 28 copies of the *RBMY* gene but only two of these are active. They argue that palindromes and gene duplication alone will not save the Y in the absence of positive selection, which does not exist and it is easier to translocate another gene copy to an autosome. Again *RBMY* and its X homologue have several autosomal copies, one of which is active in testis [48] and these act as a stand by in case the Y disappears.

The case for the disappearance of the Y thus principally rests on five arguments:

- The Y chromosome is subject to very high rate of variation and inefficient selection.
- There is evidence from across the animal kingdom and even in plants that Y (and W) chromosomes degrade inexorably.
- The Y chromosome undergoes lineage-specific degradation.
- The Y has already disappeared in some rodent lineages.
- There is next to nothing left of the original human Y and the added part of the human Y is degrading rapidly.

13.4   Are the Two Sides Close to Agreement?

Perhaps unsurprisingly, they are not. The leavers suggest that the remainers focus too much on primates, a very short evolutionary interval. The remainers suggest that the leavers fail to recognize the evidence of palindromes, lack of gene loss, and gene conversion. The parallels with the Brexit debate are astonishing. With the real Brexit on the east side of the Atlantic and the "curious and historic" (to be tactful) Presidential changes happening on the west side, we as geneticists should perhaps be flattered that something which should really only interest those who unpack the complexities of sex chromosome evolution is receiving so much public interest.

Is there any clinical importance to the question? For men undergoing ICSI, there is nothing except perhaps something to talk about in the waiting room. If their fertility problems are not caused by Y chromosome gene mutations, all this is irrelevant; while if they are, there is nothing we can do to correct a genetic deficiency at present—although with CRISPR on the horizon, who knows? Paradoxically, the degeneration of the Y will be of more interest for women than men undergoing ART. Irrespective of its potential future loss or retention, the mere fact that the Y is a degraded remnant means that there are very few "Y-specific" functions required for spermatogenesis. Indeed, in mice it has recently been shown that only two Y chromosomal genes, *Sry* and *Zfy2* are required in order to permit male meiosis and differentiation through to haploid spermatids. Moreover, both of these can be substituted by their X-linked counterparts. This opens up the intriguing possibility of in vitro production of spermatids not just from male cells but female cells, and thus an extension of ART methods to same-sex couples who would otherwise not be able to both be genetic parents to their children.

In a related manner, the "Graves prediction" of the demise of the Y chromosome inevitably raises the question (usually in the lay press) whether this means that males themselves will also disappear. In an evolutionary sense, do we need males? Those of us with a Y chromosome are usually the ones that start wars, become tyrants, and participate in violent crime far more frequently. Those without a Y do the vast majority of work carrying babies to term, nurturing and weaning them. Indeed, farm animal breeding regimes are very female biased—they only need a few sperm samples. Biologically, eliminating males would mean a completely female species reproducing parthenogenetically (there are examples of this in lizards). Part of the reason for why this is unlikely in mammals however is because of genomic imprinting. There are just too many sex-specific epigenetic "marks" on other chromosomes to make this viable. While reproduction without males is extremely unlikely without extensive development of in vitro spermatogenesis technology (as outlined above), reproduction without sperm will remain impossible.

Not wishing to dampen all this (somewhat undeserved) enthusiasm for our field therefore but there really is no serious debate about whether males (fertile or otherwise) are going to disappear. There are huge advantages to sexual reproduction among complex organisms and the majority of sexually reproducing organisms have a 50:50 sex ratio. The real argument is this: Virtually, everyone with any academic credibility agrees that the Y is degenerate X, so it has shrunk considerably. We all agree that the Y has evolved some pretty clever mechanisms to "put the brakes on." What we can't agree on is how effective the brakes are. To exemplify this, at the International Chromosome Conference in Manchester in 2011 we actually put the argument to the test, with the two Jennifers (Graves and Hughes) each arguing their own case. At the end of the debate, we asked the esteemed audience (who really should be the experts) what they thought. The divide could not have been more even: an almost exact split between leavers and remainers. Curiously however, when we broke down the vote by gender, a couple of significant and easily guessable correlations emerged. Even scientists are not as objective as we think they are.

References

1. Organ CL, Janes DE. Evolution of sex chromosomes in Sauropsida. Integr Comp Biol. 2008;48(4):512.
2. Ross JA, et al. Turnover of sex chromosomes in the stickleback fishes (Gasterosteidae). PLoS Genet. 2009;5(2):e1000391.
3. Campos-Ramos R, et al. Identification of putative sex chromosomes in the blue tilapia, Oreochromis aureus, through synaptonemal complex and FISH analysis. Genetica. 2001;111(1):143–53.
4. Griffin D, et al. Early origins of the X and Y chromosomes: lessons from tilapia. Cytogenet Genome Res. 2000;99(1–4):157–63.

5. Harvey S, et al. Karyotype evolution in Tilapia: mitotic and meiotic chromosome analysis of Oreochromis karongae and O. niloticus× O. karongae hybrids. Genetica. 2002;115(2):169–77.
6. Takehana Y, et al. Evolution of ZZ/ZW and XX/XY sex-determination systems in the closely related medaka species, Oryzias hubbsi and O. dancena. Chromosoma. 2007;116(5):463–70.
7. Ogata M, et al. The ZZ/ZW sex-determining mechanism originated twice and independently during evolution of the frog, Rana rugosa. Heredity. 2007;100(1):92–9.
8. Ohno S. Sex chromosomes and sex-linked genes. Chromosomes sexuels et genes lies au sexe, 1969.
9. Takagi N, Sasaki M. A phylogenetic study of bird karyotypes. Chromosoma. 1974;46(1):91–120.
10. Nishida-Umehara C, et al. The molecular basis of chromosome orthologies and sex chromosomal differentiation in palaeognathous birds. Chromosome Res. 2007;15(6):721–34.
11. Bachtrog D, Charlesworth B. Reduced adaptation of a non-recombining neo-Y chromosome. Nature. 2002;416(6878):323–6.
12. Benatti TR, et al. A neo-sex chromosome that drives postzygotic sex determination in the Hessian fly (Mayetiola destructor). Genetics. 2010;184(3):769.
13. Liu Z, et al. A primitive Y chromosome in papaya marks incipient sex chromosome evolution. Nature. 2004;427(6972):348–52.
14. Filatov DA. Evolutionary history of Silene latifolia sex chromosomes revealed by genetic mapping of four genes. Genetics. 2005;170(2):975.
15. Kondo M, et al. Evolutionary origin of the medaka Y chromosome. Curr Biol. 2004;14(18):1664–9.
16. Peichel CL, et al. The master sex-determination locus in threespine sticklebacks is on a nascent Y chromosome. Curr Biol. 2004;14(16):1416–24.
17. Zhou Q, et al. Neo-sex chromosomes in the black muntjac recapitulate incipient evolution of mammalian sex chromosomes. Genome Biol. 2008;9(6):R98.
18. Pala I, et al. Evidence of a neo-sex chromosome in birds. Heredity. 2012;108:264–72.
19. Carvalho AB, Clark AG. Y chromosome of D. pseudoobscura is not homologous to the ancestral Drosophila Y. Science. 2005;307(5706):108.
20. Graves JAM. The origin and function of the mammalian Y chromosome and Y borne genes–an evolving understanding. Bioessays. 1995;17(4):311–20.
21. Skaletsky H, et al. The male-specific region of the human Y chromosome is a mosaic of discrete sequence classes. Nature. 2003;423(6942):825–37.
22. Ross MT, et al. The DNA sequence of the human X chromosome. Nature. 2005;434(7031):325–37.
23. Hughes JF, et al. Chimpanzee and human Y chromosomes are remarkably divergent in structure and gene content. Nature. 2010;463(7280):536–9.
24. Hughes JF, Skaletsky H, Brown LG, Pyntikova T, Graves T, Fulton RS, Dugan S, Ding Y, Buhay CJ, Kremitzki C, Wang Q, Shen H, Holder M, Villasana D, Nazareth LV, Cree A, Courtney L, Veizer J, Kotkiewicz H, Cho TJ, Koutseva N, Rozen S, Muzny DM, Warren WC, Gibbs RA, Wilson RK, Page DC. Strict evolutionary conservation followed rapid gene loss on human and rhesus Y chromosomes. Nature. 2012;483(7387):82–6.
25. Rice WR. Genetic hitchhiking and the evolution of reduced genetic activity of the Y sex chromosome. Genetics. 1987;116(1):161.
26. Page DC, et al. Occurrence of a transposition from the X-chromosome long arm to the Y-chromosome short arm during human evolution. Nature. 1984;311(5982):119–23.
27. Saxena R, et al. The DAZ gene cluster on the human Y chromosome arose from an autosomal gene that was transposed, repeatedly amplified and pruned. Nat Genet. 1996;14(3):292–9.
28. Lahn BT, Page DC. Reposition of autosomal mRNA yielded testis-specific gene family on human Y chromosome. Nat Genet. 1999;21:429–33.
29. Rozen S, et al. Abundant gene conversion between arms of palindromes in human and ape Y chromosomes. Nature. 2003;423(6942):873–6.
30. Watanabe H, et al. DNA sequence and comparative analysis of chimpanzee chromosome 22. Nature. 2004;429(6990):382–8.

31. Hughes JF, et al. Conservation of Y-linked genes during human evolution revealed by comparative sequencing in chimpanzee. Nature. 2005;437(7055):100–3.
32. Dixson AF. Primate sexuality: comparative studies of the prosimians, monkeys, apes, and human beings. Oxford: Oxford University Press; 1998.
33. Connallon T, Clark AG. Gene duplication, gene conversion and the evolution of the Y chromosome. Genetics. 2010;186(1):277.
34. Marais GAB, Campos PRA, Gordo I. Can intra-Y gene conversion oppose the degeneration of the human Y chromosome? A simulation study. Genome Biol Evol. 2010;2:347.
35. Rozen S, et al. Remarkably little variation in proteins encoded by the Y chromosome's single-copy genes, implying effective purifying selection. Am J Huma Genet. 2009;85(6):923–8.
36. Graves JAM. Sex chromosome specialization and degeneration in mammals. Cell. 2006;124(5):901–14.
37. Graves JAM. Human Y chromosome, sex determination, and spermatogenesis—a feminist view. Biol Reprod. 2000;63(3):667.
38. Aitken RJ, Graves JAM. The future of sex. Nature. 2002;415:963–4.
39. Shimmin LC, Chang BHJ, Li WH. Male-driven evolution of DNA sequences. Nature. 1993;362(6422):745–7.
40. Charlesworth B, Charlesworth D. The degeneration of Y chromosomes. Philos Trans R Soc Lond B Biol Sci. 2000;355(1403):1563.
41. Rice WR. The accumulation of sexually antagonistic genes as a selective agent promoting the evolution of reduced recombination between primitive sex chromosomes. Evolution. 1987;41(4):911–4.
42. Graves JAM. Weird animal genomes and the evolution of vertebrate sex and sex chromosomes. Annu Rev Genet. 2008;42:565–86.
43. Bachtrog D. The temporal dynamics of processes underlying Y chromosome degeneration. Genetics. 2008;179(3):1513.
44. Sykes B. Adam's curse: a future without men. New York: WW Norton & Company; 2004.
45. Kuroiwa A, et al. The process of a Y-loss event in an XO/XO mammal, the Ryukyu spiny rat. Chromosoma. 2010;119(5):519–26.
46. Murata C, et al. Multiple copies of SRY on the large Y chromosome of the Okinawa spiny rat, Tokudaia muenninki. Chromosome Res. 2010;119:1–12.
47. Graves JAM. Recycling the Y chromosome. Science. 2005;307(5706):50.
48. Lingenfelter PA, et al. Expression and conservation of processed copies of the RBMX gene. Mamm Genome. 2001;12(7):538–45.

Index

A
Acid test, 172
Alzheimer disease, 65, 66
Antisperm antibodies (ASA), 134
ART. *See* Assisted reproductive technologies
    (ART)
ASA. *See* Antisperm antibodies (ASA)
Assisted reproductive technologies (ART), 9,
    10, 12, 17, 39, 143, 158
  paternal age (*see* Paternal age)
Asthenospermia, 130
Azoospermia, 158, 160, 162, 163

C
CFTR. *See* Cystic fibrosis transmembrane
    conductance regulator (CFTR)
Chromatin remodeling, 176–178
Clinical evaluation, male factor infertility,
    129–131
  acrosome reaction, 136
  adjunct semen and sperm tests, 133
  ASA, 134
  clinical examination, 125–126
  definition, 124
  DNA integrity, 134, 135
  endocrine evaluation, 126, 127
  hormonal profile levels, 126, 127
  incidence, 124
  medical history, 125
  miscellaneous tests, 135
  MRI, 132
  PEU, 131
  pyospermia, 133–134
  renal ultrasound, 132
  research design and method, 124, 125
  retrospective data, 124
  scrotal ultrasound (US), 132
  semen abnormalities
    asthenospermia, 130
    azoospermia, 129, 130
    OATS, 130
    teratoazoospermia, 131
  semen analysis, 127, 128
  sperm–cervical mucus interaction test, 136
  sperm viability, 134
  TRUS, 132
  vasography, 133
  zona-free hamster oocyte test, 136
CNVs. *See* Copy number variations (CNVs)
Comet assay, human sperm
  advantages, 96
  agarose distribution, 88
  cell lysis buffer, 88
  chromatin quality, 85
  comet tail measurement, 90
  description, 86
  DNA damage, spermatozoa, 86
  DNA quality, 85
  enzymatic treatment, 89
  fully automated image analysis, 90
  measurements, 90
  pH conditions, 89, 90
  protamines, 86
  semen quality, parameters, 85
  semi-automated image analysis, 90
  staining and imaging, 90
  visual inspection and classification, 90
Comparative genomic hybridization (CGH), 149
Computer-assisted sperm (CASA), 100

© Springer International Publishing AG 2018
G.D. Palermo, E.S. Sills (eds.), *Intracytoplasmic Sperm Injection*,
https://doi.org/10.1007/978-3-319-70497-5

Computer-assisted sperm morphology
        analysis-fluorescence (CASMA-F)
        technology, 102
Computerized karyometric image analysis
        (CKIA), 102
Copy number variations (CNVs), 29, 30, 34
Cryopreservation, 162, 163
Cryptozoospermia, 160–162
Cystic fibrosis transmembrane conductance
        regulator (CFTR), 26, 28

D
De novo creation of spermatozoa
    adult/prepubertal patients, 51
    autologous tissue transplantation, 54, 55
    benefit, 49
    epigenetic normality, 56, 57
    genetic integrity, 50, 52, 55
    genomic integrity and epigenetic
        regulations, 49
    germ cell transplantation and in vivo
        spermatogenesis, 53, 54
    gonadotoxic treatment, 54, 57
    ICSI, 55, 56
    in vitro spermatogenesis, 51–53
    IUI/IVF, 56
    spermatogenesis and spermiogenesis,
        50–55
DNA fragmentation index (DFI), 158
"Dominant Y" model, 187

E
Embryo aneuploidy
    FISH and CGH, 149
    IMSI and ICSI cycles with PGD, 148
    semen parameters and clinical outcomes, 149
    sex chromosome, incidence, 148
    sperm selection method, 149
Epididymal/testicular sperm, 160, 161
Epigenetics
    DNA methylation, 31, 32
    epigenetic regulators, 31
    gene mutations, 31
    nuclear proteins, 33, 34
    RNA assessment, 32, 33

F
Fetal calf serum (FCS), 51
5′-Hydroxymethylcytosine (5hmC), 176
Fluorescent in situ hybridization (FISH), 25,
        27, 28

G
Gamete intrafallopian transfer (GIFT), 9
Genetic testing
    cystic fibrosis (CF), 137
    genetic factors, 136
    Klinefelter's syndrome, 137, 138
    Y-chromosome abnormalities, 138

H
HT-Comet, 87, 91–93, 96
Human Y-chromosome
    advantages, 190
    ampliconic/repeat-rich regions, 185
    autosomal copies, 189
    biological functions, 186
    degenerative process, 183
    deletion/mutation risks, 185
    fates of Y chromosomal genes, 187
    gene order perspective, 185
    genetic degradation, 183
    Graves lab, 188
    Graves prediction, 190
    heterogametic sex chromosomes, 183
    Japanese spiny rats, 188
    leavers, 188
    loss of euchromatin (coding DNA), 184
    male generations, 187
    mating system, 186
    meiotic recombination partner, 184
    models, 187
    monotremes, 188
    MSY, 184, 185
    primates, 184
    remainers, 186, 189
    sex chromosome systems, 183
    "Y-specific" functions, 189

I
ICSI. *See* Intracytoplasmic sperm injection
        (ICSI)
International Committee for Monitoring
        Assisted Reproductive Technologies
        (ICMART), 12
Intracytoplasmic morphologically selected
        sperm injection (IMSI), 100
    advantages, 151
    clinical pregnancy and live birth delivery
        rates, 151
    Cochrane review, 151
    embryo aneuploidy, 148, 149
    fragmentation/denaturation, 143
    implantation and/or pregnancy rates, 144

IVF cycles, 143
MSOME, 143
poor ovarian response, 150
poor semen quality, 149, 150
RIF, 150 (*see also* Sperm morphology)
sperm selection, injection, 143
teratozoospermic samples, 151
Intracytoplasmic sperm injection (ICSI),
    14–17, 92, 94–96, 114
advantages, 9
ART, 9, 10
assisted fertilization techniques, 10, 11
comet sperm DNA damage
    alkaline, 94, 95
    ART outcome, 94
    chromatin quality, 92
    clinical threshold, 94
    distribution plots, 92
    DNA fragmentation, 94
    embryo quality, 95
    fertilization rates, 94
    HT-COMET, 92
    meta-analysis, 95–96
    olive tail moment, 92
    SCD, 94
    SCSA and TUNEL, 92, 94
conventional microinjection, 170
cryopreservation, 162, 163
description, 9
development, 11, 12
DFI and ART, 158
DFI mapping, 158
DNA damage, 158
ejaculated, epididymal and testicular
    sperm, 158
embryos and offspring production, 169
epididymal/testicular sperm, 160, 161
epididymides, 170
fertilization rates, 12
gamete function, 169
genetic integrity, 52
indications, 13, 14
male infertility, 9
mammalian species, 169
micromanipulation, 170
miscarriage rates and DNA fragmentation,
    159
natural intercourse, 74
oocytes, spermatozoon, 12
piezo-actuating unit, 170
popularity, 12, 13
PVP concentrations, 170
safety, 17, 18
in sea urchins, 169

semen abnormalities, 158
SMA (*see* Sperm morphology analysis
    (SMA))
sperm concentration, motility and
    morphology, 158
sperm DNA integrity, 64, 66, 72, 74–77
sperm extraction, 159
sperm injection, mouse MII oocytes,
    170, 171
sperm motility, 53
spermatozoa, 55, 56
technique
    equipment, 14, 15
    gametes, 16
    magnification, oocyte, 16
    ooplasm, spermatozoon, 17
    preparation, 15, 16
    sperm immobilization, 16
    spermatozoon, 16
    tool settings, 15
testicular *vs.* ejaculated sperm, 161, 162
    (*see also* Totipotency)
TUNEL assay, 158
Intrauterine insemination (IUI), 56, 64, 73,
    74, 77
In-vitro fertilization (IVF), 9, 10, 12, 13, 17,
    24, 26, 32, 33, 40, 43
cycles, 143
sperm DNA integrity, 64, 66, 72–74, 76, 77
In vitro spermatogenesis
testicular organ cultures, 51, 52
three-dimensional culture, single cells,
    52, 53
IVF. *See* In-vitro fertilization (IVF)

K
Klinefelter's syndrome, 137, 138
KnockOut Serum Replacement (KSR), 51

M
Male experience. *See* Male-factor infertility
Male-factor infertility, 143, 144, 146, 149
age-related fertility decline, 3
ART services, 5
barriers, 1
description, 1
fertility, masculinity and sexuality, 3
gender differences, 4
invasive methods, 5
knowledge and perceptions, 2
knowledge gaps, 2
male experience, 3, 4

Male-factor infertility (*cont.*)
   masculine hope technology, 2
   medical parlance, 2
   medicalization of reproduction, 2
   online resources, 5
   public awareness, 5
   qualitative and quantitative research, 3
   sexual dysfunction, 4
   social perspectives, 1
   social support, 5
   traditional and emergent gender
      identities, 2
   treatment experiences, 4
Male fertility preservation, 54, 55
Male infertility
   azoospermia, 25, 26
   candidate gene sequencing, 29
   CFTR mutations, 26, 28
   CNVs, 29
   DNA sequencing costs, 30
   environmental exposure, 25
   epigenetic testing, 26
   estimation, 24
   evaluation, 24
   genetic medicine, 24
   genetics revolution, 24
   genomic technologies, 29, 30
   karyotype and YCMD, 25
   obesity, 25
   physical exam, 24
   polymorphisms, 29, 34
   SNPs, 29
   sperm aneuploidy, 27, 28
   sperm DNA damage, 28
   technological advances, 23
   whole genome sequencing, 30
Membrane-targeted GFP (mGFP), 174
Membrane-targeted Tomato (mtdT), 174
Microdissection testicular sperm extraction
      (microTESE), 25, 26
Micro-epididymal sperm extraction
      (MESA), 159
Mitotic haploid parthenogenotes,
      172–174
Motile sperm organelle morphology
      examination (MSOME), 143
Mouse
   blastomeres, 171
   gamete function, 169
   ICSI, 172
   mII oocyte plasma membrane, 170
   ovulated oocytes, 171
   parthenogenetic embryos, 170

N
Neurodegenerative disorders, 65
Nuclear isolation medium (NIM), 170

O
Obstructive azoospermia, 160
Oligoasthenoteratospermia (OATS), 130

P
Palindromes, 185, 186, 189
Parkinson's disease, 65
Parthenogenetic Reprogramming of
      Nucleosomal Chromatin
      (phROSI), 175
Paternal age, 40–45
   adverse effects, 39, 40, 45
   chromosomal aberrations, 39
   ICSI and oocyte donation
      autosomal dominant disorders, 44
      confounders, 44
      effects of, 40–42
      fertility outcomes, 44
      fertilization rates, 43
      IVF cycles, 40
      mutational mechanisms, 44
      neuropsychiatric and
         neurodevelopmental
         disorders, 45
      oxidative stress, 44
      selfish selection mechanism, 45
      sperm DNA damage, 45
      sperm parameters, 43, 44
      teratozoospermia, 43
   implantation, 40
   live birth, 39, 40, 43
   maternal ageing and ART outcomes, 39
   pregnancy rates, 39, 43
Percutaneous epididymal sperm aspiration
      (PESA), 159
Poor ovarian response, 150
Poor semen quality, 149, 150
Post-coital test (PCT), 136
Post-ejaculate urinalysis
      (PEU), 131
Postimplantation phICSI embryos
   biparental genome, 174
   Cre-mediated deletion, 175
   haploid parthenogenotes, 174
   mtdT and mGFP, 174
   uniparental blastomeres, 175
Pyospermia, 133–134

R

Reactive oxygen species (ROS), 135
Recurrent implantation failure (RIF), 150
Renal ultrasound, 132
Round spermatid injection (ROSI), 52

S

Scrotal ultrasound (US), 132
"Selfish Y" model, 187
Sex determination, 183, 186
Single nucleotide polymorphisms (SNPs),
 29, 30
Sperm aneuploidy, 27, 28
Sperm–cervical mucus interaction test, 136
Sperm chromatin dispersion assay (SCD), 94
Sperm chromatin structure assay (SCSA),
 66–68, 72, 92, 94
Sperm DNA damage, 28
Sperm DNA integrity
 cancer, 65, 66, 77
 de novo mutations, 76
 DNA damage, 63–65, 76, 77
 embryonic mutations, 64
 fertility, 71, 72
 fertilization and embryo quality, 66
 flow cytometry and quality control, 67–69
 fragmentation, 63, 64
 hyaluronic acid-binding technique, 76
 intra-individual variation, 71
 IUI, 64, 73, 74, 77
 IVF and ICSI, 74, 75
 laboratories, quality control, 71
 male fertility, 71
 male health, 77
 measurement error, 69–70
 natural intercourse, 72
 neurodegenerative disorders, 65
 oocyte fertilization, 63
 oxidative stress, 76, 77
 paternal age, 64
 periodic internal test, 70, 71
 pregnancy rates, 64, 66
 SCSA, 66, 67
 semen samples, 67
 two-step hypothesis, 73, 75
Sperm extraction, 159
Sperm morphology
 blastocyst quality, 146
 chromosomal/DNA defect, 148
 clinical outcomes, 146, 147
 DNA-damaged/vacuolated
  spermatozoa, 145

DNA fragmentation
 and head vacuoles, 144
 and vacuole-free spermatozoa, 148
 head vacuoles, classification, 144
 ICM and TE comparison, 146
 IMSI/ICSI procedure, 145
 male aging, 147
 morphometrically normal spermatozoa
  injection, 144
 MSOME observation technique, 144
 semen samples, 148
 small acrosomes, 147
 spermatozoa grading, 144, 145
Sperm morphology analysis (SMA),
 102–108
 abnormalities types, 99
 algorithm performance, 113, 114
 assay performance, 101
 automated analysis, 101
 CASA, 100
 detection and analysis, 100
 digital image processing, 101
 evaluation metrics, 112, 113
 experimental data, 120
 function, component steps, 120
 image features and sperm diagnosis, 101
 IMSI, 100
 intracellular density distribution, 101
 male fertility potential, 99
 normal and abnormal sperm, 100, 111, 112
 patient recruitment and sample processing
  human sperm images, 102
  noise reduction, 102–104
  optimal tail features, 108
  shape and size, midpiece, 108
  skeleton recognition, 106
  Sobel edge detection method, 104, 105
  sperm compartment detection, 104, 105
  sperm head, 106, 108
  sperm quality, 107
 recognition of sperm parts, 117
 seminal plasma and sperm parameters, 99
 sperm components, 101, 115
 sperm images, 108
 sperm injection, 108
 sperm nucleus/head detection,
  102, 113
 typical and atypical, sperm cells, 102
Sperm penetration assay (SPA), 136
Sperm reprogramming
 mitotic haploid parthenogenotes,
  172–174
 totipotency, 171, 172

Sperm source
    and cryopreservation, 162, 163
    and ICSI, 158, 159
Sperm viability, 134

T
Teratoazoospermia, 131
Terminal deoxynucleotidyl transferase (TdT)
        dUTP Nick-End Labeling
        (TUNEL), 92–94
Testicular sperm aspiration (TESA), 159
Testicular sperm extraction (TESE), 159–161
Testicular *vs.* ejaculated sperm, 161, 162
Totipotency
    acid test, 172
    sperm reprogramming, 171, 172
Transrectal ultrasound (TRUS), 132

V
Vasography, 133

W
"Wimpy Y" model, 187

Y
Y chromosome microdeletion (YCMD),
    25, 26

Z
Zona-free hamster oocyte test, 136
Zona pellucida, 56
Zygote intrafallopian transfer
    (ZIFT), 9